Innovations in Maternal Health

Thank you for choosing a SAGE product! If you have any comment,
observation or feedback, I would like to personally hear from you.
Please write to me at <u>contactceo@sagepub.in</u>

—Vivek Mehra, Managing Director and CEO,
SAGE Publications India Pvt. Ltd, New Delhi

Bulk Sales

SAGE India offers special discounts for purchase of books in bulk.
We also make available special imprints and excerpts from our
books on demand.
For orders and enquiries, write to us at

Marketing Department
SAGE Publications India Pvt. Ltd
B1/I-1, Mohan Cooperative Industrial Area
Mathura Road, Post Bag 7
New Delhi 110044, India
E-mail us at <u>marketing@sagepub.in</u>

Get to know more about SAGE, be invited to SAGE events, get on
our mailing list. Write today to <u>marketing@sagepub.in</u>

This book is also available as an e-book.
<hr>

Innovations in Maternal Health

Case Studies from India

Edited by

Jay K. Satia, Madhavi Misra,
Radhika Arora and Sourav Neogi

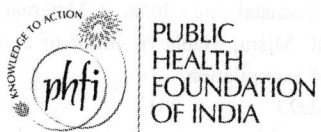

PUBLIC
HEALTH
FOUNDATION
OF INDIA

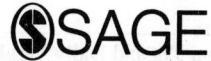 **SAGE**   www.sagepublications.com
Los Angeles • London • New Delhi • Singapore • Washington DC

First published in 2014 by

SAGE Publications India Pvt Ltd
B1/I-1 Mohan Cooperative Industrial Area
Mathura Road, New Delhi 110 044, India
www.sagepub.in

SAGE Publications Inc
2455 Teller Road
Thousand Oaks, California 91320, USA

SAGE Publications Ltd
1 Oliver's Yard
55 City Road
London EC1Y 1SP, United Kingdom

SAGE Publications Asia-Pacific Pte Ltd
3 Church Street
#10-04 Samsung Hub
Singapore 049483

Published by Vivek Mehra for SAGE Publications India Pvt Ltd, Phototypeset in 10.5/13 Times New Roman by Diligent Typesetter, Delhi, and printed at Print-O-Pack Pvt Ltd, New Delhi.

Library of Congress Cataloging-in-Publication Data

Innovations in maternal health : case studies from India / edited by Jay K. Satia, Madhavi Misra, Radhika Arora, and Sourav Neogi.
    pages cm
Includes bibliographical references and index.
    1. Maternal health services—India. 2. Postnatal care—India. 3. Maternal and infant welfare—India. I. Satia, J. K. (Jayantilal K.), editor of compilation. II. Misra, Madhavi, editor of compilation. III. Arora, Radhika, editor of compilation. IV. Neogi, Sourav, editor of compilation.
    RG965.I4I56   618.200954—dc23   2013   2013043666

ISBN: 978-81-321-1310-2 (PB)

The SAGE Team: Shambhu Sahu, Shreya Chakraborti, Nand Kumar Jha and Dally Verghese

Contents

Section B: Addressing Direct Causes of Mortality

Section C: Addressing Indirect Causes of Maternal and Newborn Mortality

Section D: Accountability of Programmes

Section E: Successful Organizations as Innovation Engines

List of Tables

List of Figures

List of Illustrations

List of Images

List of Maps

List of Boxes

List of Abbreviations

ABG	Adolescent Boys Group
AC	Air Conditioning
ACOG	American Congress of Obstetrician and Gynaecologists
ADPM	Additional District Programme Manager
AFHS	Adolescent-friendly Health Services
AGP	Adolescent Girls Programme
AKF	Aga Khan Foundation
AKF USA	Aga Khan Foundation USA
ALOS	Average Length of Stay
ALS	Advanced Life Support
AMTSL	Active Management of The Third Stage of Labour
ANC	Antenatal Care
ANM	Auxiliary Nurse Midwife
AOL	Assam Oil Limited
AP	Andhra Pradesh
APL	Above Poverty Line
ARSH	Adolescent Reproductive and Sexual Health
ARTH	Action Research and Training for Health
ARV	Antiretroviral
ASHA	Accredited Social Health Activist
ASNI	Assessing and Supporting NIPI Interventions
AWC	*Anganwadi* Centre
AWW	*Anganwadi* Worker
AYUSH	Ayurveda, Yoga and Naturopathy, Unani, Siddha and Homoeopathy
BBO	Blood Bank Officer
BCC	Behaviour Change Communication
BCG	Bacillus Calmette–Guérin (Bacille Calmette–Guérin)
BEmOC	Basic Emergency Obstetric Care
BIS	Bureau of Indian Standards
BLAC	Block-level Advisory Committees

BLS	Basic Life Support
BMC	BioMed Central
BPCR	Birth Preparedness and Complication Readiness
BPHC	Block Primary Health Centres
BPL	Below Poverty Line
BSD	*Bal Suraksha Diwas*
BSU	Blood Storage Unit
CA	Change Agents
CBHI	Central Bureau of Health Intelligence
CBMDR	Community-based Maternal Death Review
CBMS	Community-based Monitoring System
CCT	Conditional Cash Transfer
CDMO	Chief District Medical Officer
CE	Conformité Européenne (European Conformity)
CEDPA	Centre for Development and Population Activities
CEmOC	Comprehensive Emergency Obstetric Care
CEO	Chief Executive Officer
CHC	Community Health Centre
CLICS	Community-led Initiatives for Child Survival
CMO	Chief Medical Officer
C-NES	Centre for North East Studies and Policy Research
CO	Communication Officer
CRHP	Comprehensive Rural Health Project
CSHGP	Child Survival Health Grants Program
D&D	Daman and Diu
DCM	Department of Community Medicine
DFID	Department for International Development
DGUS	*Dharam Gramin Utthan Sansthan*
DH	District Hospital
DHH	District Headquarter Hospital
DHS	District Health Society
DLAC	District-level Advisory Committees
DLHS-3	District-level Household Survey-3
DM	District Magistrate
DO	Dispatch Officer
DOTS	Directly Observed Treatment Short Course
DPM	District Project Manager
DPMU	District Programme Management Unit
DPO	District Programme Officer
DQAC	District Quality Assurance Cells
ECG	Electrocardiogram
EMO	Emergency Medical Officer
EmOC	Emergency Obstetric Care

EMRI	Emergency Management and Research Institute
EMS	Emergency Medical Systems
EMT	Emergency Medical Technician
ERC	Emergency Response Centre
ERS	Emergency Response Services
FBMDR	Facility-based Maternal Death Review
FDA	Food and Drug Administration
FIGO	International Federation of Gynaecology and Obstetrics
FOGSI	Federation of Obstetric and Gynecologists Societies of India
FP	Family Planning
FP/RCH	Family Planning/Reproductive and Child Health
FP/RH	Family Planning/Reproductive Health
FP/SRH	Family Planning/Sexual and Reproductive Health
FRU	First Referral Unit
GDP	Gross Domestic Product
GE	General Electric
GMCH	Global Maternal Health Conference
GNM	General Nurse Midwife
GOG	Government of Gujarat
GoI	Government of India
GVK-EMRI	GVK Emergency Management and Research Institute
Hb	Haemoglobin
HBR	Harvard Business Review
HIV	Human Immunodeficiency Virus
HIV/AIDS	Human Immunodeficiency Virus Infection/Acquired Immunodeficiency Syndrome
HLFPPT	Hindustan Latex Family Planning Promotion Trust
HLL	Hindustan Latex Limited
HMIS	Health Management Information System
HP	Horsepower
HR	Human Resources
HSC	Health Subcentres
HTSP	Healthy Timing and Spacing of Pregnancy
I/O	Input/Output
IAH	Intersectoral Action for Health
IAS	Indian Administrative Services
ICDS	Integrated Child Development Services
ICM	International Confederation of Midwives
ICPD	International Conference on Population and Development
ICTC	Integrated Counselling and Testing Centres
ICU	Intensive Care Unit
IDA	Iron Deficiency Anaemia
IEC	Information Education Communication

IFA	Iron Folic Acid
IFPS	Innovations in Family Planning Services
IIHMR	Indian Institute of Health Management Research
IMEP	Infection Management and Environment Plan
IMNCI	Integrated Management of Neonatal and Childhood Illnesses
IMR	Infant Mortality Rate
INHP	Integrated Nutrition and Health Project
INR	Indian Rupee
IPC	Interpersonal Communication
IPD	Inpatient Department
IPHS	Indian Public Health Standards
IQ	Intelligence Quotient
ISC	Iron Sucrose Complex
ISO	International Organization for Standardization
ISQua2	International Society for Quality in Health Care
ITAP	Technical Assistance Project
IUD	Intrauterine Device
JEY	Janani Express Yojana
JHSPH	Johns Hopkins Bloomberg School of Public Health
JSY	Janani Suraksha Yojana
Km	Kilometre
KMC	Kangaroo Mother Care
KP	*Kishori* Panchayat
KVM	*Kisan Vikas Manch*
LBW	Low Birth Weight
LED	Light-emitting Diode
LHV	Lady Health Visitor
MAPEDIR	Maternal and Perinatal Death Enquiry and Response
MC	Male Communicators
MCH	Maternal and Child Health
MCHN	Maternal and Child Health and Nutrition
MD	Maternal Deaths
MDG	Millennium Development Goal
MDR	Maternal Death Review
MELA	Meet for Empowerment Learning and Advocacy
MGHN	Merrygold Health Network
MGIMS	Mahatma Gandhi Institute of Medical Sciences
MHC	Maternal Health Centres
MHT	Mobile Health Team
MHU	Mobile Health Units
MIS	Management Information Systems
MLC	Medico Legal
MMR	Maternal Mortality Ratio

MNCH	Maternal Newborn and Child Health
MNCHN	Maternal Newborn and Child Health and Nutrition
MO	Medical Officer
MoHFW	Ministry of Health and Family Welfare
MOU	Memorandum of Understanding
MP	Madhya Pradesh
MTP	Medical Termination of Pregnancy
MVM	*Mahila Vikas Mandal*
NABH	National Accreditation Board for Hospitals and Health Care Providers
NABL	National Accreditation Board for Testing and Calibration Laboratories
NACO	National Aids Coordination Organization
NASA	National Aeronautics and Space Administration
NASG	Non-pneumatic Anti-Shock Garment
NDSS	*Nav Dampati Swagat Samaroh*
NFHS	National Family Health Survey
NGO	Non-governmental Organization
NHA	National Health Accounts
NHD	Nutrition and Health Day
NHSRC	National Health Systems Resource Centre
NICU	Neonatal Intensive Care Unit
NIHFW	National Institute of Health and Family Welfare
NIPI	Norway India Partnership Initiative
NIPI–UNOPS	Norway India Partnership Initiative–United Nations Office for Project Services
NMR	Neonatal Mortality Rate
NPO	Not-for-profit Organization
NRHM	National Rural Health Mission
NSSO	National Sample Survey Office
OBGYN	Obstetrician and Gynaecologists
OCP	Oral Contraceptive Pill
OIL	Oil India Limited
OOP	Out-of-pocket
OPD	Outpatient Department
OPV	Oral Polio Vaccine
ORS	Oral Rehydration Salts
OT	Operating theatre
PCM	Phase Change Material
PDS	Public Distribution System
PFI	Population Foundation of India
PHC	Primary Health Centre
PHFI	Public Health Foundation of India
PIP	Programme Implementation Plans
PM	Post Meridiem

PNC	Postnatal Care
PNDT	Prenatal Diagnostic Techniques
PNH	Private Nursing Home
POP	Phase-out Project
PPA	Primary Programme Area
PPH	Post-partum Haemorrhage
PPP	Public–Private Partnership
PRI	*Panchayati Raj* Institutions
QA	Quality Assurance
QAC	Quality Assurance Cells
QAG	Quality Assurance Group
QAP	Quality Assurance Programme
QCI	Quality Council of India
QI	Quality Improvement
QM	Quality Management
QMS	Quality Management Systems
RCH	Reproductive and Child Health
RCOG	Royal College of Obstetricians and Gynaecologists
RCT	Randomized Control Trial
RDS	Respiratory Distress Syndrome
RH	Reproductive Health
RKS	*Rogi Kalyan Samiti*
RMP	Rural Medical Practitioners
RSBY	*Rashtriya Swasthya Bima Yojna*
RT	Referral Transportation
RTI	Reproductive Tract Infections
RTI/STI	Reproductive Tract Infections and Sexually Transmitted Infections
SC	Subcentre
SHAHN	Safdarjung Hospital Adolescent Health Care Network
SHC	Sub-health Centre
SHG	Self-help Group
SIDA	Swedish International Development Cooperation Agency
SIFPSA	State Innovations in Family Planning Project Services Agency
SNCU	Sick Newborn Care Unit
SOP	Standard Operating Protocol
SRH	Sexual and Reproductive Health
SRS	Sample Registration System
STD	Sexually Transmitted Diseases
STI	Sexually Transmitted Infections
STP	Standard Treatment Protocol
TBA	Traditional Birth Attendant
TFR	Total Fertility Rate
TN	Tamil Nadu

TNMSC	Tamil Nadu Medical Service Corporation
TPR	Temperature, Pulse and Respiration Chart
TSA	Technical Support Agency
TSRD	Tagore Society for Rural Development
TT	Tetanus Toxoid
UCSF	University of California San Francisco
UK	United Kingdom
UN	United Nations
UNFPA	United Nations Population Fund
UNICEF	United Nations Children's Fund
USA	United States of America
USAID	United States Agency for International Development
USG	Ultra Sonography
UT	Union Territories
VCC	Village Coordination Committees
VDRL	Venereal Disease Research Laboratory
VHC	Village Health Committees
VHND	Village Health and Nutrition Day
VHSC	Village Health and Sanitation Committee
VHW	Village Health Worker
VMU	Voucher Management Unit
Vox Pop	Vox Populi
WHO	World Health Organization
WHO-SEARO	World Health Organization–South-East Asia Regional Office
WRA	White Ribbon Alliance for Safe Motherhood
WRAI	White Ribbon Alliance for Safe Motherhood India

TNMSC	Tamil Nadu Medical Service Corporation
TPR	Temperature, Pulse and Respiration Chart
TSA	Technical Support Agency
TSRD	Trust Society for Rural Development
TT	Tetanus Toxoid
UCSF	University of California San Francisco
UK	United Kingdom
UN	United Nations
UNFPA	United Nations Population Fund
UNICEF	United Nations Children's Fund
USA	United States of America
USAID	United States Agency for International Development
USG	Ultra Sonography
UR	Union Regulation
VCC	Village Coordination Committees
VDRL	Venereal Disease Research Laboratory
VHC	Village Health Committees
VHND	Village Health and Nutrition Day
VHSC	Village Health and Sanitation Committee
VHW	Village Health Worker
VMU	Voucher Management Unit
Vox Pop	Vox Populi
WHO	World Health Organization
WHO-SEARO	World Health Organization–South-East Asia Regional Office
WRA	White Ribbon Alliance for Safe Motherhood
WRAI	White Ribbon Alliance for Safe Motherhood India

Foreword

Maternal and newborn mortality and morbidity remain unconscionably high despite significant progress in improving maternal and children's health.

Rapid pace of innovations and their scale-up in maternal and newborn care are critical for improved health outcomes, especially for the poor families. Many successful innovations have been undertaken by the government, civil society and private sector. Such innovations from different states in India need to be shared and replicated across the country to meet the gaps in health-care delivery at the grassroots level. These innovations are also an important source of learning which can promote further innovations, thus accelerating the pace of innovations.

The potential for faster scaling-up as well as learning for germination of further innovations is not fully realized in India because they are not well documented and shared widely.

We are grateful to John D. and Catherine T. MacArthur Foundation for providing support to the Public Health Foundation of India (PHFI) to document case studies of innovations in maternal and newborn care.

This book is a compilation of case studies which were developed. It seeks to accelerate pace of innovations by documenting contemporary innovative programmes undertaken to improve maternal and newborn care in India. 'Innovations' have been defined as 'doing what is being done differently or creating new, unique ideas and interventions'. The case studies included in this volume represent a range of innovative health programmes undertaken in different parts of India and, therefore, provide contextualized learning. Most of these programmes have been designed to reach poor and marginalized populations who face major social and geographic barriers in accessing health services. Each of the themes identified has a film accompanying it. The films capture the innovative cases which have been documented. The films and the written case studies complement each other. The set of 16 films is also a part of this book.

A landscape exercise of innovations was undertaken which led to preparation of a directory of more than 200 innovations. An analysis of directory shows that there is a need for innovations in addressing direct causes of mortality such as eclampsia or delivering optimal post-natal services. An expert advisory group helped identify the case studies that have been documented. The case studies are categorized within themes and represent a variety of programmatic approaches undertaken in different socio-cultural contexts. They provide a discussion of innovations addressing direct, indirect, distal and cross-cutting causes of avoidable mortality which cruelly end the lives of mothers and newborns. The case studies described in this book identify areas where there is a need not only for upstream research and development but also for downstream activities in terms of how to deliver these innovations to the people who can benefit the most.

This book fills an important gap in our understanding of issues in maternal and child health. The well-documented set of case studies provides a platform for further scaling up of these innovations by programme implementers at grassroots level. It is useful for those who wish to advocate for policy or programme changes. In order to enhance learning, the case study approach is a very useful tool. The intent is to use this set of case studies also for teaching and training to provide an enriching learning experience for students of public health, medical and nursing schools.

K. Srinath Reddy
President
PHFI

Acknowledgements

This book of case studies is the result of our conviction that the potential of many innovations in maternal and newborn care in India remains under-realized because of their inadequate documentation. Such documentation can be used for enabling policy advocacy, programming for the scale-up of innovations and for education of health professionals.

The John D. and Catherine T. MacArthur Foundation shared our conviction and provided generous support for this documentation of innovations without which this book would not have been possible. We are grateful to the Foundation. Poonam Mutterja, the then India representative of the Foundation, reposed faith in us for undertaking this large written and audio-visual documentation. We would like to thank her for her encouragement. Dipa Nag Chowdhury of the MacArthur Foundation provided her time and guidance throughout the documentation of these case studies. We would like to thank her for her patience and consideration towards us.

The book is a compilation of case studies of innovations which represent the work of different partner organizations and state governments in India (see the following lists of partner organizations and departments and ministries under central and state governments).

Partner Organizations
1. Action Research and Training for Health (ARTH)
2. CARE India
3. Centre for North East Studies and Policy Research (C-NES)
4. Centre for Development and Population Activities (CEDPA)
5. Comprehensive Rural Health Project (CRHP), Jamkhed
6. Department of Pediatrics, Safdarjung Hospital
7. Ekjut
8. Embrace Global
9. Futures Group
10. GVK Emergency Management Research Institute (GVK-EMRI), Hyderabad
11. Hindustan Latex Family Planning Promotion Trust (HLFPPT)
12. LifeSpring Hospitals
13. Mahatma Gandhi Institute of Medical Sciences (MGIMS), Sevagram

14. Mamta Health Institute for Mother and Child
15. Merrygold Health Network
16. Pathfinder International India
17. State Innovations in Family Planning Project Services Agency (SIFPSA)
18. Tagore Society for Rural Development (TSRD)
19. UNICEF Delhi
20. UNICEF India
21. UNICEF Madhya Pradesh
22. UNICEF Odisha
23. United States Agency for International Development (USAID)
24. United Nations Office for Project Services-Norway India Partnership Initiative (UNOPS-NIPI)
25. White Ribbon Alliance for Safe Motherhood India (WRAI)

State and Central Governments

26. Ministry of Health and Family Welfare, Government of India
27. Department of Health and Family Welfare, Government of Madhya Pradesh
28. Department of Health and Family Welfare, Government of Rajasthan
29. Department of Health and Family Welfare, Government of Tamil Nadu
30. Department of Health and Family Welfare, Government of Uttar Pradesh
31. Department of Health and Family Welfare, Government of Uttarakhand
32. Department of Health and Family Welfare, Government of West Bengal

We are indebted to them for not only did they go out of their way to make the documentation process possible for us but also, the documentation benefitted from their wisdom and wealth of knowledge on the subject.

Our Expert Advisory Group collectively guided us in this effort and individually reviewed the case studies.

Expert Committee

S.No.	Name	Designation	Institution
1.	Dinesh Agarwal	National Programmer Officer (Reproductive Health)	United Nations Population Fund (UNFPA)
2.	Kaliprasad Pappu	National Coordinator	Norway India Partnership Initiative (NIPI)
3.	Rajani Ved	Advisor Community Participation	National Health Systems Research Centre (NHSRC)

(continued)

(continued)

S.No.	Name	Designation	Institution
4.	Sanjay Zodpey	Director, Academic Affairs and Director Indian Institute of Public Health, Delhi	PHFI
5.	Dileep Mavalankar	Director, Indian Institute of Public Health, Gandhinagar	PHFI
6.	Vinod Paul	Head, Department of Pediatrics and WHO Collaborating Centre for Training and Research in Newborn Care	All India Institute of Medical Sciences (AIIMS)
7.	Jashodhara Dasgupta	Coordinator	SAHYOG
8.	Sharad Iyengar	Secretary	ARTH
9.	B.S. Garg	Dean	Mahatama Gandhi Institute of Medical Sciences
		Director	Dr. Sushila Nayar School of Public Health
		Director-Professor	Department of Community Medicine, Sewagram
		Head	WHO Collaborating Centre for Research and Training in Community Based Maternal, Newborn and Child Health, Sewagram
10.	Bulbul Sood	Country Director, India	John Hopkins Program for International Education in Gynaecology and Obstetrics (JHPIEGO)
11.	Padmanabhan	Advisor (Public Health Administration), National Health Systems Resource Centre, National Rural Health Mission	National Institute of Health and Family Welfare (NIHFW)
12.	Priya Nanda	Group Director, Social and Economic Development, Asia Regional Office	International Center for Research on Women (ICRW)
13.	B.P. Singh	Country Director	Engender Health
14.	Shireen Jeejeebhoy	Senior Associate	Population Council of India
15.	Himanshu Bhushan	Deputy Commissioner, Maternal Health, Ministry of Health and Family Welfare	MOHFW

Our deepest appreciation to them for sparing their precious time to support this effort.

We would like to record the contribution of Raj Mohan Panda, Sutapa B. Neogi and Sanghita Bhattacharya for authoring some of the case studies in the book. We thank them for the same. During the early stage of development of the case studies, Garima Pathak, Shomik Ray and Swati Saxena played an important role in conceptualizing and steering the documentation process and we thank them. We would like to acknowledge the contribution of Aditi Bam and Kumud Mohan for providing editorial support.

Our two film-making agencies—Small Screen Film and Television Pvt. Ltd and Kriti and Black-ticket Films—deserve special thanks as they took the trouble to understand each innovation and worked tirelessly with us throughout the process of documentation. We believe that the audio-visual aid accompanying each case study enriches the documentation.

We would like to thank faculty members of many medical and nursing colleges from across the country as well as non-governmental organization (NGO) and government representatives who participated in workshops, discussed the case studies and helped us revise the content. They gave us confidence that these case studies were useful and added value to the teaching and training.

We are grateful to an unknown editor whose perceptive comments helped us refine some of the case studies.

Finally, we are grateful to SAGE Publications India Pvt. Ltd for being the publishers of this book and assisting us through their editorial support.

September 2013, New Delhi

Introduction

Need for Documentation of Innovations in Maternal and Child Health

In 2005, the Government of India started the National Rural Health Mission (NRHM) with the aim of rejuvenating the health delivery system. The stress was on providing quality health care that was accessible, acceptable and affordable to all sections of the society. Besides infrastructure and human resource development, community participation and decentralization are two important components of the programme. This has enabled the state health departments and non-governmental organizations (NGOs) working in the health sector to devise innovative plans and adapt intervention strategies to tackle the local health problems.

A major goal of NRHM is to improve maternal and child health. The decline in maternal mortality ratio (MMR) over the last decade has been a slow one. MMR in India was 212 per 100,000 live births in 2007–09 (SRS 2011). Across the different Indian states, the MMR remains uneven. In states such as Rajasthan with the MMR of 318 and Assam at 390, MMR remains much above the national average. The Millennium Development Goal (MDG) for MMR for India was set at 100, but at the current rate of decline (16.8% since 1998), achieving this MDG seems impossible. Even newborn mortality and neonatal mortality figures have remained high. Infant mortality rate (IMR) for India is 47 per 1,000 live births and neonatal mortality rate is 39 for 1,000 live births (2010) with an MDG for India at 27 for child mortality by 2015. Reducing newborn mortality is crucial towards achieving this MDG child mortality.

One of the health system improvements undertaken by the government as a part of NRHM is a conditional cash transfer scheme for promoting institutional deliveries, called Janani Suraksha Yojana (JSY). In Annexure 1, we present a case study on implementation experience of JSY and its impact. The significant increase in proportion of institutional deliveries is attributed to this initiative. While this should have led to substantial reduction in maternal and newborn mortality, its impact on either has not yet been carefully evaluated.

Over the years, many NGOs have also innovated in the maternal and newborn health space with donor support. A large number of innovations have taken and are also taking place through the private sector (as well as the NGOs, private sector and government working together). Many of these innovations, including those under NRHM, succeeded in delivering promising results in addressing the health needs of the local populace. This has given rise to the possibility of replicating or adapting innovations implemented in one part of the country to other parts depending on local needs and context, towards accelerating the decline in maternal and newborn mortality.

Even though there is a huge source of learning resources available at the grassroots level, lack of proper documentation and dissemination has resulted in these successes being an untapped source of answers to similar health issues in other areas in the same as well as other states. The innovations used to effectively tackle the roadblocks faced in the field would help the public health managers to find solutions to difficult issues as well as can be used as evidence for scalability of the innovations. It would also enable public health managers to find motivation to try harder to find solutions to the problems that they face, learning from those who have been in similar situations.

Poor documentation of such efforts also does not allow for information sharing towards capacity building of current and future public health practitioners. Therefore, an urgent need was felt to strengthen competencies and build capacity of health professionals by documenting innovations which have been piloted or implemented in different parts of the country in a medium that can be used effectively for educational purposes. It is important to note here that at present, the public health curriculum in India also suffers from a lack of such documented innovations which contextualize the Indian angle for teaching and training purposes. It was felt that these innovations, when documented, had the potential to be used as very useful public health competency strengthening and advocacy tools.

Thus, these innovations in the area of maternal and newborn health in different states in India needed to be documented as case studies, such that they may be shared for skill-building and scale-up across the country to help meet the gaps in health care delivery at the grassroots level. Scale-up of some of these documented innovations is a natural course of progression. It is hoped that by documenting innovations in maternal and newborn health, practitioners may be encouraged to use similar ideas in their spheres of influence.

Therefore, in 2010, a project was undertaken by Public Health Foundation of India (PHFI), supported by John D. and Catherine T. MacArthur Foundation, to create an inventory of innovations on maternal and newborn health and document, as in-depth case studies, select innovation for competency strengthening and advocacy.

What Is Innovation in Health Care?

There are many definitions of innovations as well as of innovations in the health care sector in the literature. Omachonu and Einspruch (2010), for instance, say that health care innovations can be defined as the introduction of a new concept, idea, service, process or product aimed at improving treatment, diagnosis, education, outreach, prevention and research with the long-term goals of improving quality, safety, outcomes, efficiency and costs. Product innovations may be defined as the introduction of goods or services that are new or significantly improved with respect to their characteristics or intended uses. Process innovations are the implementation of a new or significantly improved production or delivery method. In addition, there could be innovations for creating demand (for services, products, information, etc.) or improving the functioning of the organization.

For the purpose of this book, innovations have been defined more simply as 'doing what is being done differently or doing something new'. Of course, useful innovations are those that create value benefits for the provider or user of health care.

Methodology of Documentation

Creating a Directory of Innovations

The first step in the documentation towards developing the case studies was to identify innovations taking place in the areas of maternal and newborn health care in India. In order to compile such a directory of innovations, a thorough search was undertaken where a number of NGOs and donor organizations were contacted via phone, email and personal visits, to gather information on innovative interventions for maternal and newborn health. State governments and NRHM offices were also contacted for the states in India. Extensive Internet searches were undertaken using search engines such as Google,[1] using a mix of keywords that included, among others: 'innovations maternal health' + India, 'innovations newborn care' + India, 'maternal health programmes' and 'newborn programmes'. Results from Internet-based searches were restricted to innovations undertaken/implemented in India after the year 2000. Existing directories of innovations such as the *Directory of Innovations Implemented in Health Sector* (2008), supported by Department for International Development (DFID), *Monograph on Young People's Reproductive and Sexual Health Programmes* (2009), by Population Foundation of India were also used towards developing the inventory.

Participation and information gathered at conferences such as Global Maternal Health Conference (2010) also helped in providing additions to the list of innovations in India on maternal and newborn health.

An expert group was formed to guide this project. The group comprised 16 imminent experts from the field of maternal and child health in India. Various meetings were held with the expert group which also resulted in further developing the directory of innovations.

The resulting directory of innovations had an inventory of 218 innovations. These were then classified based on the route of impact that each innovation had on maternal and newborn health. With this classification to the inventory, the directory was divided under direct, indirect, distal or cross-cutting innovations. As shown in Figure I.1, only 19% of all the innovations listed in the directory had a direct impact on causes of maternal health. Direct causes include technological innovations, blood safety and emergency referral systems among others. Innovations addressing

Figure I.1
Classification of Total Innovations in the Inventory

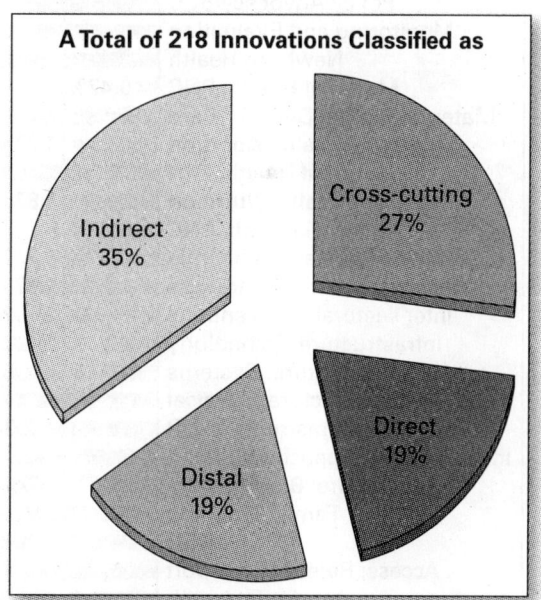

Source: Directory of innovations in maternal and newborn health created by PHFI supported by MacArthur Foundation, 2011.

[1] www.ncbi.nlm.nih.gov/pubmed; scholar.google.co.in

indirect causes of maternal mortality included innovative approaches to improve family planning, build community-based organization, monitoring and evaluation initiatives, health outreach camps, etc. Thirty-five per cent of all innovations in the directory were classified as having an indirect impact on the health indicators. The innovations clubbed as being a distal factor for maternal and newborn mortality accounted for 19% of all the innovations. These included innovations in the areas of Adolescent Reproductive and Sexual Health (ARSH), Behaviour Change Communication (BCC) and policy and advocacy. Twenty-seven per cent of innovations in the directory were listed as having a cross-cutting impact on maternal and newborn mortality. Cross-cutting themes included a mix of health systems strengthening and specific maternal health interventions.

The innovations in the directory were further reclassified as shown in Figure I.2. This classification helps in understanding the division of innovations based on themes each innovation addresses. It was seen that the maximum number of innovations (11.6%) were using policy, advocacy or BCC tools in the area of maternal health. Direct causes of maternal mortality such as postnatal care (PNC) and antenatal care (ANC) had only 0.47% of the innovations each, blood safety had 1.4% of the innovations and interventions for anaemia were again at 0.47% of the innovations in the directory.

Figure I.2
Innovation Classification in Directory

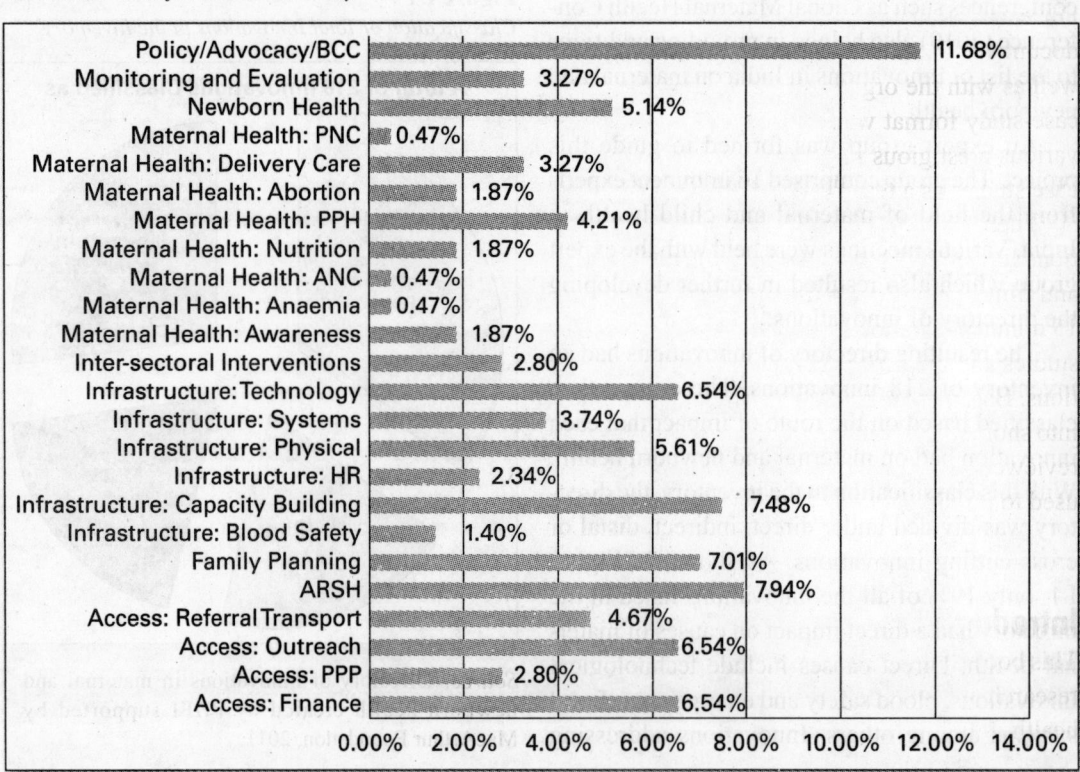

Source: Directory of innovations in maternal and newborn health created by PHFI supported by MacArthur Foundation, 2011.

A very small number of innovations (4.21%) addressed post-partum haemorrhage in the directory which is a direct cause of maternal mortality. It was also observed that there were no innovations found on eclampsia and pre-eclampsia.

Identifying Innovations for Documentation

The project team reviewed the abstracts available for each of 218 innovations in the directory. Based upon this review, it shortlisted innovations for documentation using the criteria of potential impact, feasibility of implementation, community acceptability, scalability and sustainability. A total of 23 innovations under five themes (given as follows) were shortlisted through this process:

1. Health system for Maternal and Newborn Care (Access; Quality; Availability; Affordability)
2. Addressing direct causes of mortality
3. Addressing Indirect Causes of Maternal and Newborn Mortality
4. Accountability of programmes
5. Successful innovation engines

Field Documentation

For each innovation, the relevant organizations were contacted to seek their support towards the documentation process. Secondary data and research materials available in the public domain as well as with the organizations were reviewed; the foci for the documentation were identified. The case-study format was chosen for documentation. Case study pedagogy method has been used in various prestigious institutions across the world. Annexure 2 provides a brief review of the use of case studies as a teaching method.

Then a project team member led a team of professional film-makers to the sites of the innovations for a reconnaissance visit. A team of PHFI researchers and film-makers conducted interviews and filmed the selected innovations. The footage of the shots was edited to prepare a film of about 15 minutes' duration as an audio-visual case study. Print case studies were developed. The print case studies and the accompanying films were reviewed by PHFI team members and partner organizations. Based on this, films were finalized for advocacy purposes and a few films were further edited into shorter films with duration of three to five minutes. Each case study and accompanying film was reviewed by a peer reviewer generally a member of expert advisory group. Their comments were used to refine the print versions of the case studies.

Introduction to the Book

This book on *Innovations in Maternal Health: Case Studies from India* is the result of extensive field research and documentation undertaken in order to document innovations in maternal and newborn health. It has been developed for use of four major groups of stakeholders as follows:

1. Faculty and students from public health schools, medical and nursing colleges
2. In-service training and continuing medical education

3. Government and non-government institutions
4. Public health and development practitioners

The book has been divided into five sections according to the classification of innovations documented:

1. Health system for Maternal and Newborn Care (Access; Quality; Availability; Affordability)
2. Addressing direct causes of mortality
3. Addressing Indirect Causes of Maternal and Newborn Mortality
4. Accountability of programmes
5. Successful organizations as innovation engines

Each of the five sections has been further divided into 16 sub-themes under which each case study has been categorized. Every sub-theme comprises a print case study with an accompanying film case, the print and film case studies complementing each other are to be used collectively in the classroom setting for teaching and training purposes.

In our experience of facilitating these case studies with close to 200 participants nationally over five dissemination programmes, the results have been encouraging. The formal feedbacks received have graded the materials produced as being between 'very good' and 'good' by the participants. Nearly all feedbacks received have commented on how the 'case-study method of teaching enhances learning' and is much more attractive to the facilitator as well as the student. It was found that the use of audio-visual aids while teaching helped increase information retention; participatory techniques helped in keeping students engaged in the topics under discussion. Some participants from the government and NGOs have also indicated that they will pursue scaling-up of some of these innovations in their settings.

Annexure 1: Janani Suraksha Yojana—A Case Study

Abstract

The purpose of this case is

1. To discuss implementation challenges—operational, managerial and leadership—of conditional cash transfer scheme in the context of JSY.
2. To appreciate advantages and disadvantages of conditional cash transfer scheme.

The case describes background of the scheme and discusses its impact. A programme evaluation of JSY raises several implementation issues which are briefly presented. Then experience of a district hospital is described. The case concludes with challenges in reducing MMR.

1. **Background and Rationale for JSY**

   Maternal mortality in India, although declining, remained high. During the period 2007–09, the MMR was estimated to be 212 per 100,000 live births as per Sample Registration

System (SRS), Government of India (SRS 2011). The National Family Health Survey (NFHS 2005–06) showed that coverage by maternal health services was low. Although 77% pregnant mothers had received any ANC, only 37% had accessed four or more ANC visits for pregnancies in the preceding five-year period of the survey. 38.7% of the deliveries had taken place at a health institution and 37.3% had received some PNC. Three major reasons were mentioned by respondents for not delivering in a health facility—not considered necessary, costs are too much and institutions are too far or transport not available—according to the NFHS 2005–06.

Conditional cash transfer schemes in Mexico and some other countries had shown their powerful impact on behaviour change among the poor (Lagarde et al. 2009). In 1997, Mexico launched Progresa programme with the goal of increasing the basic capabilities of extremely poor people in rural Mexico. Unlike most health programmes which focus on supply side, this programme was principally designed to affect the 'demand side'. It provided monetary incentives directly to families to help and overcome the financial barriers to the use of health services and schooling as well as to induce parents to make decisions that would bring their children more education and better health. The government provided significant levels of financial support directly to households only if the beneficiaries did their part by sending children to school and taking them to clinics for immunizations and pregnant mothers' accessed ANC and used institutions for deliveries. Progresa simultaneously sought to influence behaviour on education, health and nutrition as they are mutually reinforcing. This would also bring pressure for coordinated service delivery in these three sectors. In the health component, cash transfers were given if (and only if) every member of the family accepted preventive health services. The scheme had a striking impact on health.

In view of the aforesaid and the need to accelerate reduction in maternal mortality, Government of India initiated a scheme called JSY in 2005 under the newly created NRHM. This scheme aims at reducing maternal and newborn mortality by promoting institutional delivery where financial incentives are provided to mothers as well as to Accredited Social Health Activists (ASHAs).

2. Description of Scheme and Its Evolution

JSY is a 100% centrally sponsored scheme and it integrates cash assistance with delivery and post-delivery care. The success of the scheme would be determined by the increase in institutional delivery among the poor families. The ultimate goal of the programme is to reduce the number of maternal and neonatal deaths. The scheme began by providing the pregnant woman with ₹500 for completing ANC check-ups and then ₹900 for delivering the baby at an accredited health facility. This was later revised to provide a total amount after delivery instead of providing it in two parts. According to the current JSY guidelines, after delivery in a government or accredited private health facility, women from poor households (below poverty line) in rural areas will be provided with ₹700 (US$13) and women in urban areas will be provided with ₹600 (US$11). The high-focus states of Uttar Pradesh, Uttaranchal, Bihar, Jharkhand, Madhya Pradesh, Chhattisgarh, Assam, Rajasthan, Orissa and Jammu and Kashmir which have low rate of institutional deliveries will have all women covered under JSY irrespective of socio-economic background. Here, the cash incentives are ₹1,400 (US$25) in rural parts and ₹1,000 (US$18) in urban parts. JSY is being implemented through ASHAs at the village level. The ASHAs too receive a monetary incentive for providing help to women in receiving at least three ANC visits, immunization of the newborn baby, postnatal check-up and counselling for breast feeding.

3. Impact

According to Lim et al. (2010), JSY is the largest conditional cash transfer programme in the world in terms of the number of beneficiaries. Data suggests substantial scale-up in the past few years in terms of the number of beneficiaries' budget with an allocation of ₹15.4 billion in 2009–10. This funding, according to Lim and colleagues, is expected to provide cash transfers to about 36% of the 26 million women giving birth in India in 2010 alone. According to government reports, the number of women receiving JSY benefits in the year 2009–10 stood at 9.3 million. Although uptake of JSY varied among districts, receipt of financial assistance from JSY was associated with a significantly increased probability of receiving antenatal care and either giving birth in a facility or having a skilled attendant present at the time of delivery. Lim et al. note that JSY has probably contributed to reductions in the numbers of perinatal and neonatal deaths.

Although too early to assess impact of JSY, District-level Household and Facility Survey-3 (DLHS-3) during 2007–08 showed that 75% of the pregnant women had received any ANC, about the same as that estimated by National Family Health Survey-3 (NFHS-3) during the period 2000–05. Nearly half of the deliveries had taken place at health institutions, 9% point increase from that estimated by NFHS-3. Nearly half also had a PNC check-up within two days of delivery.

According to United Nations Children's Fund's (UNICEF) coverage evaluation survey of 2009, institutional deliveries had gone up to 72.9% which is the main indicator of success to JSY. Of these, 47% were at the public facility. The reasons for not delivering at an institution have evolved over the years. The first reason for not delivering at a health facility was that they had no time to reach the health facility, the affordability aspect has steadily reduced from 2005 to 2009 to the fourth place (see Table I.1).

The little evidence from the assessment of the effects of the conditional cash transfers in Mexico, Columbia, Nicaragua and Malawi suggests that although these programmes have led to increased use of health service, but whether they have led to improvements in health outcomes or their effects are generalizable across different settings is still not known (Lagarde et al. 2009).

4. Issues and Challenges

A programme evaluation in 2011 was conducted by the National Health System Resource Centre (NHSRC) in the eight high-focus states of Bihar, Chhattisgarh, Jharkhand, Madhya Pradesh, Orissa, Rajasthan, Uttar Pradesh and Uttarakhand, which together accounted for 84.3% and 66% of India's maternal mortality and infant mortality respectively. The two-phase study using the comparative case-study approach was conducted between April 2010 and December 2010. The first phase included a review of secondary data and a rapid appraisal of health facilities in 24 districts, three in each state. In the second phase, a subset of these districts, one per state was selected randomly and a cross-sectional survey of women who had delivered in the past year and were eligible for the JSY was conducted.

Table I.1

Reasons for Not Delivering at an Institution

Ranking of Reasons for Not Delivering at Institution		
NFHS 2005–06	DLHS 2007–08	UNICEF Coverage Evaluation Survey 2009
Not necessary	Not necessary	No time to go
Too expensive	No time to go	Not necessary
Too far/no transport	Cost too much	Better care at home
Not customary	Received better care at home	Cost too much
Husband/family did not allow	Family did not allow	Too far/no transport
Family not open	Lack of knowledge	Family did not allow
Others	Poor quality of services	Others
Poor quality of service	Not customary	Poor quality of service
		Not customary

Source: Data from NFHS 2005–06, DLHS 2007–08 and Coverage Evaluation Survey 2009.

This evaluation found that after JSY, over 50% of women who had a home delivery had now opted for an institutional delivery. Despite this increase, the study finds persistent home deliveries, about 40% in most districts studied, ranging from 7.7% to almost 63%. Women who deliver at home are more likely to be Scheduled Castes/Scheduled Tribes (SCs/STs), belong to the below poverty line (BPL) category and are non-literate or primary school dropouts. The NHSRC evaluation found that JSY excludes a significant proportion of women by virtue of criteria and these women who are excluded are those under 19 years, multiparous, poor, often with no access to a BPL card and all of those who are at higher risk of maternal and perinatal outcomes, the first two directly and the third as a proximate determinant. Messages on JSY have not reached about 40% of women who deliver at home and to those whom the message has reached, the financial incentive is much better communicated than the health and safety aspects.

Impact on Maternal Mortality

The incidence of complications in the study is about 11.9%. The experience of care seeking in the event of pregnancy complications is that women spend much greater time in a chain of referrals, with all its attendant costs and time delays before they get to the facility that provides them suitable care. The costs of care for complications, especially those requiring hospitalization, are inordinately high and are not covered by the public health programme, forcing women and families to choose the private sector care over the public sector. Even assured referral transport is much less available when complications arise than it is for a normal delivery.

Fund Flow and Streamline Procedures for Use of Funds

In the case of women who deliver in institutions, a majority of them are receiving the JSY payment, in contrast to those who deliver at home. Non-payments, however, in some districts are as high as 55% and delayed payments much beyond the actual time of discharge are common. Out-of-pocket (OOP) payments are high, amounting to ₹1,028 and including transport amount to about ₹1,400 to ₹1,600. OOP payments on home deliveries are also high, with almost 53% paying OOP payments for delivery services. The main OOP expenditures in institutional delivery are on drugs, but there are significant expenses on fees and surgery. In such a circumstance, what the JSY has accomplished has been to enable women and families overcome the financial barriers linked with the choice of institutional delivery.

Infrastructure Including Human Resources

The increase in institutional delivery is skewed, with only a few facilities taking the load of this substantial increase. Of the 5,830 institutions in 21 districts that should have managed the nearly 955,138 of expected deliveries only 852 or roughly 15% actually provided institutional delivery. The load is taken up predominantly by the facilities at the block and higher levels. Subcentres in every district provide a very small part of the midwifery services. Fewer than 20% of auxiliary nurse midwives (ANMs) were able to provide the role of midwifery and such deliveries account for less than 20% of deliveries in the district. The subcentres, located in underserved areas where ANMs conduct deliveries on a regular basis, are exceptions rather than the rule. Thus, the huge increase in institutional delivery case loads is largely taken up by the block and higher level facilities. Primary health centres (PHCs) located at the block level, community health centres (CHCs), sub-district hospital (SDH) and department of health (DH) are all providing institutional delivery services.

The increase in institutional delivery has certainly increased access to delivery by an ANM, nurse or doctor attending on the delivery. However, the study by NHSRC shows that this has not necessarily meant increased access to skilled birth assistance because most nurses and ANMs who are actually providing services were not trained in the skilled birth attendance (SBA) training. Thus practices such as the use of the partogram, active management of third stage of labour, use of injectable antibiotics, oxytocin and the use of magnesium sulphate for hypertension management, neonatal resuscitation and the identification and basic management of hypothermia and sepsis in the newborn, all of which represent the life-saving potential of SBA are not being realized.

Referral Transport

One of the issues with transport is that the family is not assured of a drop home facility. Thus families are forced to keep the vehicle waiting and pay the requisite charges and those who cannot afford to do so, use only a one-way service or hire another vehicle to take them back to home. This also creates a pressure for them to leave within six hours (pressurizing health providers to use oxytocin for augmentation), often within three hours, as the vehicle (if privately arranged) will not wait or because it would cost too much. This has, therefore, a huge health cost which is not usually counted in the three delays approach. Over 28% of women made this choice.

Regarding payment for transport, the ASHA making the transport payment is an exception rather than the rule. Of the OOP payments by the users, about 42% of families are paid less than ₹300 across 12 districts. In some districts, the figure has even gone up to ₹1,500 for transport arrangements.

Quality of Delivery and ANC

Few facilities were using standard protocols of care. The advantages of protocols were seldom realized. Misuse of oxytocin was a significant problem in many districts, but thankfully not in all. Irrational choice and use of antibiotics and intravenous (IV) fluids were also a problem. There have been significant advances made in reporting systems, but recording systems have lagged behind. Use of this information for planning and monitoring is also limited. Systems of cleanliness, hygiene and housekeeping as well as biomedical waste management are underdeveloped.

District Case Study of Ujjain District Hospital in Madhya Pradesh, India

A short drive away from the big city of Indore, one can reach the city of Ujjain, also famous for its temples. A city of 500,000 people, it mostly has agriculture and small-scale industries as its mainstay. The government district-level hospital is the major tertiary-care hospital for the entire district of Ujjain.

The hospital has a separate wing for women and maternity care. JSY was implemented in 2005 along with NRHM. The hospital at that time conducted approximately 6,800 deliveries per year. This has now increased to close to 11,000 deliveries in 2011–12 (see Figure I.3). The nodal officer in-charge for JSY at the district hospital attributes it to the JSY scheme. She goes on to say that the increase in number of institutional deliveries might be attributed to the transport facility made

Figure I.3

The Trend in Institutional Deliveries at Ujjain District Hospital (Madhya Pradesh)

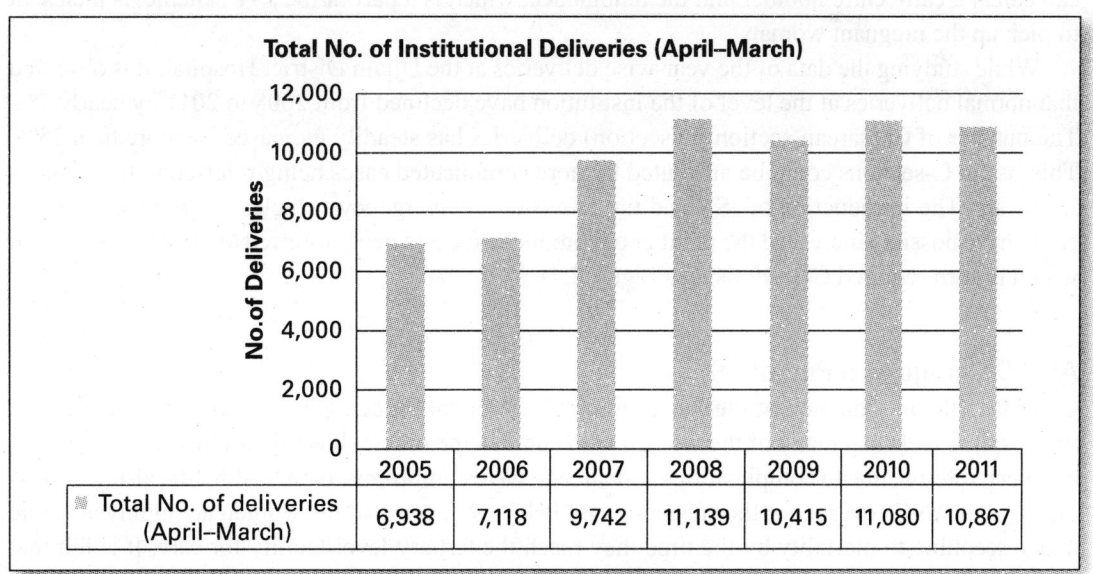

Total No. of Institutional Deliveries (April–March)

	2005	2006	2007	2008	2009	2010	2011
Total No. of deliveries (April–March)	6,938	7,118	9,742	11,139	10,415	11,080	10,867

Source: Data received from Ujjain District Hospital, Government of Madhya Pradesh, December 2012.

Figure 1.4
Year-wise Deliveries at the Ujjain District Hospital from 2008 to 2011

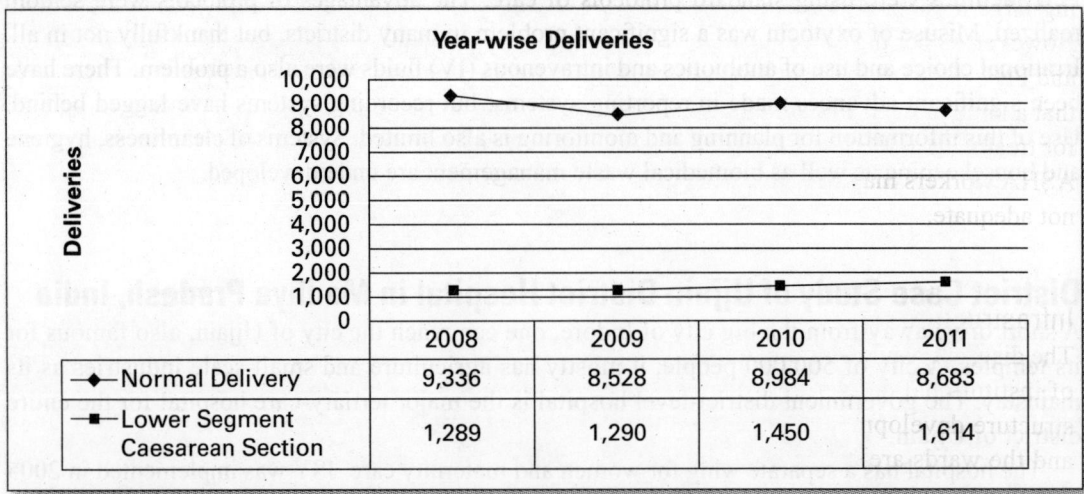

Year-wise Deliveries	2008	2009	2010	2011
Normal Delivery	9,336	8,528	8,984	8,683
Lower Segment Caesarean Section	1,289	1,290	1,450	1,614

Source: Data received from Ujjain District Hospital, Government of Madhya Pradesh, December 2012.

available to women. The transport facility, also known as Janani Express (a detailed case on Janani Express can be found in Chapter 10), brings a woman in labour to the hospital and also drops her back to her home after she is discharged. This has helped bring women from the interiors of the district to the tertiary-level hospital for institutional deliveries. The patient or the patient's family can call at a call-centre number and the ambulance, which is a part of the JSY scheme, is then sent to pick up the pregnant woman.

While studying the data of the year-wise deliveries at the Ujjain District Hospital, it is observed that normal deliveries at the level of the institution have declined from 2008 to 2011 by nearly 7%. The number of Caesarean-section (C-section) deliveries has steadily increased by more than 25%. This rise in C-sections could be attributed to more complicated cases being referred to the tertiary-level care. The introduction of JSY and the provision of emergency vehicles for women in labour could have possibly increased the number of complicated cases being referred to the district hospital which in-turn required C-sections (see Figure I.4).

ANC Coverage as a Part of JSY

Other than the introduction of the Janani Express, the nodal officer, who is also a gynaecologist at the hospital, feels that many of the women who come to the district hospital for delivery have actually been referred due to complications and already have compromised on health. She also feels that due to poor ANC coverage at the subcentre and PHC level, some of the women are highly anaemic and susceptible to mortality by the time they reach the tertiary level facility for care. It is felt that though the ASHA workers are incentivized to take women for ANC check-up, a lot more can be done in this regard.

Role of ASHA Workers

Some officials at the district hospital feel that the ASHAs are primarily responsible for bringing large number of women to the tertiary facility. This helped increase institutional deliveries. However, as per the JSY scheme, the ASHAs are also meant to encourage women to access ANC and PNC. Doctors at the district hospital feel that there remains a challenge. The doctors still find that a large number of women who are severely anaemic are being brought to the district hospital for treatment at the last stage of their pregnancy or even at the time of delivery. It is felt that the ASHA workers may not have been given appropriate training and the training they received was not adequate.

Infrastructure

The district hospital administration in-charge at the Ujjain District Hospital feels that the number of institutional deliveries at the tertiary-level hospital has gone up significantly but the infrastructure development has failed to keep pace. The hospital is now witnessing overcrowding and the wards are congested. The wait to receive treatment is also longer and the doctors and nurses are overexerting which might affect the quality of services. The hospital administration in-charge feels that the JSY scheme might have led to this situation. ASHAs have been encouraging women to come to the facility for delivery and get *protsahan rashi* which is the monetary incentive for them to bring expectant women to the facilities. Providing cash incentive has played an important role in increasing the number of women availing the JSY scheme and benefits at facility level.

Conclusion

Globally, an estimated 287,000 maternal deaths occurred in 2010, a decline of 47% from levels in 1990. At the country level, two countries accounted for one-third of the global maternal deaths: India at 19% (56,000) and Nigeria at 14% (40,000). The global MMR in 2010 was 210 maternal deaths per 100,000 live births, about the same as in India (WHO, UNICEF, UNFPA and World Bank, 2012).

Though PNC is an important part of JSY, implementation remains poor. The role of ASHAs in encouraging women to complete the PNC check-up will help complete the missing link in the implementation of JSY. It is generally seen that after delivery, most women do not return for PNC visits. This is crucial for the health of the mother and child.

A key problem in tackling maternal mortality, is how to accurately capture data and appropriately monitor it. Ascertaining the causes of maternal mortality is difficult even where there is a comprehensive registration of deaths. As most developing countries have weak vital registration and health information systems, they cannot provide an accurate assessment of maternal mortality, leave aside its causes. On the other hand, an estimate derived from the more complete vital registration systems such as those in developed countries, suffers from misclassification and under-reporting of maternal deaths. A maternal death audit was undertaken by PHFI along with Government of Uttar Pradesh. The objectives of this study were to identify the operational problems in conducting maternal death audits at community level and their potential solutions based on government guidelines and to make recommendations to the government on ways to improve maternal health services at the community and/or facility level.

The key findings were the following:

1. Places of maternal deaths were 16% in private facilities, 30% in government hospitals, 23% at home and 30% en route to a formal health facility.
2. The major direct causes of the reported deaths were: haemorrhage (38.5%), anaemia (26.3%), sepsis (14%), eclampsia (10.5%) and obstructed labour (7%).
3. The mean cost of the transport from home to facility one was ₹254, facility one to facility two was ₹1,042 and facility two to facility three was ₹910.
4. The average cost of the care in facility one was ₹3,044, facility two was ₹10,319 and facility three was ₹11,900.
5. The mean travel time between facility one, two and three was two hours.

Though the main objective of JSY is the increase in institutional facilities, in order to reduce MMR and achieve the MDGs, an outcome for success of a conditional cash transfer scheme such as JSY should also reduce MMR. In order to achieve this, factors such as quality of care and reduction of OOP should be focussed on and beyond institutional delivery, major causes of maternal deaths need to be addressed.

Annexure 2: The Case Method

What Are Case Studies?

The Merriam Webster dictionary defines a case study as, 'An intensive analysis of an individual unit [as a person or community] stressing developmental factors in relation to environment'. There are many different definitions of what a case study is. Case studies may be descriptive, explanatory or anecdotal; they may be based on stories and examples from real-life or otherwise. Cases may be based on people, organizations, events and may use varied data types and sources. They may also be of varied length, as detailed investigative cases or as shorter paragraphs. Case studies which traditionally might have been presented as just documents in print, used for teaching law, medicine and business, have now evolved into multimedia case studies, used to teach a variety of subjects. Cases can be used to illustrate

'I think of the [teaching] cases on a regular basis, remembering what others have done, relating that to the options available to me and trying to use their lessons to inform my own decisions'.

Source: Dan Schwarz, Nyaya Health, Nepal. The Global Health Delivery Project at Harvard University.

'It was really informative and set our minds to think! It gave us a framework to work upon ...'
'It was really a good method of teaching ...'

Source: Feedback from students at Indian Institute of Public Health, Delhi, 2012.

a diverse range of issues on different subjects for use in a variety of educational and research purposes. Case studies can be used in any area of study, especially in situations where instructors want to encourage students to apply what they have learnt to real-world situations.[2]

What Is the Case Method?

Over the last few decades, the case method of teaching has been used to bring in realistic examples into the classroom, to prepare students for real-world situations. One of the world's experts on the case method of teaching, C. Roland (Chris) Christensen, described the case method of teaching as 'the art of managing uncertainty', a process in which the instructor serves as 'planner, host, moderator, devil's advocate, fellow-student and judge', all in search of solutions to real-world problems and challenges (Christensen Center for Teaching and Learning).

The kind of case used in a particular class would depend on the objectives of the teaching session; typically cases used for teaching would lead to open-ended problems, towards encouraging discussion, problem-solving, decision-making and analytical thinking. Cases may often help students analyze ambiguous situations of a kind that they may face in the workplace/real-world situations. Case studies could also help study the different points of views regarding a particular problem-solving approach or situation.

Why Use the Case Method?

Unlike the lecture method in which the instructor presents lessons, points of view and information to students, the case method presents students with examples from real life or with life-like situations that don't necessarily have clear solutions, explanations or answers.

This can lead to discussions and debate that encourage analytical thinking among students, helping them study subjects from different points of view and sharpen problem-solving skills.

On the flipside, using the case method can also be challenging both for the facilitator and the student. Without a given set of rules or outcomes, effective conduct of the case method session or discussion can impact the quality of the debate and the direction in which the discussions may flow. The instructor would require to be well versed with the subject matter in order to be able to tackle the different aspects and questions that may emerge from a discussion. For students, the case method can build upon self-learning techniques, improve research and encourage debate and discussion. At the same time, it can also be a challenging task for those unfamiliar with the case method style of learning. Small groups can hamper class participation and, therefore, it is important to ensure students contribute to the discussion equally.

The case method can be used in a variety of settings and contexts; it is a useful training tool to teach subjects or topics that may be subjective in nature, require critical analysis or demand detailed evaluation and discussion.

---

[2] Boston University Center for Excellence and Innovation in Teaching. Available at http://www.bu.edu/ceit/teaching-resources/in-the-classroom/using-case-studies-to-teach/, accessed 5 August 2013.

The Case Method in Class

Unlike lectures, the case method of teaching is not based on a structured lecture-style teaching format. The presentation of the case establishes the framework for analysis. The instructors have to prepare for both the presentation and the process to guiding students through the classroom discussions, providing inputs where and if required. The instructor plays a crucial role in steering classroom discussions towards a systematic approach to analysis, '… to guide students toward the discovery of critical insights and uncovering of broader lessons through thoughtful questioning, listening and responding'.[3]

How to Conduct a Class Using the Case Method of Teaching

Since the case method of teaching is largely participant-driven with the instructor's role crucial in steering the discussion in class, there is no one way of conducting a class. Some sample plans, that may be followed while using these case studies in Indian medical, nursing and public health schools, may include the following.

Format

1. **Pre-class:** Provide students with a copy of the reading material—case study and additional readings.
2. **In-class:**
   a) Screen film.
   b) Allow 10–15 minutes for participants to reread case study (if needed).
   c) Then Begin discussion.
   d) Conclude with main points to have emerged during discussions, learnings and challenges.

Tools That May be Used by Facilitators/Instructors

Preparing to Teach

1. Know the case well so that you are able to guide discussions without conducting the session in a lecture format.
2. Know your target students (type of participants) well.[4] This will help you design the structure of the session better and guide classroom discussions more effectively.
3. Understand the subject of discussion in-depth.
4. Anticipate challenges that the classroom discussion can present to you with reference to the content related.

---

[3] Case Method in Practice: Core Principles, Christensen Center for Teaching and Learning. Available at http://www.hbs.edu/teaching/case-method-in-practice/core-principles.html, accessed on 5 August 2013.

[4] These cases are most likely to be used among medical, nursing and public health students and mid-level professionals.

5. How will you introduce-conduct-close the session.
6. Request a peer to help you with feedback in the first few sessions, this can help improve your teaching/facilitating style.
7. Depending on the make-up of participants, some students might bring to the discussion field-level experience which could help give the discussion more depth and perspective.

Classroom Tools

1. Tools available to the instructor: dialogue-debate-analytical frameworks for discussion.
2. Selecting students during discussions:
   a) Useful if some participants are dominating the discussion.
   b) To give everyone a fair chance to present their point of view.
   c) Random selection of participants may be done using rolling of dice, shuffled index cards each with a student's name, chits, etc.
3. Lead the class effectively:
   a) Ensure uniform (to the extent possible) participation.
   b) Break the ice in class to make students comfortable.
   c) Guide classroom discussion through the case and context.
   d) Facilitate discussion, control for direction of discussion, timing, engagement, etc.
4. Use a white board if needed.

Conclusion

The case method of teaching does not have a structured format to the class session. Instructors have the opportunity to explore different approaches towards conducting a classroom, enabling them to keep elements that work, reject those that don't and absorb new methods based on feedback from sessions. Knowledge of the content, target audience and ability to steer discussions will be useful in this style of teaching.

References

Baxter, P., Jack, S. 2008. 'Qualitative Case Study Methodology: Study Design and Implementation for Novice Researchers'. *The Qualitative Report*, 13(4): 544–59. Available at http://www.nova.edu/ssss/QR/QR13-4/baxter.pdf.

Buell, E.L. 1930. 'The Case Study: As a Method of Teaching Students and Graduates the Principles of Public Health Nursing'. *The American Journal of Nursing*, 30(4): 399–407. Available at http://www.jstor.org/stable/3411154.

Centre for Disease Control. Instructor's Guide for Facilitating Epidemiologic Case Studies for the Classroom. Atlanta, USA. Available at http://www.cdc.gov/epicasestudies/classroom_instructor.html, accessed on 5 August 2013.

District Level Household and Facility Survey (DLHS-3) 2007–08. 2010. International Institute for Population Sciences (IIPS). Mumbai: IIPS.

Flyvbjerg, B. 2011. 'Case Study', in N.K. Denzin and Y.S. Lincoln (eds), The SAGE Handbook of Qualitative Research, pp. 301–16. Thousand Oaks, CA: SAGE Publications. Available at http://www.sbs.ox.ac.uk/centres/bt/directory/Documents/CaseStudy4%202HBQR11PRINT.pdf.

Fritz, K. 2008. Case Study and Narrative Analysis, Qualitative Data Analysis Class Session 4. The Johns Hopkins University. Creative Commons Attribution-Non Commercial—Share Alike Licence. Available at http://ocw.jhsph.edu/courses/qualitativedataanalysis/PDFs/Session4.pdf, accessed on 5 August 2013.

Global Health Delivery Case Studies. Available at http://www.ghdonline.org/cases/qa/, accessed on 5 August 2013.

Lagarde, M., Haines, A., Palmer, N. 2009. 'The Impact of Conditional Cash Transfers on Health Outcomes and Use of Health Services in Low and Middle Income Countries'. *Cochrane Database of Systematic Reviews* (4). Article No: CD008137. DOI: 10.1002/14651858.CD008137.

Lim, S., Dandona, L., Hoisington, J., James, S., Hogan, M., Gakidou, E. 2010. 'India's Janani Suraksha Yojana, A Conditional Cash Transfer Programme to Increase Births in Health Facilities: An Impact Evaluation'. *The Lancet*, 375(9730): 2009–23.

Merriam Webster Dictionary (online). Available at http://www.merriam- webster.com/dictionary/case%20study.

National Family Health Survey (NFHS-3) 2005–06. 2007. International Institute for Population Sciences (IIPS) and Macro International. Volume I. Mumbai: IIPS.

National Health System Resource Centre (NHSRC). 2011. 'Programme Evaluation of Janani Suraksha Yojana'. New Delhi: NHSRC.

Omachonu, V.K., Einspruch, N.G. 2010. 'Innovation in Health Care Delivery Systems: A Conceptual Framework'. *The Innovation Journal: The Public Sector Innovation Journal*, 15(1).

Sample Registration System (SRS). 2011. Registrar General of India, Government of India, December 2011.

UNICEF Coverage Evaluation Survey. 2009. Available at http://www.unicef.org/india/1_-_CES_2009_All_India_Report.pdf, accessed in July 2013.

WHO, UNICEF, UNFPA and the World Bank Estimates. 2012. 'Trends in Maternal Mortality: In 1990–2010'.

Section A
Health System for Maternal and Newborn Care

Sub-themes

Access to Health Care Services in Remote Areas
Behaviour Change Communications
Financial Access to Health Care Services
Health Care Infrastructure
Human Resources
Quality Initiatives in Health Care Services
Referral Transport

Section A

Health System for Maternal and Newborn Care (Access; Quality; Availability; Affordability)

The health system, as defined by the World Health Organization (WHO), refers to all the organizations, institutions and resources whose primary purpose is to improve health and that come together to provide health care services to a population (WHO 2013). Health systems encompass a wide range of areas including leadership and governance, health information systems, health financing, human resources for health, essential medical products and technologies and service deliveries, which are brought together towards improving the health of individuals and populations equitably and affordably (WHO 2010).

This section presents 10 innovative programmes that are being implemented across India which address seven aspects of the health system. The aim of each intervention is to improve the availability, access and quality of health care services to populations in different parts of the country. Some geographical regions featured in the following case studies present poor maternal and newborn mortality indicators. The case studies in this section demonstrate innovative approaches used for health system strengthening with emphasis on improved delivery of services for maternal and newborn health.

The section begins with two unique models of mobile boat clinics implemented in different riverine areas, the Sunderbans in the state of West Bengal and islands on the Brahmaputra in the state of Assam. The Tagore Society for Rural Development (TSRD) in the Sunderbans region presents a three-tier model towards providing health services in inaccessible areas. Boat clinics in different locations are operated alongside land-based doctors clinics that are further supported by 144 field clinics which provide primary health services by nurses. The Centre for North East Studies and Policy Research (C-NES) operates a fleet of large boats which can reach remote islands on the Brahmaputra and a fleet of smaller ones for islands closer to the mainland, ferrying medical doctors, nurses and programme managers to different islands for health camps that provide primary health care services with maternal and newborn health services, immunization and family planning.

Health outcomes often require interventions which target influences on health both inside and outside the health system. The next case study on Reproductive and Child Health, Nutrition and AIDS (RACHNA) programme by CARE India features the use of behaviour change communication strategies implemented under the programme which were used to improve nutrition, demand generation, family planning services and other behaviours which impact maternal and newborn health.

Financial access is often a barrier towards accessing maternal and child health services; limitations of the public health sector in terms of providing free health services range from the ability of people to pay to access those services (transport, out-of-pocket (OOP) expenses on medicines, etc.) and often the perception of the quality of health care services that are provided free of cost. This case study looks at financial access to maternal health through the Sambhav Voucher Scheme which provides vouchers (coupons) that enable BPL families to access health care services through private providers and cover antenatal care (ANC), postnatal care (PNC), newborn care, family planning and some other services.

The case study on innovative health care infrastructure exclusively for maternal health covers two initiatives by LifeSpring Hospital Private Limited and Merrygold Health Network that aim to provide quality, affordable clinical-level reproductive health care along with outreach and referral services at low-costs.

The shortage of human resources in the Indian health system is well documented. This case study features a cadre of non-clinical health workers in India (called Yashodas) introduced at public maternity hospitals to improve the quality of health care services delivered to clients using the facility for maternity services. The Yashoda worker's primary role is to support the hospital staff in the pre and post delivery care of a mother and her newborn through counselling and support with labour, breastfeeding and immunization.

Long-term success of initiatives to encourage institutional deliveries and strengthen health system services also depends on the quality of care a woman and her family receive at the facility level. Quality of care includes clinical and non-clinical aspects of health care from biomedical waste management to high standards of disinfection and hygiene in the labour room, hygiene and sanitation at the facility, training of paramedical staff and much more. The case study on the Quality Assurance Programme (QAP) illustrates the first stages of implementation of the programme in West Bengal and uses data from a completed programme in the state of Odisha to demonstrate the impact of QAP on maternal and newborn health indicators.

Emergency transport services—in rural and urban areas—can play a significant role in reducing delays in accessing as well as in encouraging delivery at the facility level. This case study features two models of emergency transport services, the Janani Express and GVK-EMRI service from Madhya Pradesh and Andhra Pradesh, which demonstrate the use of basic and comprehensively constructed emergency transport vehicles (ambulances) and support systems that help in taking women in labour in rural, semi-rural and urban areas to the facility level for deliveries.

References

World Health Organization. 2010. Key Components of a Well Functioning Health System. Available at http://www.who.int/healthsystems/EN_HSSkeycomponents.pdf, accessed on 5 August 2013.

World Health Organization. 2013. Q and A: Health Systems. Available at http://www.who.int/topics/health_systems/qa/en/index.html, accessed on 5 August 2013.

Access to Health Care Services in Remote Areas

1. Ships of Hope: Mobile Boat Clinics in the Riverine Areas of Assam (C-NES)
2. Three-tier Outreach Model for Hard to Reach Areas: The Sunderbans

1

Ships of Hope: Mobile Boat Clinics in the Riverine Areas of Assam (C-NES)

Radhika Arora

As the mid-sized boat approaches the sandy islands in the river Brahmaputra, activity on-board picks up pace. Cardboard cartons packed with medicines and other supplies are piled on the deck along with tables and chairs, ready to be carried ashore. The helmsman uses a long bamboo pole to estimate the depth of the water as the boat approaches the sandy shores, shouting out instructions to steer the boat in the right direction. There is sudden silence as the engine is cut-off and the boat, carrying a team of medical personnel, supplies, community health worker and the boat-crew, slowly drifts ashore.

Context

Located in the North Eastern part of India, Assam is one of the largest and most populous states in the North East. The topography of the state includes valleys, hills and rivers. One of Asia's most important rivers, the Brahmaputra, flows through the state, covering a distance of approximately 1,800 miles (see Image 1.1). The river is dotted with small habited islands called *sapori*s or *char*s, depending on which part of Assam you're in. Heavy rains, especially during the monsoon season, are characteristic of the climate of this region. The geographical and climatic conditions of the state often make parts of it, especially the river islands inaccessible, flood prone (the region accounts for 9.4% of India's total flood-prone area) and cut-off from transport and communications, making the provision of health care services difficult in ordinary circumstances and almost impossible in times of natural disasters or extreme climate conditions. Access to and from the islands which is difficult throughout the year is made worse during the monsoon season.

Image 1.1
Satellite Images of the Majuli Islands

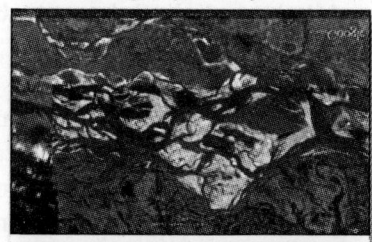

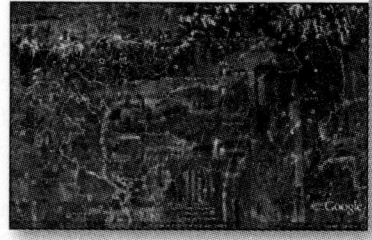

Source: Courtesy Google Maps (March 2011)

Almost 10% of the population of Assam (Gogoi) lives on the 2,300 remote islands on the Brahmaputra in upper Assam. Access to health care, education, sanitation and even basic infrastructure facilities such as electricity and potable water is a challenge in this region (Forrey et al. 2007–08). Assam has some of the worst health indicators in the country. The infant mortality rate (IMR), i.e., 58[1] and maternal mortality ratio (MMR), i.e., 390 (SRS 2007–09) are higher than the national average. Bringing health care to people is a challenge, especially during the monsoon season which often causes floods on the mainland; the problem of access is even more severe for the residents of the remote *sapori*s where flooding often cuts them off of communication and access.

Sanjoy Hazarika, founder of Centre for North East Studies and Policy Research (C-NES), decided to use local skills and resources to reach out to populations living in large riverine islands on the Brahmaputra, by using boats and the idea for having mobile boat clinics to take basic health care services, with emphasis on maternal and newborn health to the marginalized populations living on the islands on the Brahmaputra river in Assam, was born.

Introduction to the Innovation

In 2004, C-NES under the guidance of Sanjoy Hazarika won the World Bank Development Marketplace 2004 award for their innovative sustainable boat clinic initiative to deliver health services to the people living on the islands in Assam. The idea was to design a boat which would be large enough to carry teams of medical personnel, medical equipment and supplies.

Using the grant, C-NES worked with local boat makers to develop the first prototype mobile boat clinic christened *akha* which means 'hope' in Assamese.

Akha—the ship of hope—was started in 2005 and continues to serve populations in upper Assam today. The organization now owns seven boats and operates another eight boats which are taken on rent, but operated by C-NES.

The initiative is unique because it's one of the first initiatives of its kind to reach out to island populations. The boat itself is unique

---

Voices from the Islands: Morigaon District, Assam

'We had to face great difficulties prior to boat clinic services, it was very difficult to take a patient to the hospital, we had to hire boats and sometimes that patient had to be taken along with other passengers which was troublesome. The help of boat clinic services is giving us satisfaction especially for the pregnant women. The village environment has improved. Earlier people did not understand about health care, now with the services of boat clinics the awareness levels of the people have improved. Whatever you are saying is very good and you are doing good work. We should take part in making the communities aware about the messages that you are spreading.

We have to hire boats to carry the serious patients to civil hospital which is located far away and we have to face lot of difficulties. This *char* is Hamur *char* and civil is located to the west of Lahorighat. There are financial constraints; we are poor people, if you give us money to carry the patient to hospital we may not get boats in the time of need resulting in death of the patient before reaching the hospital. The pregnant women die before reaching the hospital.'

Source: Interview, ©PHFI, July 2011 (Vox Pop, Islander Morigaon District, Assam).

---

[1] Our Women and Children—Present Status of Infant Health. Chief Minister's Vision for Women and Children in Assam 2016. Available at http://online.assam.gov.in/documents/218378/2d2df305-bfd4-46f5-86aa-10fcec046fa7, accessed on 5 August 2013.

in its design and the use of indigenous talent and materials, as well as in its ability to carry crew members, house a basic laboratory for on-the-spot testing and other services for days at a stretch.

The innovation was appreciated by the Governments of India and Assam; today the boat clinics are operated with support from the National Rural Health Mission (NRHM), Assam.

The Clinic

The boat clinics aim to visit every island at least once every month. The riverine islands are spread out across a large area on the Brahmaputra. C-NES boats are docked at mainland areas across Kamrup District, Dibrugarh, Tinsukia and Jorhat. Depending on the location of the islands that need to be visited, a programme for the month is drawn up at the head office located in Guwahati in consultation with community workers and local staff. Two types of boat clinic operations are run. These are day boats and long-stay boats. In addition, there are also referral boats. See below:

1. **Kinds of boats:**

   a) **Day boats:** Mobile boat clinics that leave for day trips from the mainland. These boats ferry doctors and supporting medical staff to islands, usually located in lower Assam, for day-long health camps. Some of these boats are taken on a lease-basis by C-NES.

   b) **Long-stay boats:** These boats are larger, often based on the prototype and usually owned by C-NES. They ferry medical personnel and other crew members to islands that are further away from the mainland. Once on-board crew members spend two to four days travelling from one island to another before making their way back to the mainland. Health camps are held at islands during the day. The camp is typically wrapped up by mid-afternoon and the crew makes their way to the next island before sunset, where they dock and set-up camp for the next health camp, the next morning. This enables them to visit islands that are four to seven hours away by boat.

   c) **Referral transport boats:** Sometimes row boats are earmarked for emergency transport from the islands to health care centres on the mainland. This is essential for health emergencies, especially pregnancy-related cases. Boat clinics are not available 24×7 to the populations on the islands.

2. **Design of boats:** Keeping in mind the distances that the boat will serve and the fact that the crew would need to live on-board for days on end, the boat clinics needed to combine functionality with comfort; made by local boat makers, the boats were made in the style of other local boats, using better designed diesel engines (120 hp, diesel reconditioned truck engines, unlike irrigation pumps used by local country boats). These engines gave the boats better power and improved navigation in the river areas.

   For the medical personnel and crew members, who often spent days at a stretch on the river, the boats offer cabins, toilets and kitchen facilities.

   The boats are also equipped with basic laboratory services which offer blood testing facilities and a pharmacy that stocks essential drugs and vaccines. Solar energy is used to power the refrigeration facilities required to stock supplies on board.

A typical boat clinic unit comprises (C-NES, Annual Report 2009–10)

a) two medical officers per boat,
b) two auxiliary nurse midwives (ANMs),
c) a general nurse and midwife (GNM),
d) pharmacist,
e) laboratory technician,
f) community worker,
g) boat crew: pilot/navigator, engineers, boat operator and cook.

3. **Operations:** Apart from the boat crew, the programme managers, ground officers and community health workers play a crucial role in bringing health care services to the islands. Administrative and operational decisions are taken at the offices on the mainland (Guwahati and local offices), but it's the community workers and the district programme officers (DPOs) that mobilize government health workers and the populations on the islands, informing them about the health camp schedule and encouraging attendance to the camp, especially for maternal and newborn care and immunizations. The district programme officer (DPO), C-NES community worker and the Accredited Social Health Activist (ASHA) worker play an important role in informing the islanders of the camp.

Services Provided

The most important service that the mobile boat clinics provide is access to basic health care services in areas where there was almost none. The focus of the clinics, especially under the NRHM, is to bring maternal and newborn care to the island populations. Some health services provided and utilized by the community are as follows.

Services for improved maternal and newborn health

- Antenatal care (ANC) and postnatal care (PNC)
- The clinics are not equipped to conduct surgeries; but they have conducted safe deliveries
- Tetanus toxoid (TT) vaccines to pregnant women
- Distribution of iron and folic acid (IFA) tablets

> **Voices from the Islands: Naogaon District**
>
> From evening she was mentioning about her headache. I gave her pain killers. After mentioning to me about her headache two–three times, she was attacked by Tetanus. Immediately, we poured water to her head. She got relief for a while when we did that. She was attacked by Tetanus thrice that time. A local quack was called immediately who examined the case and referred her to be taken to the nearest hospital. We searched for the boat to carry her to the hospital. By then it was 10 PM. We managed a boat to carry her and it took two hours to reach the ghat on the other side. We had to wait for an hour at the ghat for the hospital ambulance which never came. Then we managed a hand cart and carried her to the hospital which took another two hours' time. She was administered saline at the PHC and was advised by the nurse to take her to Morigaon civil if not cured. At 4.30 AM when we were taking her to a hospital in Dhing in Naogaon District she passed away.
>
> *Source:* Interview, ©PHFI, July 2011.

- Information on nutrition, pregnancy and childbirth and importance of vitamins and breast-feeding

Immunization services for vaccination

- Basic immunization and follow-ups

Family Planning services for improved contraception and birth spacing

- Information and awareness on family planning
- Access to family planning services and methods

Services available on board the boat clinics

- Laboratory: basic testing facilities for anaemia, malaria, etc., available on-board
- Medical supplies: essential medicines and vaccines are carried on-board for use and distribution during health camps

Information education communication activities

- The boat clinics are also used to spread awareness on sanitation, hygiene, safe drinking water, immunization, family planning, malaria control, etc.

Monitoring information systems

- The boat clinics conduct monitoring services towards the submission of monthly reports to the NRHM

Training and capacity building as part of the clinic work

- Training of medical personnel on the boat clinics is conducted regularly
- Opportunity for young medical graduates to work on mobile boat clinics as part of their rural posting

Common health care needs the boat clinic services address

- Fever, stomach ache and diarrhoea (Akha)
- Distribution of oral rehydration solution (ORS)

Key Strategies

Partnership

The boat clinics function as a result of a partnership between C-NES, UNICEF and the Government of Assam (NRHM).

Target group

- Tribal and non-tribal communities living on the 2,300 islands of the river Brahmaputra
- Focus on women and children

Scaling up and Sustainability

In May 2005, Akha–the Ship of Hope—was launched as the first boat clinic by C-NES to deliver health services to the people living on the *sapori* of the Brahmaputra river in Assam. The first boat was launched with the help of district health and administration organizations as well as assistance from local non-governmental organizations (NGOs), business and Oil India Limited and Assam Oil Limited.

Akha was a success; the initiative was noticed by the government as well as international organizations such as United Nations Children's Fund (UNICEF) which now supports the initiative along with the government. With the support of the NRHM under the Government of Assam (through a public private partnership), the Akha boat clinic initiative was scaled-up in a phased manner with the addition of boats and other resources to the services.

> **Voices from the Islands: The Impact**
>
> 'After the boat clinic services and doctors, people have benefited a lot. We did not know that pregnant women have to be given injections for TT, now they are getting these services every month.
>
> We have no other option but to reside in the *char* areas. We are poor people and we cannot buy land in the mainland areas where the land rates are very high.'
>
> *Source:* Interview, ©PHFI, July 2011.

In the first phase—2008—of the partnership between C-NES and NRHM, along with UNICEF's support, was expanded to reach out to populations in five districts of Assam—Dibrugarh, Tinsukia, Dhemaji, Morigaon and Dhubri. The second phase of the initiative took place in 2009 with services being extended to five more districts—Lakhimpur, Jorhat, Sonitpur, Nalbari and Barpeta. Three more districts—Kamrup, Goalpara and Bongaigaon—were included under the boat clinic initiative in 2010. The initiative which started with one boat in 2005 inaugurated its sixth boat at the time of writing this note in March 2011. Work on a seventh boat is underway. The project aims to cover 10 lakh people who live on the *sapori*s on the Brahmaputra by 2012 (C-NES, Annual Report 2009–10).

Concluding Remarks

Less than a decade after they started, the mobile boat clinics have taken health care services to some of the most hard to access areas of the country. Similar initiatives are ongoing in other parts of India also to address issues of social and geographic exclusion.

The boat clinics bring health care services once a month to each island. While this service does take essential basic health services to populations in remote areas it is still insufficient in times of emergencies that may be related to disease, injuries, pregnancy and childbirth among others. Given the location and circumstances, the team does the best it can to provide basic health services and preempt any health care need of the population. A referral mechanism is in place for emergency services as well as for those who need higher level of health care, such as smaller boats to ferry emergency maternal cases to mainland or to transport emergency medical cases to the mainland in times of flooding when the larger boats might not be able to access the smaller islands safely.

There are many constraints faced by the medical team on the boats and the boat crew, from braving extreme weather conditions such as thunderstorms, choppy river water and extreme rain, to walking for miles on soft sand under a hot sun on dry summer days when the river water recedes from the islands.

Ushering in Changes

Aboard a boat ferrying doctors, nurses, field workers and medical supplies across the river Brahmaputra in the state of Assam, a doctor recalled a visit by a 60-year old who seemed to be perfectly healthy. The 'patient' had not come to the doctor for a medical consultation, but to see what a doctor looked like. He had, in his entire life, never seen a doctor.

Such stories are not unusual. Up until 2005, access to health care services was almost negligible for approximately 25 lakh people living across 2,500 river islands on the river Brahmaputra, in Assam.[2] In 2005, the Centre for North East Studies introduced the first boat clinic. In 2008, C-NES along with the NRHM, Assam expanded upon the boat clinic initiative under the Boat Clinic Project. Now, C-NES along with the NRHM operate an extensive fleet of around 15 boats that provide basic health services, essential maternal and child care services, family planning, laboratory facilities and other health services to the island communities.

The boat clinics have brought to the islands health services that were previously unavailable or inaccessible to most. In addition, awareness levels on health care services were low. In the period between 2008 and 2012, under the partnership between C-NES and the NRHM, 10,385 health camps were conducted in the intervention areas, providing health checkups to almost 832,325 people. Around 44,355 women received antenatal care. Postnatal care, immunization and nutrition interventions and awareness were other important services delivered successfully by the boat clinics under the partnership. Intervention districts show high levels of awareness on health services such as ANC (61%), immunization (80% aware of BCG vaccination).[3]

Nutrition, awareness and addressing anaemia, family planning and improving referrals are other areas of work being conducted through the boat clinics. In the few years that this innovative approach was implemented to provide health care services to populations living in remote areas, utilization of the clinics was high at about 95.4%, with the majority accessing services for immunization and antenatal care.[4]

---

[2] Dr. Chiranjeev Bhattacharjya. Utilization of Boat Clinic Services in the Char Areas of Nalbari District.
[3] Information from C-NES.
[4] Dr. Chiranjeev Bhattacharjya. Utilization of Boat Clinic Services in the Char Areas of Nalbari District.

Sources:

Based on data provided by C-NES in June 2013.

Dr. Chiranjeev Bhattacharjya. Utilization of Boat Clinic Services in the Char Areas of Nalbari District. Centre for North East Studies. Unpublished.

References

Annual Report 2009–10. Centre for North East Studies and Policy Research (C-NES).

Forrey, G., D'Cruz, J.J., Gvetadze, N. and Goswami, R. 2007–08. 'Delivering Primary Health Care and Education to the Brahmaputra River Islands: A Case Study of the Akha: Boat of Hope'. Knowledge Community on Children in India. Government of India and UNICEF. Available at http://blog.lib.umn.edu/gpa/globalnotes/India%2007%20AKHA%20BOAT%20ASSAM.pdf, accessed on 5 August 2013.

Gogoi, M. 'Dodhia: A Mishing Island in Brahmaputra'. UNICEF India. Available at www.unicef.org/india/emergency_3243.htm, accessed in September 2011.

Sample Registration System (SRS). 2007–09. Office of Registrar General of India. Special Bulletin on Maternal Mortality in India 2007–09. Available at http://www.censusindia.gov.in/vital_statistics/SRS_Bulletins/Final-MMR%20Bulletin-2007-09_070711.pdf, accessed on 5 August 2013.

2

Three-tier Outreach Model for Hard to Reach Areas: The Sunderbans

Sourav Neogi

Background of the Sunderbans

The Sunderbans, a unique biosphere reserve of mangrove forests and one of the global heritage sites, are located in the extreme south of West Bengal (an eastern Indian state) and Bangladesh, the neighbouring country. The entire area is surrounded by tidal rivers or estuaries from north and south and by innumerable narrow tidal creeks from east to west creating a beautiful but inhospitable terrain. The area outside the reserve forest (54 islands), home to about four million people spread over 19 administrative blocks, is the human face of the Sunderbans and epitomizes abject poverty, deprivation and acute struggle against geographical challenges (see Map 2.1). It is, however, important to note that the geographical challenges vary across blocks. People, who live in the 'remote' Sunderbans—the blocks adjacent to the forest area or the Bay of Bengal—face more serious problems compared to those who live in the 'peripheries' (and closer to Kolkata) (Kanjilal et al. 2010).

Map 2.1
Sunderbans

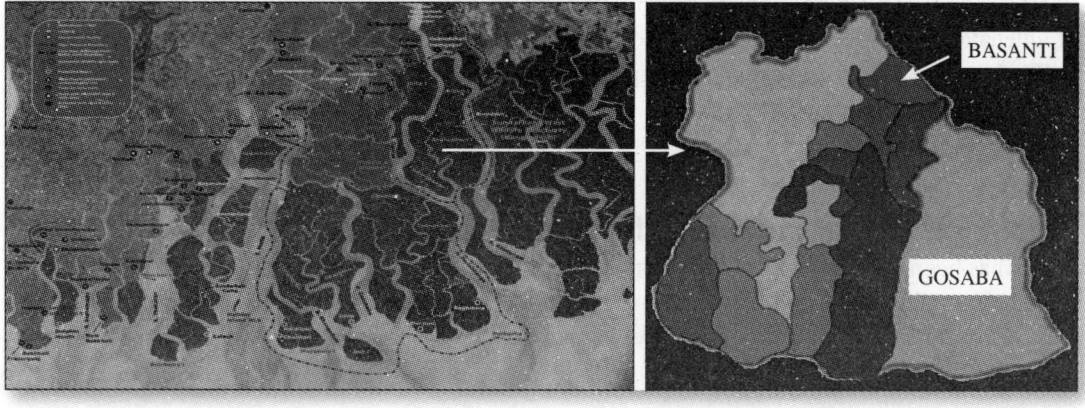

Source: Google Maps 2011.

Health Services Are Scarce—How to Reach out?

Formal health services are scarce in Sunderbans and government services are severely inadequate. Through this case study we would like to highlight the measures that have been taken by Tagore Society for Rural Development (TSRD) to reach the far flung islands to provide health services. Many obstacles, however, are still present and would need greater effort and support to overcome them.

Formal Service

TSRD has been working in the Sunderbans since 1969. Formal health service providers are limited and can be counted on the fingertips in any block or tehsil. Government is the largest health provider through community health centres (CHCs), primary health centres (PHCs) and subcentres. Unfortunately even with these facilities in place, availability of formal care is limited by large-scale absenteeism among doctors and paramedics. Thus for the four million people spread over 19 administrative blocks, TSRD's health facilities are among the reputed service providers in the community. TSRD's services focus by and large on reproductive and child health services although first-hand emergency services have been provided by the health assistants (nurses).

Informal Services

Informal health services are provided in substantial measure, the providers being well dispersed and popular in the community. Absolute dominance of rural medical practitioners (RMP) in the outpatient care market has been found. Sixty-two per cent (Kanjilal et al. 2010) of outpatients were treated by RMPs who practise by rampantly providing irrational combinations including steroids and modern medicines without any formal medical training.

Maternal Health Care Situation in the Sunderbans

Maternal health care utilization at institutions is low in the Sunderbans. According to the Future Health Systems Research Programme report published in 2010, only 29% delivered their last child at a public or private health facility (Kanjilal et al. 2010). However, most of these institutional deliveries (about 71%) were conducted at government hospitals. It is interesting to note that utilization of antenatal care (ANC) is quite high (see Table 2.1), yet institutional deliveries are not common. Difficult terrain and broken chain of transportation—especially in the least accessible islands—seem to force the mothers to deliver at home.

Tagore Society for Rural Development: Rangabelia Project

TSRD has been serving people of the Sunderbans for the last three decades. It started with the individual effort of Tushar Kanjilal which later on transformed into a social development movement. In 1967, Tushar Kanjilal joined the Rangabelia High School as headmaster and to his dismay, within a

Table 2.1
Service Statistics of Clinics

District South 24 Parganas	Basanti Block		Gosaba Block	
Total population	274,577		236,191	
Total no. of remote villages under the cover of MHC services	26		34	
Population in these villages	96,379		158,559	
	Apr 09–Mar 2010	Jan–Mar 2011	Apr 09–Mar 2010	Jan–Mar 2011
Time Period				
Total no. of ANC cases examined	5,300	2,251	8,618	2,716
• No. of 1st ANC check-up	1,720	647	2,346	651
• No. of 2nd ANC check-up	1,325	542	2,153	615
• No. of 3rd ANC check-up	2,255	1,062	4,119	1,450
Total no. of PNC cases examined	708	240	1,118	331
Pregnancy complication—Anaemia	219	182	413	168
Pregnancy complication—hypertension	6	9	15	10
Pregnancy complication—Eclampsia	18		48	
No. of pregnant mothers given injection TT 1st dose	1,471	463	1,454	429
No. of pregnant mothers given injection TT 2nd dose	1,335	480	1,276	360
No. of children received BCG vaccine	1,774	454	1,407	467
No. of children received Measles vaccine	1,607	428	2,348	484

Source: MIS Data TSRD.

short time he realized that one-fourth of the students were coming to school on an empty stomach. This was the beginning of a journey of a man with a mission. At the age of 37, he started a comprehensive development programme in three villages and today it has spread to a large part of the Sunderbans. At the beginning, the Rangabelia Comprehensive Rural Development Project focussed on agriculture and tried to free poor villagers from the clutches of moneylenders. Nowadays, it delivers a spectrum of development interventions from agriculture to health initiatives (TSRD 2010).

In this case study we will be focussing on the health interventions of TSRD.

Comprehensive Health Project under the Rangabelia Project

In 1978, this health project started in a small public club room at Rangabelia; during those years the team was primarily working with the villagers to make them aware about their own health and hygiene. Later, the project identified and provided training to a few literate village girls about health and hygiene issues and after the training these girls started working with villagers to educate them on health issues. Presently in 2 blocks (Basanti and Gosaba) out of 13 blocks of South 24 Parganas district, there are 72 health workers, 18 health assistants and 3 supervisors working with the villagers. When they started working on the demand side (from the communities) of health care, they realized that there was a huge gap in the supply side (health facilities) of health care. With this understanding in 1985, a comprehensive health centre, i.e., a hospital building with 25 beds and other important facilities came up.

As discussed earlier, the Sunderbans are a group of isolated islands covered on all sides by saline river water where the only mode of transportation is by boat set against this tough physical terrain, TSRD has been working with the poor over the last three decades by providing them medical services in their islands.

Health Facilities under Tagore Society for Rural Development

TSRD started with only one health care facility; however, currently TSRD has two health facilities in the Sunderbans which take care of the supply side of health care. Recently, a few government health facilities have also come up in nearby areas, which have definitely increased access to health services for the villagers. However, many residents of the Sunderbans still prefer to come to TSRD health facilities because of the quality and round-the-clock services available in these facilities.

- **Rangabelia Hospital (20-bedded hospital)**: The hospital provides both preventive and curative health services to the islanders. Activities undertaken by the hospital authority are training, awareness generation and health check-ups, besides operating mobile health clinics which serve the Gosaba and Basanti Blocks. However, the main services provided by the hospital authority are the residential hospital services and the treatment of patients at a minimum cost. The authority calls specialist doctors from Kolkata to provide the best possible treatment to patients. The hospital has provision for services including X-ray, electrocardiogram (ECG) and pathology.
- **Community Delivery Centre**: The Community Delivery Centre was started in 2008 under a public–private partnership initiative with the NRHM, West Bengal. This has been established with the objective of serving pregnant women of below poverty line (BPL) categories in the nearby islands. This particular facility functions 24×7 and two doctors, two paramedics and two staff nurses are also available round-the-clock. The services are provided free of cost to the patients. In case of complications, pregnant women have been referred to the tertiary level facilities (district hospital) located in the mainland. Transports for the referrals include mechanized boats, *dola*s, vans and ambulance.

Three-tier Outreach Model

Due to the nature of the terrain, most parts of the Sunderbans areas are inaccessible, many hours of travel required to reach a health facility, which is time consuming and expensive for people. The importance of a comprehensive outreach model for the poor villagers is great in a place such as the Sunderbans. This is especially true from the maternal health point of view, since almost 70% of the deliveries are still happening at home. Reaching these mothers at the right time is very important and especially in Sunderbans where formal services are scarce. Due to the difficult terrain, doctors and paramedical staff are not keen to stay on these islands. This makes the situation much more difficult and challenging for the programme implementers.

Figure 2.1
Interlinkages between Three-tier Outreach Model

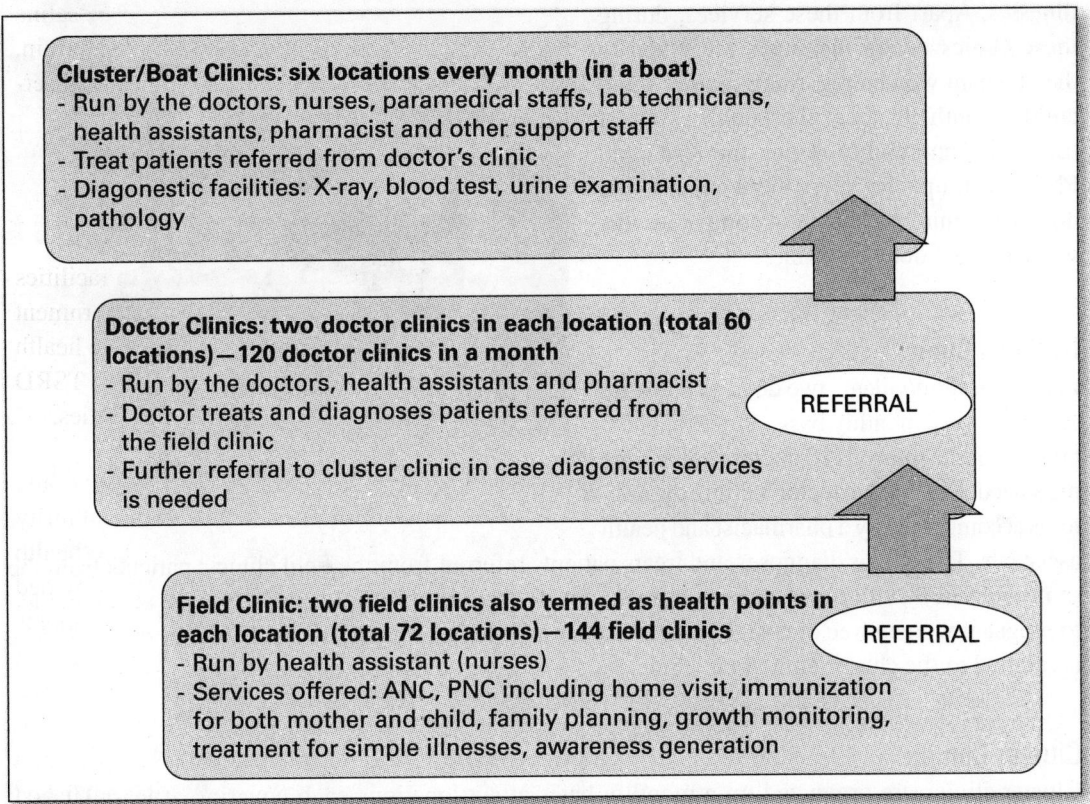

Cluster/Boat Clinics: six locations every month (in a boat)
- Run by the doctors, nurses, paramedical staffs, lab technicians, health assistants, pharmacist and other support staff
- Treat patients referred from doctor's clinic
- Diagonestic facilities: X-ray, blood test, urine examination, pathology

Doctor Clinics: two doctor clinics in each location (total 60 locations)—120 doctor clinics in a month
- Run by the doctors, health assistants and pharmacist
- Doctor treats and diagnoses patients referred from the field clinic
- Further referral to cluster clinic in case diagonstic services is needed

REFERRAL

Field Clinic: two field clinics also termed as health points in each location (total 72 locations)—144 field clinics
- Run by health assistant (nurses)
- Services offered: ANC, PNC including home visit, immunization for both mother and child, family planning, growth monitoring, treatment for simple illnesses, awareness generation

REFERRAL

Source: PHFI.

With the mandate to provide medical check-ups for the children and pregnant women and emergency medical services in the inaccessible areas of the Sunderbans, TSRD set up a three-tier outreach model with support from the West Bengal Government.

The outreach model consists of field clinics, doctor clinics and cluster clinics. A description of each is given in Figure 2.1. The three clinic types are interlinked and work with active referral and follow-up from one tier to another.

The three-tier model enables the efficient use of limited resources by conducting periodic health check-ups at the primary level and ensuring timely referrals for those who need it.

Field Clinics

Every month, 144 mobile camps/field clinics are held at 72 points covering 60 villages of Gosaba and Basanti Blocks. Field clinics are run by the health assistants who are from the village and have been trained by the TSRD medical doctors and nurses on a periodic basis on the key health issues. During the field clinics, the health assistants conduct ANC and postnatal care (PNC) including home visits, immunization for mother and child, family planning and treatment for general illnesses. Apart from these services, during these clinics health messages are given to the pregnant women regarding mother's and cnild's health. In case, the health assistant finds any abnormality during the ANC and PNC check-up s/he refers the woman to the doctor's clinic. S/he also accompanies the woman to the doctor's clinic.

Doctor's Clinic

In each location/village, two doctor clinics are organized on a monthly basis. Since there are 60 locations, a total of 120 doctors' clinics are organized. During the doctor's clinic the doctor is accompanied by a pharmacist and health assistants. The doctor diagnoses and treats patients referred from the field clinics; patients from the same and nearby villages also visit for treatment. At the doctor's clinic, medicines are also provided to pregnant women free of cost. In case, the doctor feels that the patient needs further diagnosis she is referred to the cluster clinic/boat clinic.

Image 2.1
People Accessing Services on the Boat Clinic

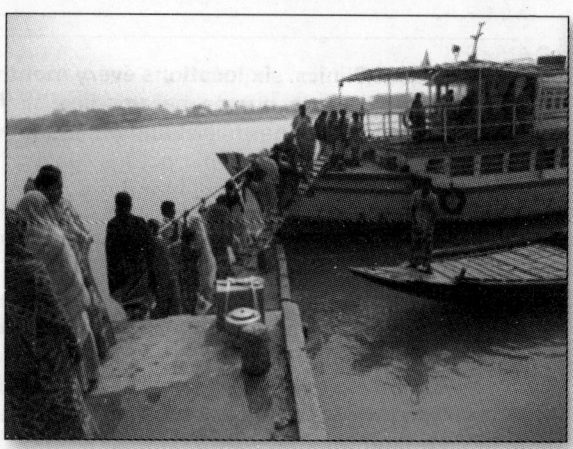

Source: Image credit – Sourav Neogi, ©PHFI, July 2011.

Cluster Clinics

Cluster clinics are organized on a monthly basis at six locations each covering at least 10 to12 villages. These cluster clinics are also known as boat clinics as they are organized on a boat. Apart from the main boat, there are two small boats available which escort patients from the river bank of the island to the main boat (see Image 2.1). The main boat stays in the main river because of its large size and it cannot go close to the river bank. In the cluster clinic, the patients are accompanied by the health assistants. Mainly patients referred from the doctors' clinics visit these clinics, but people with other ailments also visit. Besides the doctors, nurses, paramedical staff, lab technicians, health assistants, pharmacists and other support staff also participate in these clinics. Diagnostic facilities such as X-ray, blood test, urine examination and pathology services are available in this clinic.

Deliveries are not conducted in these clinics. For deliveries, the pregnant women are instructed either to visit Rangabelia Hospital or the community delivery centre.

Service Statistics

A few key service statistics of these clinics are given in Table 2.1. TSRD is working in two blocks of South 24 Parganas. It submits statistics every quarter to the Ministry of Health and Family Welfare, Government of West Bengal.

Key Characteristics of the Organization

Dedicated Manpower

In order to explain the features of the project, we have to mention the dedicated and self-motivated manpower of TSRD. Several employees/workers have been associated with TSRD for last 20 years or more. Many of them have mentioned that through their work they are contributing back to the society and this motivates them to work for the organization.

Multi-sectoral Approach

TSRD is not only working on health; it works on other developmental issues as well such as agriculture, education, livelihood activities, deforestation, cultural activities and many more. Due to the range of services they provide, which affects the life of large number of people staying in the Sunderbans, the people are also motivated to join hands with them to bring about positive change.

Challenges

In this section of the case study, we are trying to highlight the issues that an organization faces when it comes to implementing/providing health care services to remote populations. TSRD is facing many challenges these days which, at times, hinder their work. A few key challenges are mentioned as follows:

- **Electricity**: Large parts of island still do not have electricity. Hence, electrical diagnostic equipment fails to work in the health facilities.
- **Difficulty in referral**: In case of complications, people are referred to the tertiary hospitals. But due to poor bumpy condition of the roads (brick roads) patients face a lot of difficulty. On the islands, hand-pulled rickshaw is the mode of transportation for everything, including patient transportation (see Image 2.2).
- **Financial crisis**: The project is totally dependent on external funding mainly from government and donor agencies. The government, at times, does not increase the allocation of funds for manpower and drugs which creates a financial crisis for the project implementers. Many of the health assistants, even after

Image 2.2
Patient Being Taken on Cycle Rickshaw to Boat Clinic for Referral

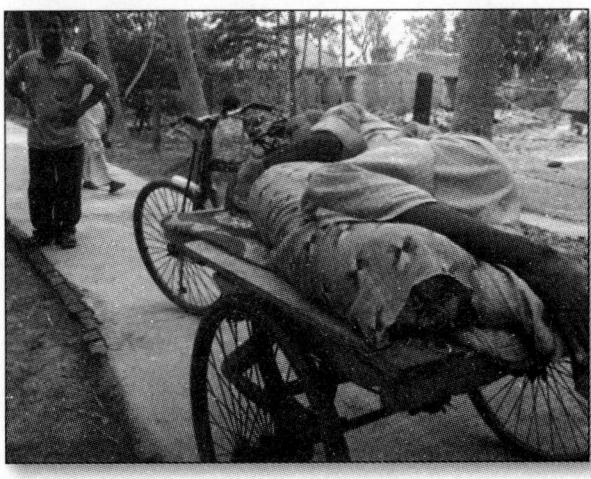

Source: TRSD.

working with the organization for more than 10 years, get less than ₹100 per day (which is less than the minimum daily wage).

Post-storm Aila: There was no cultivation taking place for the last two years after storm Aila struck the island. Due to the storm, salt water from the sea came into the agricultural lands in the Sunderbans, which left the lands infertile. Agriculture is the main occupation for many people. This has left people in deep crisis.

References

Kanjilal, B., Mazumdar, G.P., Mukherjee, M., Mondal, S., Barman, D., Singh, S. and Mandal, A. 2010. Health Care in the Sundarbans (India): Challenges and Plan for a Better Future. Supported by Future Health Systems Research Programme. Submitted to Department for International Development.

Tagore Society for Rural Development (TSRD). 2010. Rangabelia Project Document Brochure. West Bengal. Available at http://tsrd.org/achive.html.

Behaviour Change Communications

3. Innovation in Behaviour Change Communication: The RACHNA Project

3

Innovation in Behaviour Change Communication: The RACHNA Project[1]

Raj Mohan Panda and Sourav Neogi

Maternal Health Situation in India

Millennium Development Goal (MDG) 5 focusses on improving maternal health and aims to reduce the maternal mortality ratio (MMR) by 75% between 1990 and 2015. Globally, overall maternal mortality has declined from 409,100 deaths in 1990 to 273,500 in 2011. Out of the 273,500 global maternal deaths in 2011, India accounts for 50,648, around 19% of the global burden (Lozano et al. 2011). Maternal mortality varies by region and state in India, being higher in the eastern and central regions and lower in north-western and southern regions (Mavalankar 2000). Common causes of maternal deaths in developing countries such as India are largely preventable. Maternal and neonatal mortality are influenced by factors such as poverty and other social factors such as the position of women in the society, access to health care, traditional practices, as well as the overall level of development in the region. Women's education, age and parity also have a strong influence on maternal and neonatal mortality and morbidity.

As depicted in Figure 3.1, maternal health outcomes are directly and indirectly affected by factors at different levels. In the past, efforts to improve maternal health have focussed more on issues within the health system; however, this requires strategic efforts that address issues both inside and outside the health system. According to the framework above, household and individual behaviours can also be major factors for improving maternal health outcomes. These factors include appropriate use of household resources for women's and children's health, nutrition behaviours, health care demand (for contraception, antenatal care (ANC), etc.), as well as social factors such as early marriage and pregnancy (Chatterjee et al. 2009). To promote healthy behaviour, it is essential that families have adequate knowledge of healthy practices as well as the ability to act on this information. Risks during pregnancy and newborn care are exacerbated by inappropriate behaviours as well as by limited

[1]The authors acknowledge the contribution made by Dr Musa and Dr Kurian towards the completion of this case study.

Figure 3.1

Pathways to Improve Maternal Health Outcomes

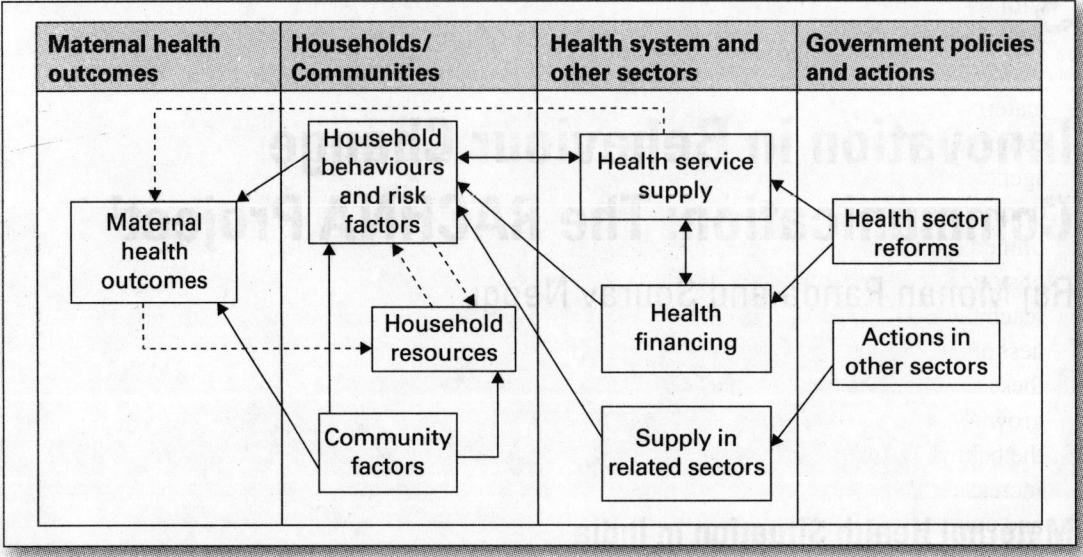

Source: Claeson et al. (2001).

household resources. Issues such as food security, poor maternity care, dysfunctional systems of providing nutritional and social security also contribute to the problem. There is evidence to show that malnutrition is more common among the children of illiterate mothers as well as in low socio-economic populations.

Access to health care services also influences maternal health outcomes. The National Family Health Survey-3 (NFHS-3) conducted during 2005–06 shows that only 62.4% of ever married women respondents living in urban areas and even fewer 27.7% of rural women respondents have received the WHO-recommended four antenatal visits. The District Level Household Survey-3 (DLHS-3) conducted during 2007–08 indicates an overall improvement in access to maternal care (if three or more antenatal check-ups are taken as proxy) in the post National Rural Health Mission (NRHM) period, perhaps more for the high focus states (with poor health indicators) than the non-high focus states (which had better health indicators) (Nair and Panda 2011). Apart from access to care, community factors such as gender norms and stereotypes, myths and misconceptions about practices, social cohesion, access to community services and cultural practices can have a direct bearing on maternal health outcomes. The interplay of all these factors critically affects the way a household member behaves and if the factors are negative, they result in poor maternal health outcomes. Maternal nutrition during the pre- and postnatal periods is extremely important for safe motherhood as well as infant feeding. A balanced diet, as well as vitamin and mineral supplementation, improves birth outcome and maternal well-being. Being underweight contributes to poor maternal health and birth outcomes. Pregnant women are particularly vulnerable to anaemia due to increased requirements for iron and folic acid. Anaemia during pregnancy is a significant problem in developing countries. In India, for example, the prevalence of anaemia among pregnant women is estimated at almost 50%.

Anaemia is a life-threatening complication for women during pregnancy and puts them at risk of dying from even small amounts of blood loss during the pregnancy and post-partum period. Women with severe anaemia are particularly at risk and have a 3.5 times greater chance of dying than those without anaemia (Lule et al. 2005).

Community mobilization and awareness can play an important role in generating demand for maternal health services, as well as improving access to the services. Birth preparedness is a key component of globally accepted safe motherhood programmes and is widely promoted by international agencies. An area in which community interventions can be of value is in increasing birth preparedness (birth planning) and complication readiness, helping a family know where or from whom (identify trained birth attendants [TBAs]) to seek help and provide access to funds or transportation during an obstetric emergency. These interventions will help in addressing the delays (deciding to seek care and reaching services) that contribute to maternal morbidity and mortality. Increasing community aware-ness about the signs of emergency obstetric complications and motivating families to seek help when these emergencies are identified. These can greatly improve a woman's chance of survival. There is growing evidence that well-designed behaviour change interventions can be effective in producing the behaviour required for achieving desired health objectives. These interventions do not focus on increasing knowledge alone, but also to extend contextual factors such as the behaviours of family and community. Such an intervention is called behaviour change communication (BCC). These are designed to promote, elicit, support and stimulate specific behaviour change via communication. In the context of maternal health, BCC strategies can play a key role in promoting certain attitudes, knowledge, skills and capacity. For example, in many parts of India, there are certain beliefs and practices regarding food during pregnancy, both on how much and what to eat. There is a tendency by communities to encourage the pregnant mother to eat less ('eating down') so as to have a small baby and, thus, have an easy delivery. This reduces the woman's already meagre average daily food intake and discourages the intake of nutritious items such as meat and leafy vegetables during preg-nancy. BCC strategies that use various reinforcing messages through multiple channels that target both men and women can be effective in removing such misconceptions and myths.

BCC is a research-based, consultative process of addressing knowledge, attitudes and practices through identifying, analyzing and segmenting audiences and participants in programmes and providing them with relevant information and motivation through well-defined strategies, using an appropriate mix of interpersonal, group and mass media channels, including participatory methods (Government of Uttar Pradesh 2008). The term BCC specifically refers to community health seeking behaviour. In order to roll-out a BCC campaign for a targeted population, development of a com-munication strategy is a prerequisite. Development of a communication strategy consists of three phases, the first phase involves formative research to understand the audience and the messages they would need, the second step is to refine the messages and design a BCC strategy and the last phase is implementation and monitoring. Along with developing an appropriate communication strategy based on local cultural strengths, building the capacity of the people/staff who implement the strategies need the utmost attention. Clear and repetitive messages communicated to the local people have a lasting impact. Those efforts which are sustainable usually help to encourage healthy behaviour and improve access to health services. Mass media plays an important role in creating awareness and influencing beliefs, attitudes and practices. It is important to involve mass media in BCC strategies for rural audience as it can be an effective instrument in influencing social norms

(Ramakrishnan and Arora 2010). It is also important to include other development partners, including government schemes and their strategies aimed at behaviour change. BCC has an important role to play in community mobilization, however, it should be noted that there are other challenges facing the system which also affect behaviour and in such cases BCC has a limited role to play. A poorly functioning public distribution system (PDS), social exclusion of certain castes, gaps in functioning of the Integrated Child Development Services (ICDS) and chronic poverty of families also contribute hugely to the malnourished state of women and children in this country. These factors need to be considered while designing BCC programmes.

Reproductive and Child Health, Nutrition and AIDS (RACHNA) which was one of the biggest projects in maternal neonatal and child health and nutrition (MNCHN) in India was administered by CARE India for many years, in different phases. Many of the components of RACHNA were mini projects by themselves and over time have influenced several interventions in the area of MNCHN. We studied the RACHNA project and although we could showcase the case study for many things relevant in the area of maternal and newborn health, we wanted to focus on one major strength and legacy for which RACHNA would be remembered. The analysis we did from secondary literature as well as discussions with the people who have worked in RACHNA (CARE India) helped us understand that one of the fundamental pillars of RACHNA was its BCC strategy. RACHNA's BCC strategy helped in promoting healthy behaviours in the communities that the programmes targeted, as well as in strengthening the ICDS training cadre at the block level. This helped in decentralizing the training as well as creating a pool of trained personnel at different levels in the ICDS system. RACHNA facilitated the widespread dissemination of BCC materials in communities through adopting and strengthening several existing government platforms. These efforts and other innovations helped institutionalize many of these 'best practices' in MNCHN. These practices which were developed throughout RACHNA's implementation cycle continue to be championed even today as a part of both ICDS and the NRHM. This case study documents RACHNA through a lens which focusses primarily on its BCC component.

Box 3.1: The RACHNA Programme: An Innovation in BCC Addressing Antenatal, Delivery and Postnatal Care (PNC)

The RACHNA programme of CARE India included two United States Agency for International Development (USAID)—supported projects: the second phase of Integrated Nutrition and Health Project (INHP-II), which focussed on child health and nutrition and the *Chayan* project, which supported interventions for promoting birth spacing and the prevention of transmission of HIV/AIDS among groups at high risk. INHP-II built upon the lessons and experiences of the first phase was implemented in 747 ICDS blocks in 78 districts across nine states from October 2001 to December 2006 to complement the maternal and child health and nutrition (MCHN) efforts of the ICDS and the Ministry of Health and Family Welfare (MoHFW) programmes. To achieve its goal of 'sustainable improvements in the nutrition and health status of seven million women and children', INHP-II adopted a two-track approach. First, supporting service providers to improve the quality and coverage of MCHN services and systems and second, engaging communities to support better infant feeding and caring practices and sustain activities for improved maternal and child health and survival. The implementation was facilitated by small programme teams of CARE, located at the district, state, national levels and working

(Box 3.1 Continued)

(Box 3.1 Continued)

closely with the functionaries of the ICDS programme and MoHFW and also with a range of partners, including local non-governmental organizations (NGOs) and community-based organizations. The main strategies were strengthening of existing systems, BCC and capacity building. In July 2002, the *Chayan* project was added to INHP-II and along with a few other, smaller health projects run by CARE-India. The rural component of *Chayan* (*Chayan* rural) supported the strengthening of family planning services for birth spacing and the prevention and management of reproductive tract infections and sexually transmitted infections (RTI/STI). It operated in 29-INHP-II districts in four out of the nine INHP states—Uttar Pradesh, Rajasthan, Chhattisgarh and Jharkhand. *Chayan* rural aimed at increasing contraceptive prevalence rates in men and women in the reproductive age groups as well as increasing awareness and treatment seeking behaviours for RTIs and was operationally integrated with INHP-II. The urban component of *Chayan* (*Chayan* urban) attempted to increase safe sex practices and treatment of RTI/STI/HIV among high-risk groups, especially female sex workers, truckers and migrants. It also included interventions for promoting life-skills and awareness on RTI/STI/HIV prevention among youth, implemented in selected urban blocks of ICDS.

- INHP was a 14-year project of which the first phase (INHP I) was implemented between October 1996 and September 2001 and INHP II between October 2001 and September 2006.
- INHP III: The Phase out Project (POP) was carried out between October 2006 and December 2010. The three-year POP was designed to consolidate lessons from INHP I and II and to enable integration of good practices for sustained improvement of health and nutrition outcomes, into government programmes (Annexure 1).

The implementation of the programme was facilitated by teams of CARE, located at the district, state and national levels. These teams worked with ICDS functionaries and the health department at various levels and advocated convergence and improvements in service delivery. At the field level, this was facilitated by several community-based organizations and NGOs.

The project worked around three approaches:

1. Strengthening of existing systems
2. BCC
3. Capacity building

Source: Information received from Care India by PHFI.

RACHNA Project: BCC Component

One of the main initiatives under the RACHNA project was strategizing and implementing BCC strategies (Working Papers Series, Executive Summary and Papers 1–12).

Important components of the BCC strategy are listed as follows:

- **Interpersonal Communication**
  RACHNA facilitated the development and uptake of interpersonal communication (IPC) materials which helped in identifying practices for families and communities to adopt healthy behaviours. The actual behaviour change came about over time as a result of consistent and correct behaviour change messages using context-specific BCC techniques. Greater dialogue on health and nutrition issues between health care communication professionals and families created enabling conditions for behaviour change. Prioritized home contact practised by the service providers, namely *Anganwadi* Workers (AWW), *Mitanin* (village volunteer)

and auxiliary nurse midwives (ANM), during key contact periods of the life cycle[2] helped reinforce critical messages that contributed to behaviour changes. Communication materials supported the messages that were targeted towards individuals and families. The communication was one-to-one and targeted towards understanding individual household situations and supporting the individual behaviour change process.

- **Regular Monthly Stakeholder Meeting (Village Health and Nutrition Day)**
  Meetings were organized at the village level to discuss various health and nutrition issues and on fixed days, pregnant and lactating women and mothers of children under the age of three years, came to the *Anganwadi* Centre (AWC) to receive their take-home ration and health services. These meetings became useful platforms for ICDS and health staff to come together and discuss issues and the model was adopted by the NRHM to constitute its village health and nutrition days (VHND). VHNDs are now institutionalized across the country. The themes and issues for discussion were decided based on the seasonal calendar, for example, in the rainy season there would be emphasis on diarrhoea management. Apart from interpersonal communication being carried out by the service provider, there were media campaigns (wall paintings and hoardings) to disseminate messages to a wider audience.

The initiatives included:

1. **Mass Communication Campaigns**: Rural Mass Communication Campaigns were organized in select pockets (villages, *gram panchayats*, sectors) about the high incidence of malnutrition and mortality. These were organized periodically with the involvement of the civil society and local NGOs. Print aids, audio-visual aids and culturally accepted mediums were used. In order to access difficult to reach areas, RACHNA also facilitated Meet for Empowerment Learning and Advocacy (MELA) which was organized with the support of different government departments and agencies on a periodic basis. Nutrition demonstrations and health and nutrition education sessions were some of the activities conducted under the MELA initiative.
2. **Consultations/Engagement with *Panchayati Raj* Institutions (PRIs)**: Regular engagement with PRIs was carried out through periodic orientation (structures training) and quarterly *gram sabha* and *janpad* meetings to enhance their understanding on key issues related to malnutrition and child survival. Audio-visual and print aids (effective medium of communication) were used. Under the project, PRIs supported the service providers and also held them accountable for non-delivery of the services.

What Makes the RACHNA Programme Innovative?

1. Engaging with Multiple Constituents

INHP established change agents (CAs) in order to have a cadre of volunteers at the community level to improve MCHN outcomes. This was aimed at expanding utilization of services

---

[2]Key contacts during life cycle: fourth month, sixth month, ninth month of pregnancy, first-day visit, visit during first week of birth, visit during first month, visit during sixth month of the child, visit during ninth month of the child.

by minimizing exclusion and, more importantly, by promoting and sustaining the critical behaviour change needed to impact MCHN outcomes. Initially, local NGOs were contracted to recruit, train and support the CAs, but when the programme went to scale, responsibility for all facets of the CA cadre from recruitment to maintenance was handed over to the ICDS, the health systems and the PRIs. For quite some time now, there has been increasing realization of the importance of community engagement and community-centered approaches for sustainable societal changes. Lasting and widespread behaviour change is best brought about when societal norms and values change in the community as a whole. INHP-I recognized that building capacity of communities and individuals is as important in addressing unhealthy behaviours as it is dealing with supply side issues for reaching short-term nutrition and health targets. INHP-II continued with this conviction and recognized that simultaneous engagement of the health system and communities is basic to achieving programme objectives. The impact hypothesis of RACHNA also highlights the importance of complementary and synergistic interaction between the system and community processes for achieving stated programme objectives.

2. Working with Existing Systems

It was recognized that 'the government has the largest and the most important infrastructure dedicated to making nutrition and health improvements, therefore, influencing and supporting the government system to adopt and replicate best practices is critical' (INHP 2001). The programme was operationally defined as 'identification and scale-up of best practices through government partnership and capacity building'. None of the technical interventions that RACHNA promoted were new to the existing national programmes, ICDS and reproductive and child health (RCH). In supporting the national programme for a chosen set of interventions, RACHNA's aim was to help the programmes prioritize interventions that had the highest likelihood of impact. The RACHNA project started doing this through identification of best practices,[3] for scale-up. To identify best practices, key stakeholders across the state were involved. After identifying the best practices, a demonstration site (Anderson et al. 2006)[4] was created to implement them. Based on the learnings from the demonstration site, in order to replicate these practices in other parts of the country, an operational strategy with well-defined concepts was prepared. During the second phase of the project (INHP-II), the best practices have been implemented in the replication. The learning experiences during implementation were systematically incorporated into the government system. Capacity building was undertaken to scale-up best practices across the state.

3. Multiple Approaches to Capacity Building

This included partnership, top-down organizational, bottom-up organizational and community approaches, each of which had the potential to contribute to capacity building in its own right and in consort with the others. Evidence from scientific literature suggests that multiple approaches lead to more effective capacity building and this programme wisely incorporated multiple approaches into its structure.

---

[3]Each Phase of INHP had a set of best practices. The lessons from INHP-II and best practices have been brought out in 12 Working Papers series and they can be found: http://www.careindia.org/healthcare-0. The lessons from INHP-III and best practices can be found at http://www.careindia.org/sites/default/files/pdf_file/08.

[4]Used as a learning ground and platform for fresh innovations.

4. Increasing Convergence between the ICDS and RCH Programmes

One of the RACHNA programmes' areas of focus and impact was to increase the use of services, as well as to improve health behaviour. To increase the use of services and improve health behaviours was a major strategy and accomplishment of RACHNA. The most effective innovation was the monthly nutrition and health days (NHDs). At these NHDs a take home food ration (THR) for pregnant and lactating women and children (6–36) months was used as an incentive to increase participation for immunization, antenatal check-up, micronutrient supplementation and weighing/growth monitoring services at the AWC. An impressive measure of community involvement is that community-based organizations or PRIs participated in nearly half of all NHDs.

The monthly NHDs were also effective because they became the focal point for intersectoral convergence between ICDS, MoHFW and the PRIs. RACHNA strategy, thus, focussed on strengthening systems while working on national priorities and programmes which were crucial for creating sustainable results. CARE has successfully built a strong and influential working relationship with ICDS at all levels. This was uniformly observed across all the states. The AWWs felt that the training they received from CARE refreshed their knowledge and renewed their focus on key interventions important for improving maternal and child health outcomes. A proper functional health system is a very significant factor in the ability of the ICDS programme to achieve its objectives. Convergence at all levels is vital for an efficient referral, preventive and curative health care. The partnership with the PRIs was strengthened over the years. This led to better collaboration between ICDS and the health delivery system. One of the results of this improved collaboration has been better immunization coverage. RACHNA's effort to bring two vertical government service delivery systems to converge helped strengthen service delivery and is a remarkable achievement in itself. District-level advisory committees (DLAC) and block-level advisory committees (BLAC) were two convergence and coordination forums at the district and block levels for ICDS and the health department, which helped build convergence at different levels of service delivery. These forums were engaged in periodic monitoring of process, identification of neglected areas and analysis of data and taking decisions to operationalize convergent processes.

5. Capacity Building Strategy of RACHNA

This focussed on strengthening of 'on-the-job performance' of the ICDS and health functionaries. Central to the capacity building was the development of training teams at all levels, from the district up to the sector. The block training team was particularly successful in reaching out and troubleshooting on various issues during and after the training. The cascade training concept which involves the health system and ICDS officials at the block level is an example of a sustainable approach to development. It is important to note here that CARE enjoyed a good working relationship with the ICDS department and to some extent the health department by virtue of long standing partnerships. As a result of their initial role as a donor of food aid, they enjoyed certain privileges of trust and had a good knowledge of the entire sector. This experience and relationship was one of the strengths that they capitalized on while implementing these best practices. It is important to remember this factor as many of the best practices focus on suitable and sustainable partnerships. It is by virtue of their early and long standing engagement with ICDS that CARE was able to achieve many of its objectives. New approaches and tools introduced by rural RACHNA in 2005, including improved AWW home visits, better supervision and using sector meetings for in-service training hold promise for better health and nutrition outcomes.

Best Practices

Best practices were envisaged as solutions to operational challenges in bringing the two key stakeholders—systems and community—together to improve infant survival and reduce maternal malnutrition. The best practices were seen as specific processes that would help the health systems and ICDS improve the quality and coverage of maternal and neonatal services on one hand and mobilize communities to demand improvements in service delivery and sustain behaviour change on the other hand. These best practices helped build training capacity in the ICDS/health system in BCC as well as promoted the uptake of BCC messages in the community. In this section, we summarize some of the best practices.

Best Practice No. 1: Change Agents

CAs were created to promote nutrition and health promoters at the community level, to serve as a link between service providers and communities and to positively influence both service delivery and behaviour change. These CAs received monetary incentives in exchange for their services to the community. They were also acknowledged by the community as champions of change. RACHNA invested in their training.

Best Practice No. 2: Convergence through Nutrition and Health Days (NHD)

NHDs constitute a mechanism for convergent service delivery, an intervention designed to reach the most marginalized sections of the community with health and nutrition services and simultaneously as an event to provide a forum for community involvement in monitoring health and nutrition services. NHDs are an effective innovation and the only best practice that still continues as part of sectoral strengthening approach. Continued engagement of the PRIs and other community-based organizations helped improve the level of convergence between AWWs, ANMs, lady health visitors (LHVs) and the community. The sectoral strengthening approach by CARE was also an important innovation for convergence among these groups and the effort to involve community participation in promoting the BCC strategy is highly commendable. ICDS functionaries acknowledged that CARE had helped strengthen the convergence between the ICDS and health at the community level and the NHDs were an effective means to do so at the village level.

Best Practice No. 3: Community-based Monitoring System

The main objective of community-based monitoring system (CBMS) is to mobilize and empower communities and to manage the health and nutritional status of women and children. A CBMS is a set of tools/visuals that has evolved through a participatory process. This enables families and community groups to monitor their health practices and take steps to adopt healthy behaviours. Providing a set of tools to self-monitor on all critical parameters of care during the antenatal and newborn period is a good example of how RACHNA developed and implemented simple tools at the individual and community level across the country. Linking this with the village map to continuously track information on key parameters such as pregnancy, malnutrition, left-outs and dropouts was an important step towards development of a comprehensive tool for empowerment, self-regulation, development of social cohesion, reduction of social exclusion and promotion of equity and public accountability.

Best Practice No. 4: Strengthening Supervisory System to Improve BCC Intervention

The success of a BCC strategy or activity depends on many factors. The RACHNA project used IPC as a communication tool to bring positive change in behaviour. To support this BCC strategy, prioritized home visits were planned by health workers to package key behaviour messages at critical time of the pregnancy period. Proper training and a supportive supervisory system helped build confidence in front-line health workers to produce the desired outcome. In the third phase of INHP-III, the best practices were standardized in order to facilitate the system to maintain quality and take it to scale. Standardization in the areas of fixed nutrition and health days, prioritized home visits, supportive supervision and structured sector strengthening, helped existing systems achieve better maternal and child health outcomes.

In 2006, the final evaluation report of the RACHNA programme found that the programme had an impact on national and state policies and that the lessons learned are relevant to improving performance in the Government of India programmes such as ICDS, RCH and NRHM. The key findings in the report also stressed that the rural RACHNA programme, despite its impact on increasing the use of services, had less success in changing behaviours, except in the area of newborn care. Further improvement is needed in AWWs' and ANMs' counselling skills and in the availability of more culturally specific job aids on small doable actions for improving complementary feeding practices. Better communication of the advantages and side effects of family planning methods using job aids would be valuable. The report also recommended that specific components of the programme continue and listed the following innovations as having the greatest value.

1. Strengthening community-based organizations/PRIs for demand generation and increasing accountability and convergence of ICDS and RCH systems for achieving intended health and nutrition outcomes.
2. Improving nutrition in pregnancy and lactation and in children under two, especially infant and young child feeding and hygiene practices.
3. Improving supervision, capacity building and BCC.

Annexure 1

Table 3A.1

Evolution of INHP over 14 Years

Phase	Geographic Areas and Coverage	Objectives	Technical Interventions	Programme Strategies
INHP I (1996–2001)	• Seven states (AP, Bihar, MP, Orissa, UP, Rajasthan and West Bengal) • 937 blocks • 119,215 AWCs • 6.63 million population	To improve the health and nutritional status of women and children, especially girl children.	• Targeted supplementary feeding for children of 6–24 months and pregnant/lactating women. • Iron and folic acid supplementation for pregnant women. • Complete immunization of children under one and pregnant women. • 10% areas: Early and exclusive breastfeeding and timely, adequate complementary feeding practices. • Target: Pregnant women, lactating mothers, adolescent girls and children under two years.	• Promoting convergence of services at the community level (especially MHFW and ICDS services). • Encouraging technical and process innovation. • Building community ownership. • Demonstrating best practices. • Promoting capacity of government, communities and NGO partners. • Promoting replication of best practices.
INHP II (2002–06)	• Nine states (AP, Bihar, Chhattisgarh, Jharkhand, MP, Orissa, UP, Rajasthan and West Bengal) • 747 ICDS blocks • 78 districts • 6.85 million population • 94,592 AWCs	Vulnerable families achieve sustainable improvement in the nutrition and health status of seven million women and children in 805 ICDS blocks across eight states by 2006.	• Supplementary feeding for children under six years and pregnant women and lactating mothers. • Maternal and child immunization. • Infant feeding. • Vitamin A supplementation. • Newborn care at the community level. • Chayan Project (HIV-AIDS, RTI/STI and Family planning) added under umbrella Reproductive and Child Health Nutrition and AIDS (RACHNA) programme. • Target: Pregnant women, lactating mothers, adolescent girls and children under three years.	• Innovation and demonstration for behaviour change through NGO partnerships. • Replication of proven best practices through government partnership and capacity building. • Effective use of food. • Strategic alliances for organizational learning and advocacy. • Promotion of gender equity. • Synergy with other projects.

(Table 3A.1 Continued)

(Table 3A.1 Continued)

Phase	Geographic Areas and Coverage	Objectives	Technical Interventions	Programme Strategies
INHP III (2007–10)	• Eight states (AP, Chhattisgarh, Jharkhand, Madhya Pradesh, Orissa, Rajasthan, UP and West Bengal) • 1,297 blocks • 96 districts • 234,891 AWCs • 15,544,000 participants (this includes all the target population directly reached in the operational areas inclusive of supplementary nutrition participants)	Achieve sustained reduction in infant mortality and child malnutrition in targeted areas.	• Essential nutrient actions. • Community-based essential newborn care and ANC. • Primary immunization. • Target: Pregnant women, mothers with children under three years of age, with greater focus on under two years. • Operational and management intervention priorities to fill capacity gaps in the systems at different levels. • Enhance accountability mechanisms for sustainability of effective programming after the phase-out.	• Consolidation and systematic phasing out of programme through system strengthening, community participation, enhancing nutritional focus of the ICDS with policy dialogues, replication of best practices in AP and Chhattisgarh. • Techno-managerial and operational assistance to ICDS at district levels in replication blocks of PPA districts taking leadership in adopting/adapting INHP good practices. • Responsive technical, managerial and operational assistance for continued support to replication process in AP and Chhattisgarh. • Advocacy and sector-wide support to influence policies and larger ICDS and RCH programmes.

Source: Authors' own.

References

Chatterjee, M., Levine, R., Murthy, N. and Seshadri, S.R. 2009. 'Sparing Lives: Better Reproductive Health for Poor Women in South Asia'. World Bank Publication. Available at http://siteresources.worldbank.org/SOUTHASIAEXT/Resources/Publications/448813-1231439344179/sparinglives.pdf, accessed on 5 May 2012.

Government of Uttar Pradesh. 2008. 'Behaviour Change Communication (BCC) Strategy for NRHM in Uttar Pradesh'. Department of Health and Family Welfare, Govt. of Uttar Pradesh. Available at http://www.sifpsa.org/digitization/bcc_strategy_uploading.pdf, accessed on 25 March 2011.

Integrated Nutrition and Health Project (INHP). 2001. Development Activity Proposal. CARE, India.

Lozano, R., Wang, H., Foreman, K., Rajaratnam, J., Naghavi, M., Marcus, J., Lindgren, L., Lofgren, K., Phillips, D., Atkinson, C., Lopez, A. and Murray, C. 2011. 'Progress towards Millennium Development Goals 4 and 5 on Maternal and Child Mortality: An Updated Systematic Analysis'. *Lancet*, 378: 1139–65; published online on 20 September 2011. DOI:10.1016/S0140-6736(11)61337-8.

Lule, E., Ramana, G., Ooman, N., Epp, J., Huntington, D. and Rosen, J. 2005. 'Achieving the Millennium Development Goal of Improving Maternal Health: Determinants, Interventions and Challenges'. Health, Nutrition and Population. Washington, DC: World Bank. Available at http://siteresources.worldbank.org/HEALTHNUTRITIONANDPOPULATION/Resources/281627-1095698140167/LuleAchievingtheMDGFinal.pdf, accessed on 29 March 2012.

Mavalankar, D. 2000. 'State of Maternal Health in India'. Available at http://www.azadindia.org/social-issues/maternal-health-in-india.html, accessed on 30 March 2011.

Nair H. and Panda R. 2011. 'Quality of Maternal Health Care in India: Has the National Rural Health Mission Made a Difference?' *Journal of Global Health,* 1(1): 79–86.

Ramakrishnan N. and V. Arora. 2010. 'Media Perspectives on Partnerships to Address Family Health in Northern India'. Availabale at http://medind.nic.in/jah/t10/s1/jaht10s1p93.pdf, accessed on 21 April 2012.

Working Papers Series: RACHNA Programme. 2010–2006. Executive Summary. What We Have Learnt So Far. Available at http://www.careindia.org/healthcare-0, accessed in April 2012.

Working Papers Series: RACHNA Programme. 2010–2006. Paper 1: What RACHNA has Done So Far. Available at http://www.careindia.org/healthcare-0, accessed on 22 April 2012.

Working Papers Series: RACHNA Programme. 2010–2006. Paper 2: Methods Used for Assessment in RACHNA Programme. Available at http://www.careindia.org/healthcare-0, accessed on 25 April 2012.

Working Papers Series: RACHNA Programme. 2010–2006. Paper 3: Enhancing Newborn Care. Available at http://www.careindia.org/healthcare-0, accessed on 28 April 2012.

Working Papers Series: RACHNA Programme. 2010–2006. Paper 4: Changing Infant and Child Feeding Behaviours. Availabe at http://www.careindia.org/healthcare-0, accessed on 28 April 2012.

Working Papers Series: RACHNA Programme. 2010–2006. Paper 5: Widening Coverage of Micronutrient Supplements. Available at http://www.careindia.org/healthcare-0, accessed on 28 April 2012.

Working Papers Series: RACHNA Programme. 2010–2006. Paper 6: Supplemental Feeding Its Role in a Large-scale Maternal and Child Nutrition and Health Programme. Available at http://www.careindia.org/healthcare-0, accessed on 28 April 2012.

Working Papers Series: RACHNA Programme. 2010–2006. Paper 7: Widening Coverage of Primary Immunization. Available at http://www.careindia.org/healthcare-0, accessed on 28 April 2012.

Working Papers Series: RACHNA Programme. 2010–2006. Paper 8: Deepening Access to Spacing Methods. Available at http://www.careindia.org/healthcare-0, accessed on 28 April 2012.

Working Papers Series: RACHNA Programme. 2010–2006. Paper 9: HIV Prevention in Vulnerable Indian States. Available at http://www.careindia.org/healthcare-0, accessed on 12 May 2012.

Working Papers Series: RACHNA Programme. 2010–2006. Paper 10: Working with Systems Lessons from INHP. Available at http://www.careindia.org/healthcare-0, accessed on 12 May 2012.

Working Papers Series: RACHNA Programme. 2010–2006. Paper 11: Engaging Communities to Improve Health and Nutrition Outcome: The Role of Community Volunteers in INHP. Available at http://www.careindia.org/healthcare-0, accessed on 12 May 2012.

Working Papers Series: RACHNA Programme. 2010–2006. Paper 12: A Cost Analysis of the RACHNA Programme. Available at http://www.careindia.org/healthcare-0, accessed on 15 May 2012.

Financial Access to Health Care Services

4. Increasing Financial and Physical Access for Service Delivery: Sambhav Voucher Scheme

4

Increasing Financial and Physical Access for Service Delivery: Sambhav Voucher Scheme

Sourav Neogi

Maternal and child health care is extremely important in countries faced with high infant and maternal mortality. India had the largest number of deaths at 68,000 accounting for one-eighth of all maternal deaths in the world (World Development Report 2012). There are variations in maternal mortality by region and state in India. Without healthy mothers, our children will either fail to survive or will survive lacking the advantages of maternal support. Proper maternal and child health services are, therefore, critical for the survival and well-being of pregnant women, women who have recently delivered and the newborn.

Financial Access to Maternal Health

Access to health care with equity and universal coverage is critically linked with public financing of health care services. Countries with near universal access and relative equity in access to health care have organized health care systems where public financing accounts for over two-thirds of health care spending (WHO 2012, Duggal 2005). However, in India the dominant role of the private sector in health care system is well known, both in health provision and financing. India is one among the developing countries where households spend a disproportionate share of their consumption expenditure on health care. Results from the survey suggest that for the year 2001–02, households' out-of-pocket (OOP)

Benefit of Voucher Scheme: A Testimony by a Beneficiary

'We are labourers and have to earn to stay alive; from where we will get money to go to a private facility for delivery and in the government facility the services are not up to the mark; through the Sambhav Voucher Scheme we were able to deliver at private facility; ASHA supported us throughout.'

Source: Interview transcripts of husband of AzraBano; she is a beneficiary under the Voucher Scheme; Kalsi Village, Uttarakhand, ©PHFI, July 2011.

health expenditure is estimated to be ₹72,759 crores which accounts for 3.2% of the GDP at current market price (GoI 2005).

In India, however, other than supply side issues, factors such as cost of the services, financial status of the family and distance from the health facility lead to a low level of utilization of maternal health services among poor women. Despite the governments' efforts and favourable policies aimed at improving service provision, utilization rates for maternal health services are very low among the poor (Sharma et al. 2005). Included under the umbrella of financial access are transportation costs, wage loss, OOP costs, etc. Another important dimension is seeking care in private sector due to overcrowded government facilities. Husband of a beneficiary under the voucher scheme rightly cited the reasons for not availing the maternal health services earlier in government and private health care facilities and how the voucher scheme has transformed them (see the box titled 'Benefit of Voucher Scheme: A Testimony by a Beneficiary').

A study conducted by IFPS Technical Assistance Project (ITAP) funded by United States Agency for International Development (USAID) in UP found that the average time for a woman to travel to the nearest source for institutional delivery was 84 minutes in rural areas, compared to 11 minutes in urban areas (USAID 2008). Similarly, in Uttarakhand the Health and Population Policy clearly states that 'all efforts will be made to reach people in the remotest inaccessible areas'. The state policy recognizes that more than 75% of the population lives in rural areas and villages in non-contiguous hilly areas and that more than 50% of the population lives in areas not accessible by roads.

Another important deterrent for the poor is opportunity cost (wage loss) of hospital care for the patient and caregivers (Mavalankar 2010). People who are daily wage earners are more vulnerable when they need to go for hospital care, as they not only spend on health services but also lose their wage for that day. Especially in case of deliveries, where women are usually accompanied by a male member of the family, there is greater loss as it means losing the wages of both the woman and those accompanying her.

Of all the people hospitalized in India, in a year about 24% are pushed below the poverty line (BPL) because of hospitalization costs, as per National Sample Survey (PwC 2010). According to a study conducted by USAID in UP, one major factor that may prohibit or delay a BPL household's decision to use family planning/reproductive and child health (FP/RCH) services is monetary cost (USAID 2008). Numerous women interviewed during field visits reported having incurred substantial debt to pay for an institutional delivery and that the loans often came with exorbitant rates of interest. According to study findings, more than 90% of UP households made some payment at the time of delivery. Median payments were ₹400, 1,284 and 2,962 for deliveries in a home, a public sector facility and a private sector facility respectively. The median payment per delivery for rural and urban households was ₹450 and 800 respectively. Only the highest income quintile had median expenditures per delivery of about ₹1,500 with the remaining quintiles' median expenditures ranging from ₹350 to 500, suggesting that households in all quintiles but the highest quintile elects home deliveries either because of the high monetary and/or time costs (USAID 2008).

As per NSSO 60th round data (year 2004) in India on an average ₹1,169 and ₹2,806 was spent per childbirth in the rural and urban areas respectively. The cost of delivery in private hospital was as high as ₹4137 in rural as compared to ₹5480 in urban. As per the report, expenditure involved in the case of availing of antenatal care (ANC) services was more than that of the postnatal care (PNC) services, in both rural and urban areas. The average expenditure on ANC and PNC was ₹499 and ₹404 respectively in rural areas. The corresponding values in the urban areas were ₹906 and

₹596. These costs create an additional burden for the household and discourage people from avail-ing maternity health services. The situation for women in Uttarakhand is much more alarming. In Uttarakhand, the Health and Population Policy also recognizes disparities in household expenditures on health care. Often, households allocate a higher proportion of financial resources for men's health needs as compared to women's health needs. Similarly, disparities in dietary intake place women at a disadvantage relative to men. A recent study indicates that families are often unwilling to allocate more than minimal resources to the preventive care and treatment of women (Schuler et al. 2002).

Schemes and Financial Support

The National Rural Health Mission (NRHM) was launched in 2005 in order to provide equitable, affordable and quality care for the poor residing in rural areas. Under NRHM, Janani Suraksha Yojna (JSY) was introduced, in order to increase the institutional delivery rate. JSY planned to accomplish its goal by giving cash incentives to pregnant women who attended antenatal clinics and went for institutional deliveries. Introduction of the JSY scheme into the health system in India proved to be one of the main reasons for the increase in the institutional delivery rate; which increased signifi-cantly in the last few years across the country (Lahariya 2009). The institutional deliveries to total deliveries increased from 56.7% in 2006–07 to 78.5% in 2010–11 (GoI 2011).

Problems began to arise when facilities became overcrowded resulting in service quality being compromised. As there is a significant presence of private facilities in urban areas, the government felt that this could be a potential option for public–private partnership (PPP) where private facilities could provide institutional delivery services for the poor with the financial support from the government.

Strong Presence of Private Sector

A large proportion of Indians seek private health care, therefore, linking the public and private sectors would give mothers a choice of where to go for their health care needs. In addition to strengthen-ing the public sector efforts to improve health, the Government of India (GoI) has also articulated strategies for improving health services and outcomes through the development of PPP models. PPPs are attractive as they can draw on the strengths of the private allopathic sector (which has greater numbers of human resources, facilities and technology) and may be designed and implemented in ways that improve access/equity and efficiency of essential health services, increase provider choice and enhance the quality of care.

Sambhav Voucher Scheme

The Sambhav Voucher Scheme was designed as a PPP for provision of high-quality family planning and reproductive health services. The voucher scheme was component of the Innovations in Fam-ily Planning Services (IFPS) project, a collaborative effort of the GoI and USAID. The ITAP was implemented by Futures Group, India and partners. The goal of the voucher scheme is to reduce inequities in reproductive health care by enabling access to services, while empowering the below poverty line (BPL) population to choose their own provider (Futures Group 2009). It was designed and implemented to enhance selective RCH and FP services amongst BPL families. The scheme uses an innovative approach to allow BPL families to gain access to critical reproductive health and family

Table 4.1

Vouchers for Equity in Reproductive Health

	Uttar Pradesh	Uttarakhand	Jharkhand
Pilot phase	Agra and Kanpur	Haridwar	Gumla and Dhanbad
Beneficiaries	All BPL families and slum dwellers	All BPL families	All BPL families
Service coverage	ANC, delivery, PNC, FP and RTI/STI	ANC, delivery, Neonatal complications, PNC and FP	FP
Started	Jan 2007–Agra Nov 2008–Kanpur	May 2007	End Sept 09–Gumla End Oct 09–Dhanbad
Scaled-up	Kanpur, Allahabad, Varanasi, Agra and Lucknow	Haridwar, Dehradun, Udhhamsingh Nagar, Nainital and Almora	
Scaled-up services started	October 2009	September 2009	

Source: Project documents shared by USAID and Futures Group in 2011.

planning services in private health care facilities. Ultimately, BPL families are enabled to access free-of-cost health services in reputable private health facilities. The scheme offers the following services: ANC, delivery, PNC, newborn care, sterilization, oral contraceptive pills, condoms, intrauterine contraceptive devices (IUCDs) and institutional deliveries including treatment for complications.

The scheme was implemented in three states in India. Table 4.1 is a snapshot of the scheme in these states.

In this case study, we discuss the Sambhav Voucher Scheme designed for the state of Uttarakhand as a PPP intervention. Uttarakhand has three distinct regions; the upper Himalayas, mid-Himalayas and foothills/plains. The Himalayan region being predominately mountainous, access to health services is particularly difficult. The voucher scheme was launched in five districts including Haridwar and Dehradun where a comparatively strong private sector is present and people from other districts can visit these districts to access services under the scheme. In rest of the eight districts, the private sector presence is negligible.

A few key indicators for Uttarakhand compared to all-India figures are presented in Table 4.2.

Table 4.2

Some Key Indicators for Uttarakhand

S.N.	Item	Uttarakhand	India
1	Total fertility rate (SRS 2008)	NA	2.6
2	Infant mortality rate (SRS 2008)	44	53
3	MMR (SRS 2004–2006)	440	254
4	Mothers who had at least three antenatal visits for their last birth (%) (NFHS–3)	44.8	50.7
5	Institutional births (%) (NFHS–3)	36.1	40.8

Source: SRS 2004, 2006, 2008, NFHS-3 2005–06.

Sambhav Voucher Scheme Phases

The scheme was launched in 2007 and has been running for five years in Uttarakhand. However, it has undergone many changes over the years. The five years can be subdivided into three phases: Pilot Phase, Scale-up Phase 1 and Scale-up Phase 2; each phase is described in the following paragraphs.

Pilot Phase (2007–09)

The Pilot phase was launched by the health minister and health secretary of the state. It got underway immediately as the accredited social health activists (ASHAs), who play a key to its implementation, had already received training about the services and benefit available under the scheme. While the scheme was meant for the BPL families, many of them did not possess a BPL card. Thus, at the initial pilot stage it was decided that the *pradhan* (village chief) would give a written certification of their status. Later, however, it was decided to allow only proper BPL card holders to receive services. The scheme was initially implemented in two blocks in Haridwar District covering a population of 0.51 million of rural blocks (Imlikheda and Bahadrabad). Dharam Gramin Utthan Sansthan (DGUS),[1] a local non-governmental organization (NGO) managed the programme. At the pilot stage, the package of reimbursements by the government to private providers for a normal delivery was ₹2,200 and ₹8,000 for caesarean. ASHAs received ₹600 for referrals and accompanying the pregnant woman for delivery. DGUS, the programme management unit, managed to form positive relations with both the private nursing homes and government functionaries. Thus, monetary transactions operated properly and reporting was timely. Figure 4.1 shows the operational model.

Scale-up Phase 1

The Government of Uttarakhand decided to expand the scheme in five districts (Almora, Dehradun, Haridwar, Nainital and Udham Singh Nagar) of the state. The scale-up Phase 1 began in 2009 and continued till March 2011. Recognizing the limited number of private providers in other areas, the state decided to make all BPL holders, regardless of their district of residence, eligible for services provided by the accredited private nursing homes in the five districts. Several changes were made in the Scale-up Phase from the Pilot stage. Deliberations between GoI and Government of Uttarakhand led to modifications of the rates piloted. The package rate for private facilities at the Scale-up Phase 1 was ₹2,690 for both normal and caesarean deliveries. This decision was based on the Chiranjeevi Scheme (Annexure 1) being implemented in the state of Gujarat where private facilities get ₹1,800 for each delivery. ASHAs' remuneration went down from ₹600 to just ₹200. Due to lower remuneration and reimbursement rates, ASHAs did not actively promote the voucher scheme as was done during the Pilot Phase. Private nursing homes and hospitals started receiving

---

[1]According to proposed project, the district magistrate/chief medical officer (DM/CMO) was to recruit the staff for voucher management. The District Project Manager (DPM) was to be responsible for the whole project. It was around this time that the DPM resigned and due to the approaching elections there was a blanket ban on recruitment. This absence of a DPM necessitated that an NGO (Dharam Gramin Utthan Sansthan) would perform all the roles related to programme management.

Figure 4.1
Pilot Phase Operational Model

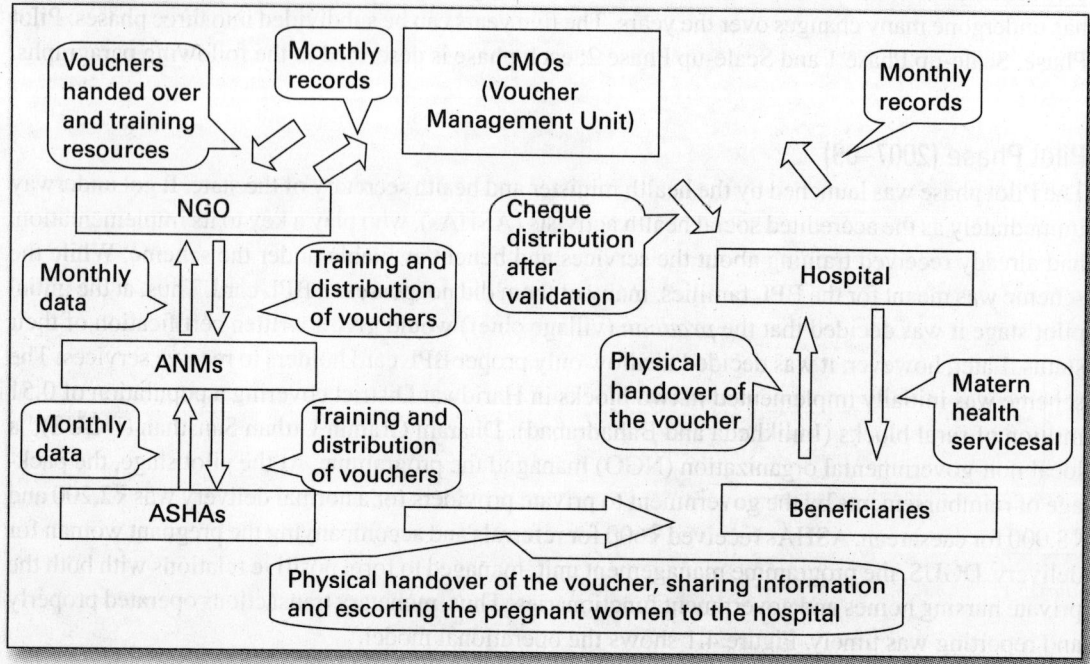

Source: PHFI, 2011.

complicated cases and the cost of their speciality care increased significantly. The lower rates for providers and remuneration for ASHAs, as well as the challenges in promoting the scheme to a larger client base, were identified among the reasons for poor performance. The stakeholders' roles also shifted with the NGO no longer being a part of the scheme and the funding was handed over solely to ITAP.

Scale-Up Phase 2

Based on the feedback shared on the scale-up initiatives by key stakeholders a revised scale-up plan was prepared. The Scale-up Phase 2 began in May 2011 and is presently in place. In the revised plan, the package rate was increased. Since in Scale-up Phase 1 the number of institutional deliveries was relatively low, new rates were introduced more in line with the cost of providing services without increasing losses. As in the Pilot Phase, under this phase, the providers now receive reimbursement for the type of delivery provided rather than an averaged amount. Under the revised package, private nursing homes receive ₹3,200 for normal deliveries and ₹5,500 for caesareans. The remuneration of the ASHAs was also increased to ₹350 in rural areas and ₹200 in urban areas. The operational model is presented in Figure 4.2.

The major structural difference between the Pilot and Scale-up Phase was that the programme management was carried out by an NGO at the Pilot Phase and is being carried out by the district programme management unit (DPMU) at the scale-up stage. Also, at the Pilot Phase the vouchers

Figure 4.2
Scale-up Phase 2 Operational Model

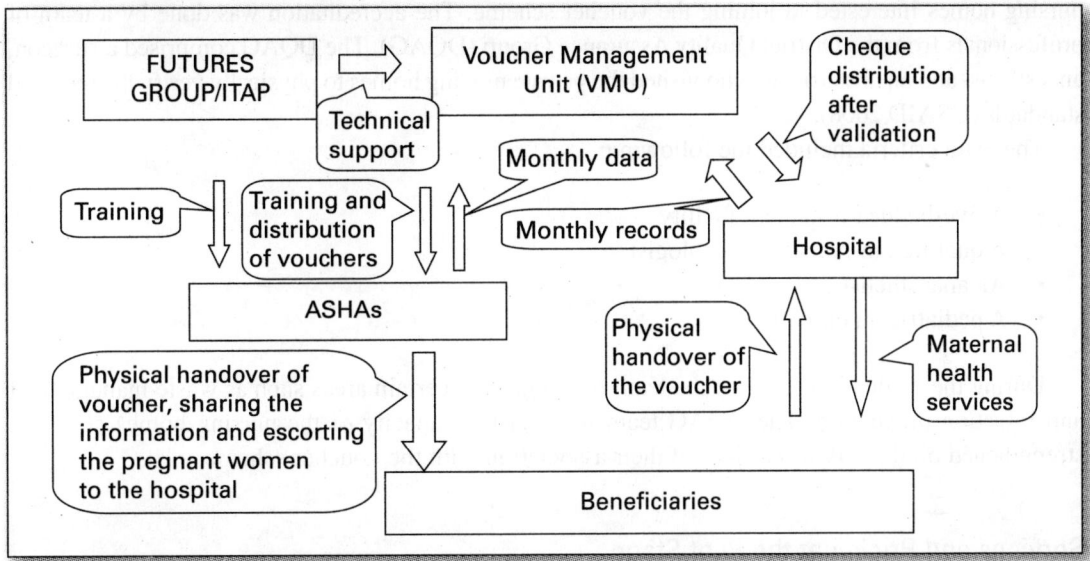

Source: PHFI, 2011.

were initially distributed to the auxiliary nurse midwives (ANMs) and they distributed the vouchers to the ASHAs. At the scale-up stage, the vouchers are distributed to ASHAs directly by the DPMU.

Key Features

Establishment of Voucher Management Unit by the Voucher Management Agency

According to initial specifications for the project, the DM/CMO was to recruit the staff for the voucher management unit. The district project manager (DPM) was responsible for the whole project for the district. Under the guidance of the DPM, the NGO (DGUS) started performing all the roles related to implementation of the scheme. DGUS recruited two block coordinators and one programme co-ordinator during the Pilot Phase. However, the DPM's post was vacant during that time and DGUS played the role of the programme management (USAID 2009).

DGUS was responsible for dealing with the private nursing homes and the government functionaries for monetary transactions and timely reporting. They also monitored the implementation of the scheme at the ground level.

Setting Quality Standards

The first task was setting accreditation standards and identifying potential private facilities. Public health standards, as laid out by the Uttarakhand Government, were reviewed and essential requirements for providing reproductive health services were identified. These standards were taken into consideration by ITAP when developing the essential quality standards which were used for accrediting private nursing homes interested in joining the voucher scheme. The accreditation was done by a team of professionals from the District Quality Assurance Group (DQAG). The DQAG comprised a surgeon, anaesthetist and an obstetrician who visited the private nursing homes to physically verify the required standards (USAID 2008).

The main criteria included the following:

- A five-bedded in-patient facility
- A qualified in-house gynaecologist
- An anaesthetist
- A pediatrician on-call

During the evaluation process, the team found gaps in certain areas such as waste management and infection prevention. The DQAG team felt that the capacity of the nursing homes could be strengthened on these issues as part of their association with the voucher scheme.

Services and Pricing at the Pilot Stage

In order to decide which services needed to be included in the scheme and the package rate for these, a consultative process was organized in one block each in Roorkee and Haridwar and their adjoining towns. Once the services were finalized, they were individually priced (see Table 4.1). The services included under the scheme are as follows:

- ANC
  - Ultrasound
- Institutional deliveries including complications
- PNC
- Newborn care, neonatal and child care
- FP services
  - Sterilization
  - Oral pills and condoms
  - IUCD insertion
- Diagnostic tests

Based on the negotiations with the selected private providers in the presence of representatives from the Directorate of Health and Family Welfare, Uttarakhand, the following prices were fixed for each of the services at the Pilot stage (see Table 4.3).

In addition:

- In case of complications, referrals to higher facilities would be arranged. Travel will be arranged and the cost would be reimbursed by government.
- Supply of medicines will be ensured by the government sector.

Table 4.3
Service Package Rate Fixed by Private and Government Service Providers

Service Package	Rate	Remarks
ANC (minimum three visits, inclusive of tetanus toxoid injections [TT] and iron folic acid [IFA] provided by government).	₹100 (total)	Cost remains same if the visits exceed three visits.
Routine lab investigation	₹500	Haemoglobin (Hb), urine, Venereal disease research laboratory (VDRL), blood sugar, human immunodeficiency virus (HIV) will be conducted by qualified pathologist.
Normal delivery	₹2,200	Inclusive of medicine, stay, routine stomach wash, oxygen excluding meals.
Ultrasound	₹150 per examination	
PNC	₹100	Expected to be two visits inclusive BCG, Polio, pills, condoms and counselling.
IUD	₹100	Multi-load supplied by government.
Sterilization Ligation	₹1,500 ₹2,000	For ligation instruments provided by government.
Complication during ANC period	₹500	If outpatient department (OPD) service is required and it includes stay and medicine.
Delivery (caesarean) with Eclampsia with PPH	₹8,000 ₹8,000 + 2,000 ₹8,000 + 1,000	All services are inclusive of medicines and stay but if blood is required then its cost will be ₹500 per bottle with replacement. If replacement is not found then government would provide help.
Child care		Two–seven days hospital stay.
Respiratory Distress Syndrome (RDS)	₹2,500	Two–five days.
Photo Therapy	₹1,000	
Neonatal Complication	₹500	
Incubator Cost	₹500	

Source: USAID (2008).

Voucher Scheme Key Player Roles

Chief Medical Officer

The role of the CMO is to build systems for establishment of the voucher management unit by ensuring space, furniture, stationery and essential office infrastructure through the DPM's unit budget in consultation with the district nodal officer and the additional district project manager (ADPM). The CMO has to establish systems of management of vouchers and create financial systems for advancing and/or reimbursement of funds to private hospitals. They also conduct periodic quality audits of the accredited facilities to ensure quality of services and preside over all meetings related to the Sambhav Voucher Scheme.

Non-governmental Organization

Pilot Stage

The NGO was an integral part of the Pilot Phase. In the absence of a DPM, the NGO performed all roles related to programme management (training community-level health workers, conducting monthly meetings, collection of data, reporting, etc.). The NGO was brought in as an interim arrangement for a period of six months, however, the health department felt that a dedicated staff of an NGO could manage and monitor the voucher scheme activities well. Therefore, it was decided to make the NGO the voucher management unit (VMU).

Accredited Social Health Activist

ASHAs play a key role in the scheme. Their main roles are to raise awareness, preparation of micro-plan for women during pregnancy, distribute vouchers, arrange for transportation, accompany the pregnant women and report client feedback. An ASHA is also the most essential link for the functioning of the scheme as she connects BPL families to health facilities. ASHAs cover all five districts and identify the BPL beneficiaries within the project implementation areas.

Beneficiaries

Primary beneficiaries are women in the age group of 15 to 49 years, who are pregnant or have a new-born up to six weeks from delivery and men (husbands of eligible women). All beneficiaries must be identified as BPL by showing proof of a BPL card, Rashtriya Swasthya Bima Yojana (RSBY) card or health card; issued by the Department of Health and Family Welfare, Government of Uttarakhand.

Private Nursing Homes

The hospitals must provide a package of cashless services, maintaining quality standards and equity. The private nursing homes (PNH) maintain approved information systems (record select districts and blocks) and submit periodic reports to the VMU. PHN submits vouchers to VMU for reimbursement.

Results from the Pilot Phase

In 2006, ITAP carried out an in-depth baseline study covering FP/reproductive health (RH) areas to find out the vital indicators of the community. After implementation of the project for three years, an evaluation was carried out and data gathered on the vital indicators. An improvement on the vital health indicators was seen after comparison of the end-line evaluation and baseline figures. Some significant achievements/results are highlighted in Table 4.4.

It is evident that ANC coverage increased by almost 5% in the three-year period. However, the improvement may not be attributed exclusively to the Sambhav Voucher Scheme; as a similar improvement has happened for both BPL and non-BPL families, whereas the Sambhav Voucher Scheme only targets and works with the BPL families.

Table 4.4

Percent of Pregnant Women Who Received No ANC Care

	Baseline 2006	Endline 2009
BPL	87.5%	92.3%
Non-BPL	87.3%	92.3%

Source: Baseline and end line study report shared with PHFI by Futures Group in 2011.

Increase in access to ANC care, institutional delivery and use of modern contraceptives methods among women from BPL households was recorded.

Full ANC coverage has always been a challenge for the policymakers; it is a key indicator to improve maternal health outcomes. It is evident from Table 4.5 that ANC coverage has increased significantly among BPL families from 5.9% to 10.6%. However, among non-BPL families the rate of improvement is lower.

Table 4.5

Percent of Pregnant Women Accessing Full ANC Care

	Baseline 2006	Endline 2009
BPL	5.9%	10.6%
Non-BPL	12.4%	15%

Source: Baseline and end line study report shared with PHFI by Futures Group in 2011.

Institutional delivery is a key process indicator and is considered to be the most relevant indicator to understand the status of maternal health. The institutional delivery percentage has improved significantly from less than 29% to 47% among BPL families. Even among non-BPL families, the rate of improvement is encouraging. In Uttaranchal, the JSY scheme benefits are extended to all women (not restricted to BPL women). Hence, even among non-BPL women, the institutional delivery rate has increased significantly over the years.

Table 4.6

Percent of Women Who Availed Institutional Delivery

	Baseline 2006	Endline 2009
BPL	28.9%	47%
Non BPL	30.8%	46.7%

Source: Baseline and end line study report shared with PHFI by Futures Group in 2011.

Institutional Delivery by Place of Delivery

The baseline figures indicate a preference of people to go to private health facilities in comparison to government health facilities for delivery. However, at the baseline stage more non-BPL families

Figure 4.3

Institutional Delivery Public/Private Sector

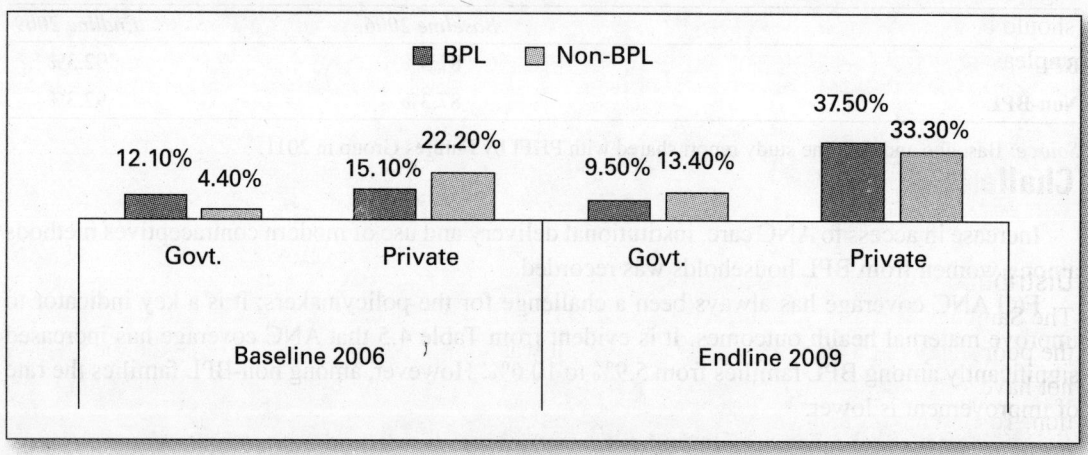

Source: Baseline and end line study report shared with PHFI by Futures Group.

were availing delivery services from private health facilities in comparison to BPL families. The end line data clearly suggests that more BPL families are availing delivery services from private health facilities due to the implementation of the Sambhav Voucher Scheme. In 2006, 12.1% of BPL families were using government health facilities; but in 2009 the percentage dropped to 9.5%. In 2006, 4.4% of non-BPL families used to go to a government health facility for delivery. Non-BPL families are not covered under the Sambhav Voucher Scheme. After introduction of the JSY scheme, non-BPL families started accessing delivery services from government health facilities and in the three-year period the percentage increased threefold from 4.4% to 13.40% (see Figure 4.3).

Learnings

Variations among State/Districts Should Be Taken into Account

District-to-district health situations vary greatly, state-to-state health systems and schemes can arguably differ even more. What works for one district may not work for another.

At the scale-up stage, the Chiranjeevi Scheme was considered to decide the package rate; without considering the differences between Gujarat and Uttarakhand. A strong private presence at the district level was key to the success of the Chiranjeevi Scheme; however in Uttarakhand, the private health facilities are very few. Hence, the existing private health facilities do have a lot of control in the market.

Important Factors to Consider While Scaling-up a Model

The purpose of a Pilot Phase is to put to test what has been hypothesized and created. After finding that the pilot was successful, the Scale-up Phase is expected to replicate the model. In this scheme, however, the pilot was ignored and a new model was brought in without being put to the test. Learning from such a scenario is that if a budget or facet of a project is going to be replaced, another pilot should be carried out instead of scaling-up the changed and untested model. This can avoid a lot of unpleasant surprises and impair the optimum success of the initiative.

Challenges

Distribution of BPL Cards/Identification of BPL

The Sambhav Voucher Scheme is meant for BPL families, the idea being, to benefit the poorest of the poor segment of the population. However, it was found that many poor families in the state do not have a BPL card and, therefore, such families would not be able to access services or information. To circumvent this, while the scheme requires the beneficiaries to have a BPL card to receive the voucher coupon, certification from the *pradhan* was accepted in the Pilot Phase. However, once the Scaling-up Phase occurred, such certification was not accepted as it was seen that in many cases instead of true BPL status, local community-level politics became the grounds for the *pradhan*'s certification (USAID 2008).

Number of Deliveries Reduced Due to Lowering of the Package in the Phase 1 Scaling-up

At the Scale-up Stage, the package was significantly lowered, based on the Chiranjeevi experience (Annexure 1: Chiranjeevi Scheme) and a flat rate was established for all types of deliveries. This made the private health facilities less interested in the scheme and some dropped out altogether. Deliveries went down from about 1,900 a year (a total of 3,341 deliveries in 21 months) (Voucher Exchange Workshop 2009) at the Pilot stage to 459 a year at the Scaling-up Phase. Ultimately, the package was revised in consultation with the government.

Parallel Scheme: Janani Suraksha Yojana versus Sambhav Voucher Scheme

The purpose of the Sambhav Voucher Scheme is to make institutional delivery services accessible to BPL families through PPP and to enhance RCH services by means of ANC, delivery and neonatal care, postnatal and FP services. Under the scheme, JSY benefits were not given to the patients. The key message bearer to the community for both JSY and Sambhav Voucher Scheme was the ASHA. Hence, it was left to the ASHA to decide/convince the family members whether to avail the benefits under the JSY or the Sambhav Voucher Scheme.

Annexure 1: Chiranjeevi Scheme

Unavailability of obstetricians and gynaecologists in the government health system was a major challenge for the Government of Gujarat (GoG). Various studies indicated that there were more obstetricians and gynaecologists available in the private sector than in government sector. Hence, in order to increase access to institutional delivery the GoG announced the Chiranjeevi Scheme under the PPP in April 2005. The objective of this scheme is to reduce high maternal and infant mortality by encouraging private medical practitioners to provide a defined package of maternal health services in remote areas for the poor. This is done by providing financial protection to these families and covering their OOP costs incurred on travel to reach the health care facility. The scheme was launched in December 2005 in five districts, i.e., Banskantha, Dhod, Kutch, Panchmahal and Sabrkantha. Each of the five pilot district governments provides local management of the scheme. Subsequently, the project has been scaled-up across the state.

The package of services includes ANC, ultrasound, delivery, medicines and reimbursement of transportation costs, *dai* services and blood transfusion in the case of complicated deliveries (see Table 4A.1). The scheme also provides financial support to the accompanying person to compensate for the loss of wages. The scheme uses several mechanisms to target BPL families, the main mechanism being the BPL card.

BPL households are eligible to receive free services in the benefit package from a panel of any one of the private nursing homes or private hospitals by showing their BPL card at the time of service. In the event that poor households do not have a BPL card, they are considered eligible for free service if they obtain an authorization letter from the sarpanch or the Municipal Corporation. Only one of the five districts has issued a Chiranjeevi card.

Table 4A.1

Details of the Financial Package under the Chiranjeevi Scheme

Services, Procedure and Benefits	Cases Per 100 Deliveries	Cost (₹) Per Procedure	Total Payment (₹) Per 100 Deliveries
Normal delivery	85	800	68,000
Complicated cases			
Eclampsia/forceps/vacuum/breech	3	1,000	3,000
Septicemia	2	3,000	6,000
Blood transfusion	3	1,000	3,000
Caesarean section	7	5,000	35,000
Pre-delivery visit (ANC)	100	100	10,000
Other costs			
Investigation	100	50	5,000
Sonography	30	150	4,500
NICU support	10	1,000	10,000
Food	100	100	10,000
Dai **(accompanying person)**	100	50	5,000
Transport (cash payment to mother)	100	200	20,000
Total	100		1,79,500

Source: Bhat et al. (2009).

The GoG contracted out the covered services to private gynaecologists. The GoG obtained inputs from Federation of Obstetric and Gynaecologists Societies of India (FOGSI) representatives to arrive at a uniform reimbursement for each of the services in the package. To reduce any financial incentive for providers to 'induce demand' for caesarean sections, the same amount is paid for each delivery regardless of the procedure performed. In 2006, the reimbursement was estimated as ₹179,000 for 100 deliveries (assuming 85% would be normal deliveries and 15% would be complicated deliveries including 7% caesarean sections). Thus, providers are paid ₹1,790 for each delivery in a private facility. Out of which, they have to pay ₹50 to a *dai* and ₹200 to the patient for transportation. In cases where the private practitioner provides the delivery service in a public facility, s/he is reimbursed ₹440 for services (Bhat et al. 2007). To develop this package and PPP, lot of consultations were done with various stakeholders by the GoG. The health commissioner and his team visited many districts personally to meet and convince private providers to join this programme. The health commissioner monitors the scheme personally to ensure that it works smoothly and payments are made on time.

References

Bhat, M., Mavalankar, D., Singh, P. and Singh, N. 2009. 'Maternal Health Care Financing: Gujarat's Chiranjeevi Scheme and Its Beneficiaries', *Journal of Health, Population, and Nutrition*, 27(2): 249.

Bhat, R., Mavalankar, D., Singh, P. and Singh, N. 2007. Maternal Health Financing in Gujarat: Preliminary Results from a Household Survey of Beneficiaries under Chiranjeevi Scheme. Indian Institute of Management. Available at http://www.iimahd.ernet.in/publications/data/2007-10-06Bhat.pdf, accessed in August 2013.

Duggal, R. 2005. *Public Health Expenditures, Investment and Financing under the Shadow of a Growing Private Sector.* (CEHAT: Review of Health care in India, pg. 225) Available at http://www.cehat.org/publications/PDf%20files/r51.pdf, accessed in 2011.

Family Health Survey (NFHS-3), 2005–06. International Institute for Population Sciences (IIPS) and Macro International. 2007. National Family Health Survey (NFHS-3), 2005–06: India. Volume I. Mumbai: IIPS.

Futures Group. 2009. Voucher Scheme for Equity in Health—India Experience—Voucher Exchange Workshop, 8–11 September. Nairobi, Kenya.

Government of India (GoI). 2011. 'Family Welfare Statistics in India'. Statistics Division, Ministry of Health and Family Welfare, GoI.

GoI. 2005. Background Papers of the National Commission on Macroeconomics and Health Financing and Delivery of Health Care Services in India, Ministry of Health and Family Welfare, GoI. Available at http://www.who.int/macrohealth/action/Background%20Papers%20report.pdf, accessed in March 2011.

Lahariya, C. 2009. Cash Incentives for Institutional Delivery: Linking with Antenatal and Postnatal Care May Ensure 'Continuum of Care' in India. Available at http://www.ncbi.nlm.nih.gov/pmc/articles/PMC2763661/, accessed in March 2011.

Mavalankar, D. 2010. 'State of Maternal Health in India'. Available at http://www.azadindia.org/social-issues/maternal-health-in-india.html, accessed on 30 March 2011.

National Sample Survey Organisation (NSSO). 2006. Morbidity, Health Care and Condition of the Aged, NSSO 60th Round (January–June 2004) Report No. 507 (60/25.0/1). Available at http://mospi.nic.in/rept%20_%20pubn/507_final.pdf.

PowerPoint Presentation by Futures Group on Sambhav Voucher Scheme.

PricewaterhouseCoopers (PwC). 2010. 'Access to Health Care : Challenges and Solutions'. Available at http://www.cuts-ccier.org/cohed/pdf/Access_to_Healthcare.pdf, accessed in April 2011.

Ruth, S., Schuler, L., Bates, and Khairul, M. 2002. 'Reconciling Cost Recovery with Health Equity Concerns in a Context of Gender Inequality and Poverty: Findings from a New Family Health Initiative in Bangladesh'. *International Family Planning Perspectives*, 28(4): 196–204.

Sharma, S., Smith, S., Sonneveldt, E., Pine, M., Dayaratna, V. and Sanders, R. 2005. 'Formal and Informal Fees for Maternal Health Care Services in Five Countries: Policies, Practices and Perspectives'. POLICY Working Paper Series No. 16. Available at http://www.policyproject.com/pubs/workingpapers/WPS16.pdf, accessed in February 2011.

SRS Bulletin Sample Registration System. 2008. Registrar General, New Delhi, October. Available at http://censusindia.gov.in/Vital_Statistics/SRS_Bulletins/SRS_Bulletins_links/SRS_Bulletin_October_2008.pdf.

USAID. 2008. 'Vouchers to Improve Access by the Poor to Reproductive Health Services—Design and Early Implementation Experience of a Pilot Voucher'. Scheme in Agra District. Health Policy Initiative, Uttar Pradesh, India. Available at http://pdf.usaid.gov/pdf_docs/PNADP969.pdf, accessed on 5 August 2013.

USAID. 2009. 'The Accomplishment Haridwar Voucher'. New Delhi: Futures Group International.

World Development Report. 2012. 'Gender Equity and Development'. Washington, DC: World Bank. p. 78. Available at http://siteresources.worldbank.org/INTWDR2012/Resources/7778105-1299699968583/7786210-1315936222006/Complete-Report.pdf, accessed on 5 August 2013.

WHO. 2002. 'World Health Report 2001'. Geneva: WHO.

Suggested Reading

Sudhakaram, V. 2009. Institutional Deliveries in India—A Socio Economic and Cultural View. Available at http://www.articlesbase.com/womens-health-articles/institutional-deliveries-in-india-a-socio-economic-and-cultural-view—808672.html, accessed in June 2011.

Health Care Infrastructure

5. LifeSpring Hospital Pvt Ltd.
6. Merrygold Health Network

5

LifeSpring Hospital Pvt Ltd.

Madhavi Misra

Background

In India, maternal mortality and morbidity levels remain among the highest in the world. According to the District Level Household Survey-3 (DLHS-3) (2007–08), 53% of Indian women did not receive any care at birth by doctor/nurse/lady health visitor (LHV)/auxiliary nurse midwife (ANM)/ other health personnel. Urban Andhra Pradesh with an urban population of nearly 28 million (Census of India 2011) has only 35,000 beds in government health facilities as per Central Bureau of Health Intelligence (CBHI) 2010. Services available at government hospitals are lower in cost but their quality may not be satisfactory, one of the reasons why only a handful of government facilities cater to a large population in urban India. The other issue with government hospitals is of privacy of patients who avail these services. Private hospitals, on the other hand, have what are referred to as super specialists and are often of better quality as perceived by a majority of the people. This, however, comes at a huge financial cost for the patients, especially the urban poor.

Context

It has been estimated that globally, by 2015 more than half of the population in developing countries is projected to live in urban areas. From 2000 to 2030, the world's urban population is projected to grow at an average annual rate of 1.8%, nearly double the rate expected for total population growth (United Nations 2008). The urban population growth will be particularly rapid in less developed regions, averaging 2.3% per year during this period. Almost all of the world's population growth is expected to take place in the urban areas of less developed regions. There is a great need, therefore, to offer good quality services in urban areas at a cost that the common man can afford.

According to the National Family Household Survey-3 (NFHS-3), Eight Cities Report (2009), it was found that 40% of the very poor in the city of Hyderabad accessed health services from the public health care system as compared to 63% in Chennai (Gupta et al. 2009). This meant that 60% of the very poor in Hyderabad were accessing health services from private medical providers. This results in high out-of-pocket (OOP) payments being incurred by the poor. According to Garg et al. (2005), the World Health Organization (WHO) and National Health Accounts (NHA) estimate that OOP payments account for 80% of total health expenditure in India as compared to an average of 65% in low and middle-income countries.

Hospitals in the city of Hyderabad charge anywhere between ₹50,000 to ₹80,000 per delivery. Thus families belonging to the lower socio-economic strata find it difficult to avail these expensive services and are forced to use the services of the government hospitals, which are struggling to meet the needs of the ever growing patient load. This situation has raised three basic needs for health care for the poor:

1. Need for good quality of clinical care
2. Need for affordable care
3. Need to focus on maternal and childcare

In order to provide an alternative to the government health delivery system and in competition to private hospitals, the chain of LifeSpring Hospitals was set-up in December 2005. The aim was to fill the existing void of care by providing high quality yet low-cost maternal health care. Women have been increasingly voicing a need for better quality of care for maternal health services. LifeSpring is a joint venture with a 50–50 partnership between HLL Lifecare Ltd, a public sector company in India (see Box 5.1), and Acumen Fund (see Box 5.2).

Its model rests on building a chain of small-sized (20-bedded) hospitals across India.

The concept of LifeSpring took birth in 2003 and got its shape by 2005. It was started by Anant Kumar, CEO of LifeSpring Hospitals, who was working for Hindustan Latex Limited (now HLL Lifecare), one of the world's largest producer of condoms. In this capacity, Kumar travelled to hospitals around the country visiting women who had just undergone childbirth to learn about family planning practices and contraceptive use. Over time, it became apparent that women were not satisfied with the level of care received at government hospitals and many felt their experience would have been better at a private clinic. Based upon this feedback, Kumar approached the board members of HLL

Box 5.1: HLL Lifecare Limited

This was launched in 1966, with its incorporation as a corporate entity under the Ministry of Health and Family Welfare, Government of India. HLL was set-up in Kerala, for the production of male contraceptive sheaths for the National Family Welfare Programme. HLL commenced commercial operations in 1969 in Thiruvananthapuram. It went on to produce blood transfusion bags, Copper T intrauterine devices (IUDs), surgical sutures and hydrocephalus shunt. HLL has grown today into a multi-product, multi-unit organization addressing various public health challenges. HLL is a Mini Ratna and upgraded as a Schedule B Central Public Sector Enterprise.

Source: Text adapted from http://www.lifespring.in/current-investors.html, http://www.hlfppt.org/ and http://acumen.org/, accessed on 5 August 2013.

Box 5.2: Acumen Fund

The mission of Acumen Fund is to create a world beyond poverty by investing in social enterprises, emerging leaders and breakthrough ideas. Its vision is that one day every human being will have access to the critical goods and services they need, including affordable health, water, housing, energy, agricultural inputs and services, so that they can make decisions and choices for themselves and unleash their full human potential. This is where dignity starts; not just for the poor but for everyone on earth. They have more than 44 thriving enterprises helping tens of millions of people across the world. In India, the Acumen Fund has more than 10 investments in innovative enterprises, including some in health.

Source: Text adapted from http://acumen.org/, accessed on 5 August 2013.

with a proposal to open a clinic providing high-quality, affordable maternal and child health care services to low-income families in Hyderabad's sprawling urban slums. The clinic would bridge the divide between the low-cost, but overstretched government hospitals and the high-quality, high-price private clinics. In 2005, with financial support from HLL, the first LifeSpring Hospital opened in Moula Ali, a suburb of Hyderabad.

LifeSpring Hospitals aim to be the leading health care providers, delivering high quality, affordable maternal health care to lower income mothers across India. Their goal is to be the lowest cost operator with customer-focussed service and their motto 'LifeSpring CARES' embodies an approach whereby each LifeSpring employee is courteous, attentive, respectful and enthusiastic, leading to a safe environment for customers.

LifeSpring Beneficiaries/Customers

LifeSpring focussed on the working poor who are usually not covered by government social insurance schemes. The LifeSpring philosophy is that an expectant mother is not a patient, who needs treatment because pregnancy is not a disease, but is a client who is availing services being offered by LifeSpring. Thus LifeSpring does not refer to women coming to the hospital as patients but as clients or customers. The clients are viewed as active participants in their own health who have the right to demand affordable and dignified care and not as passive recipients of free services. The story of Mallika (see Box 5.3) shows the profile of the beneficiary and their experience at LifeSpring Hospital. Each LifeSpring hospital caters to women and families in its 5–7 km radius, known as the catchment area. The hospitals are usually set-up in localities which have inhabitants from the lower socio-economic strata, thus the target clientele being women and their families who earn between ₹3,000 to 7,000 per month. The majority of women availing services from LifeSpring, have education levels of up to class 10 and are unemployed. The husbands of these women are usually auto-drivers, construction workers or micro entrepreneurs. Earlier, these families were accessing maternal health facilities at government hospitals or at private facilities but because of the high-quality and low-cost services offered by LifeSpring, they can now shift to this chain.

> **Box 5.3: Story of Mallika**
>
> Mallika works at a well-known super-speciality hospital of Hyderabad. For her first pregnancy, Mallika realized she could not afford the super-speciality hospital she worked at and, thus, used the facilities of a government hospital during her delivery. Her experience was not up to her satisfaction at the government facility. For her second pregnancy, she decided not to use a government facility. Mallika has been introduced to LifeSpring Hospital and is very happy that she can now get quality care at an affordable price. She regularly visits the hospital and is satisfied with her experience.
>
> *Source:* From an interview conducted with Mallika at LifeSpring Hospital, Moula Ali, Hyderabad in 2011.

LifeSpring offers high-quality services at a low price, thus making maternal health care affordable for the urban poor. Each consultation was originally priced at ₹75 and now marginally increased to ₹80. A normal delivery costs ₹4,000 in the general ward, ₹5,500 in the semi-private ward and ₹7,000 in the private ward. A normal delivery package is all inclusive and includes a two-day stay, medicines, vaccinations and a baby kit consisting of a baby robe and a blanket. A caesarean section costs ₹9,000 for the general ward, ₹12,000 for the semi-private ward and ₹16,000 for the private ward. The typical length of a hospital stay after caesarean section is five days. These services are offered at prices that are 30 to 50% less than other private hospitals in metros such as Hyderabad.

Interface with Government

The state and central governments are both encouraging the efforts of LifeSpring. All new facilities of LifeSpring are usually inaugurated by a high-level government functionary. LifeSpring is exploring the idea of using old buildings belonging to the government and besides this, till recently was getting vaccines at a subsidized rate from the government.

Cost-effective Model

Infrastructure

Each LifeSpring Hospital building is usually taken on lease. LifeSpring does not believe in purchasing land and creating infrastructure by constructing. It identifies unused or vacant buildings from private developers for use. For example, one LifeSpring Hospital is an unused residential apartment building. This helps in reducing capital costs.

Services

Another interesting fact about LifeSpring in Hyderabad and adjoining areas of Hyderabad is that it does not own and operate ambulances. All 12 LifeSpring Hospitals together have only one ambulance for their internal use. The reason for not owning and operating ambulances is because when an ambulance is required, LifeSpring uses the services of the state-run Emergency Management and Research Institute (EMRI) ambulance service, thus piggybacking on an existing facility provided by the state. It is estimated that the cost of operating each ambulance in Andhra Pradesh annually is upwards ₹10 lakhs and by using the EMRI services in times of need, LifeSpring saves on this cost for each of its hospitals.

The services offered at LifeSpring include normal deliveries and caesarean sections. The doctors include gynaecologists, obstetricians and paediatricians. The hospitals are equipped with a labour room and an operation theatre for caesarean sections. Each hospital has a pharmacy and laboratory attached to it. Each customer has the flexibility to sign up to avail antenatal care (ANC) and postnatal care (PNC) facility at a nominal cost of ₹80. Till recently, the programme involved a nurse from the hospital visiting the woman at home for an ANC or PNC visit. Due to financial viability, this programme has now been done away with.

Usually, the pharmacies and laboratory services are outsourced to well-known external agencies. For instance, the chain of pharmacies set-up at each LifeSpring Hospital keep kits ready for delivery and only charge when purchased. This way LifeSpring does away with pilferage and wastages and is not responsible for day-to-day management of the work of a pharmacy or for medicine supply, etc.

Specialization for Doctors

LifeSpring's focussed specialization in maternal health care enables the chain to focus on lowering costs and increasing productivity at its 12 existing locations. LifeSpring has successfully optimized the utilization of its most expensive asset—its doctors. On an average, each hospital employs two full-time and two on-call doctors. Each LifeSpring doctor performs four to five deliveries per week, in comparison to the one to two deliveries a week by a doctor at private clinics, thus providing them with a non-monetary incentive of improving their skills. At each hospital, a doctor is put in charge of monitoring protocol adherence among staff. Such high volume enables optimal utilization of a doctor's time. In addition, Lifespring doctors are not expected to perform administrative functions that most other hospitals require. By relieving doctors of this function, they are able to spend more time with customers, perform surgeries and deliver babies. The story of Dr Nabhat Lakhani (see Box 5.4) explains what motivates doctors to work at LifeSpring Hospitals. The clinical team works closely to ensure high quality of services. These doctors in turn report to the director of clinical quality. Regular teleconferencing between all the LifeSpring Hospitals and the director of clinical quality ensures efficient results.

> **Box 5.4: Story of Dr Nabhat Lakhani**
>
> Dr Nabhat Lakhani joined LifeSpring Hospital as a consulting doctor after a short stint in the private sector. She feels that LifeSpring is filling the gap between government facilities and the private sector which is out of the reach of many. She feels that maternal mortality is highest among people of lower socio-economic strata and they usually go to the government hospital to avail services. They are not looked after very well at the government hospital. LifeSpring has provided an alternative to that at an affordable cost. This motivates Nabhat to work at LifeSpring.
>
> *Source:* From an interview conducted with Dr Nabhat Lakhani at LifeSpring Hospital, Hyderabad, 2011.

Role of Nurses

The nurses at LifeSpring play a very important role unlike at other private or government hospitals. They double up as administrators. This reduces overhead expenditures by eliminating an entire unit of administrators and accountants. The nurses are trained to carry out billing and attend to the reception section of the hospitals. The nurses were also involved in fieldwork till recently. Here, in addition to her daily duties, each nurse was bound to do two days of fieldwork each week. This involved the nurse visiting the 5–7 km catchment area and meeting those LifeSpring customers who had signed up for ANC and PNC services.

Outreach System

Each LifeSpring Hospital has outreach workers attached to it. These lady fieldworkers make house-to-house visits and encourage married women who are either pregnant or otherwise eligible to access the services offered at the LifeSpring Hospitals. These outreach workers serve as an extended arm of the hospitals and help in spreading awareness about their services to the people in the nearby community. This system works on a results basis where the outreach workers are given a certain sum of money for bringing clients to the hospitals. LifeSpring also focusses on community outreach programmes to educate the community. Each hospital conducts community health camps on a monthly basis. The camp involves education by a doctor and offers a free prenatal check-up for new customers, free paediatric consultations and vaccinations.

Referral System

As a policy, no complicated case is ever admitted by the hospital. Such cases are identified and referred early on to nearby private facilities. The clients are advised to access services from an affiliated charitable hospital where prices are already pre-fixed. A LifeSpring Hospital is a low-cost model and, thus, does not have an intensive care unit (ICU) or a neonatal ICU on its premises. Cost-effectiveness is achieved by referring complicated cases to other hospitals early on, thus minimizing investment on expensive equipment.

Cost of the Model

As stated by the Anant Kumar, 'LifeSpring is still a work in progress'. This is a for-profit model. There is cross selling of additional services to patients who require specialist health care in gynaecology, obstetrics and paediatrics. The venture broke even after 20 months of operation, thus, making it financially sustainable. In addition to the revenue generated from deliveries, additional income is attributed to family planning services, outpatient doctor consultation fees and the rent received from the outsourced laboratory and pharmacy. Standardized kits for surgery and use of generic drugs purchased in bulk result in procedures being affordable for users. All the processes that have been mentioned lead to cost cutting and, thus making, LifeSpring a viable, profit-making venture.

LifeSpring hires less-expensive ANMs in addition to general nurse midwives and has developed a strict standard of clinical protocols and other procedures to enable clarity of tasks and ensure that staff and resources are used efficiently. It is a midwife-led model and though the doctor-nurse ratio is the same as in the private clinics, the utilization of the nurse workforce is 2.5 times higher.

Quality Control at LifeSpring

At LifeSpring, quality consists of three elements.

1. Clinical excellence
2. Customer care
3. Efficient operations

For Lifespring, good quality care means no mortality, no morbidity and an increase in patient satisfaction. All of the approximately 180 processes identified at LifeSpring are standardized and written. Training is designed for each of these processes whereby a new person who joins can undergo the training which makes it easy to enter the system. Non-clinical processes, such as fumigation techniques, keeping the operation theatre and labour room sterile and cleaning methods, are standardized. Clinical procedures such as labour management and induction of labour are standardised as well. The hospitals have strict guidelines for clinical and non-clinical quality work standards. To maintain quality care and hospital safety, LifeSpring has partnered with the Institute for Health Care Improvement, based in Cambridge, USA and follows the Royal College of Obstetricians and Gynaecologists (RCOG) and American Congress of Obstetrician and Gynaecologist (ACOG) standard guidelines which are somewhat modified to suit the needs of Lifespring.

This low-cost venture has reaped vital rewards through a stringent focus on training and development. Today, training is the backbone that has equipped Lifespring to scale-up successfully. The training focusses on the following:

- How to remain low cost and profitable?
- How to ensure standardized and consistent services across all locations?
- How to ensure that staff is well trained and well mannered at every level?

Training is imparted on 180 processes. E-learning training modules are used to ensure efficient and standardized training delivered. These are deployed on moodle training software in order to be accessible. LifeSpring received a grant from the Rockefeller Foundation to create 50 videos. Trainings are imparted to all employees, doctors, nurses, administrators and corporate staff. Even outsourced staffs such as security guards and ayahs are trained. LifeSpring developed several in-house videos as well. This way the quality of trainings is of a set standard and no one is able to deviate from what is being taught. Even during the expansion of LifeSpring chain from one to 12 hospitals, the quality of training to all staff has remained uniform.

Incorporation of User Feedback

LifeSpring constantly incorporates user feedback from clients. This is not always paper-based but also involves interpersonal communication. For instance, feedback received was about long out-patient department lines for clients and a long wait for billing. After analyzing the situation, it was realized that the nurses, who manage the reception and computerized billing system, were not well acquainted with the system. Thus, a training programme was devised whereupon all the nurses were trained on how to use the billing system and monitor the reception desk. The billing system itself was simplified and the registration system which had five to six steps was reduced to two to three steps.

Scale-up

Key motivationg factors behind the decision to scale-up the LifeSpring strategy have been the large social impact that it has created and also its financial sustainability.

For three years, LifeSpring worked at perfecting the operations in the first hospital. After this, it began its expansion to other neighbourhoods surrounding Hyderabad, with financial support from HLL Lifecare and Acumen Fund. By 2012, the chain had grown to 12 hospitals located in high density, low-income areas. It aims to open 100 such hospitals by 2017 and expand its geographic reach to other states across the country.

LifeSpring hopes to receive recognition from National Accreditation Board of Hospitals (NABH) soon.

Challenges Faced along the Way and Solutions Sought

After setting-up the first hospital, LifeSpring's main challenge was how to efficiently run a chain of hospitals. As a strategy, LifeSpring began to set-up its hospitals in clusters, close to each other, though serving different geographic areas. This way, the amount of time required to travel to each location would reduce. For their expansion plans, when scaling-up outside Hyderabad, LifeSpring plans to use a similar strategy. Another challenge was how to ensure quality of services and keep patient satisfaction levels high and maintain the same quality in each hospital. This was done by creating high-quality protocols. Virtual classroom training and using portals such as media training vidoes for training all employees was done. Protocols are usually written in English and ayahs and security guards who do not understand English can go through the visual training programme. Some modules were also translated for their benefit. Such as, the training in biomedical waste management in the local language together with a video helped the employees responsible for this task to get trained and carry out their responsibilities efficiently. LifeSpring spent its resources and time in creating detailed protocols for these tasks and then transformed these into online training programmes for its employees.

References

Census of India 2011. Office of the Registrar General and Census Commissioner, Ministry of Home Affairs, Government of India. Available at http://www.censusindia.gov.in/2011-prov-results/prov_results_paper1_india.html, accessed on 5 August 2011.

District Level Household and Facility Survey (DLHS-3) 2007–08. 2010. International Institute for Population Sciences (IIPS). Mumbai, India: IIPS.

Garg et al. 2005. Health and Millennium Development Goal 1: Reducing Out-of-pocket Expenditures to Reduce Income Poverty—Evidence from India, Equitap Project, Working Paper 15, May 2005.

Kamla Gupta, Fred Arnold and H. Lhungdim. 2009. Health and Living Conditions in Eight Indian Cities. National Family Health Survey (NFHS-3), India, 2005–06. Mumbai: International Institute for Population Sciences; Calverton, Maryland, USA: ICF Macro.

United Nations. 2008. World Urbanization Prospects: The 2007 Revision Highlights. New York: United Nations.

6

Merrygold Health Network

Madhavi Misra

Introduction

Uttar Pradesh (UP) is the most populous state in India accounting for 16.5% of the population of India (GoI 2011). More than 70% of the births in UP are not assisted by any doctor/nurse/lady health visitor (LHV)/auxiliary nurse midwife (ANM)/other health personnel. According to 2007–09 figures, UP is, therefore, burdened with high infant mortality, with an estimated infant mortality rate (IMR) of 63 per 1,000 live births and maternal mortality ratio (MMR) of 359 per 100,000 live births (SRS 2007–09). In 2007–09, the national IMR was estimated to be 50 per 1,000 live births and MMR of 212 per 100,000 live births (SRS 2007–09). The unmet need for family planning is 21.9% in UP whereas the unmet need for family planning in all of India is 12.8%. More than 73% of mothers in UP did not receive the three antenatal care (ANC) visits for the last birth (National Family Health Welfare 2005–06).

Given the scenario of dismal health and demographic indicators, an urgent need was felt to provide access to affordable and quality health care to women in UP.

Social Franchising for Health

Franchising has been defined as:

> A form of business organization in which a firm which already has a successful product or service (the franchisor) enters into a continuing contractual relationship with other businesses (franchises) operating under the franchisor's trade name and usually with the franchisor's guidance, in exchange for a fee.[1]

Social franchising is an attempt to use franchising methods to achieve social rather than financial goals, influencing the service delivery systems of the private sector in a manner similar to what social marketing has adapted traditional outlets for commodity sales (Monatgu 2002).

[1]'What is a Franchise?' Available at http://www.investorwords.com/2078/franchise.html, accessed on 2 August 2013.

There were various reasons why privatization was considered important for the development of reproductive health (RH) services. These services had to provide 'more with less' because governments were required to develop an expanding array of high-quality services. Demand for RH services was also rising because of the increasing number of people in the reproductive age group, the rising need for preventive services, increasing education and awareness of RH needs and the growing human immunodeficiency virus (HIV) epidemic.

Today, various forms of privatization are being pursued in the provision of RH services. Governments across the world in lower and middle income countries have engaged in contracting of services—contracting both in and out—often with the non-profit sector in their countries as the provider (Ravindran et al. 2011).

Franchising is a hybrid business structure somewhere between a market and a firm in the study of organizational economics. Franchisors and franchises typically engage in a contractual exchange, with a regular transfer of goods or services between the two, similar to what would occur in a market with long-term contracts. As a part of this contract, the franchisors strictly regulate many of the activities of the franchise—standardizing retail outlet design and colour, the range of goods and services offered and acting to assure quality and prices (Lafontaine 1992).

Merrygold Health Network

Merrygold Health Network (MGHN) emerged as one of the answers to address UP's maternal mortality. The different units of MGHN are shown in Figure 6.1. It has been able to successfully spread and establish itself all across UP since its inception in 2007. United States Agency for International Development (USAID) and State Innovations in Family Planning Project Services Agency (SIFPSA) have developed this innovative social franchising programme through consultations with various

Figure 6.1
Different Units of Merrygold Health Network

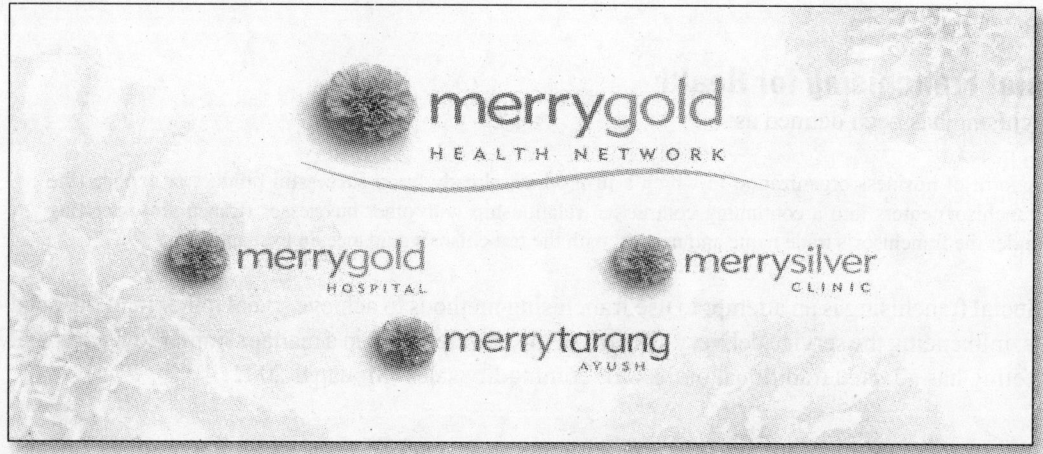

Source: Adapted from information taken from http://merrygold.org.in/MGHN.htm and interviews of employees.

Figure 6.2
Merrygold Health Network Model

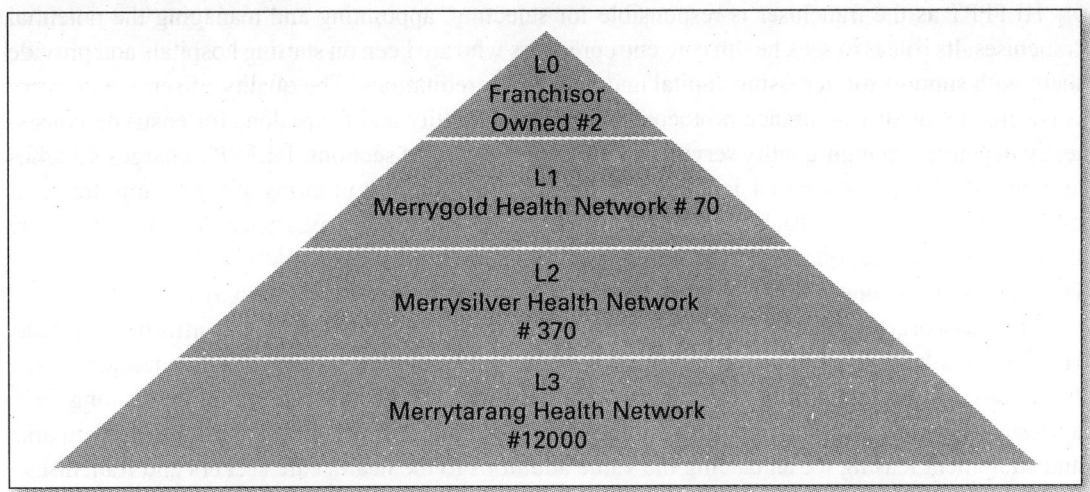

L0
Franchisor
Owned #2

L1
Merrygold Health Network # 70

L2
Merrysilver Health Network
370

L3
Merrytarang Health Network
#12000

Source: Adapted from organization documents and information received from the organization.

national and international experts. Hindustan Latex Family Planning Promotion Trust (HLFPPT) implements this public–private partnership (PPP) for delivering maternal health services and is supported by USAID and SIFPSA. HLFPPT has developed, managed and sustained the MGHN.

The MGHN aims to provide high-quality maternal and child health services at affordable prices. This network currently comprises the following franchise private providers—7,020-bedded Merrygold Hospitals, 700 Merrysilver clinics and 10,000 Merrytarang workers—as described in Figure 6.2. This network of providers aims to provide varied package of services at affordable prices. Currently, MGHN covers 36 of the 71 districts of UP and 469 of the 834 blocks, which means that MGHN is present in more than 50% of districts and blocks.

How Does This Model Work?

The franchisers (Merrygold Hospitals) own the L0 (level 0)-tier hospitals and operate these themselves (see Figure 6.2). These hospitals provide maternal, newborn and family planning services including comprehensive emergency obstetric care. These services include:

1. ANC
2. Delivery care
3. Post-delivery care
4. Child care
5. Family planning

These are also referred to as model referral hospitals. There are only two L0 hospitals, one in Agra and the other in Kanpur. These are 20-bedded hospitals managed and run by HLFPPT and the Merrygold brand itself. The Merrygold Hospital's own hospital model was difficult to replicate across the state so the franchise model was initiated.

HLFPPT as the franchiser is responsible for selecting, appointing and managing the potential franchises. Its role is to seek health care entrepreneurs who are keen on starting hospitals and provide them with support for accessing capital and needed accreditations. The quality of service delivery is ensured by quality assurance protocols and periodic quality audits are done for ensuring consistency in delivering high-quality services to the underprivileged sections. HLFPPT charges ₹3 lakhs as franchising fee from the L1 level franchises and gives support in terms of marketing, training, developing network, outreach activities, medical audits and quality assurance. Merrygold sets up the franchises' entire information technology (IT) system. It provides software to all the Merrygold Hospitals and is capturing all the data from the field at one point (see Figure 6.3).[2]

This network provides high-quality maternal and child health services at affordable prices. HLFPPT conducts process audits for ensuring that quality of care standards is maintained by the franchises. As the franchising network expands, HLFPPT has been focussing on developing linkages such as with community health insurance schemes, low-cost generic drug marketing networks and equipment leasing for enhancing the value additions to the health care seekers and franchises.

The franchiser is the owner and originator of the brand and policies. In the MGHN, HLFPPT is the franchiser and HLFPPT's functions can be categorized as:

- Creating access to products and services for improving reproductive and child health through social marketing and franchising.
- Developing programmes for HIV prevention among populations with highest risk of contracting HIV.
- Providing technical assistance in public health programmes.
- Programming new technologies for public health.

Figure 6.3
Benefits of Social Franchising

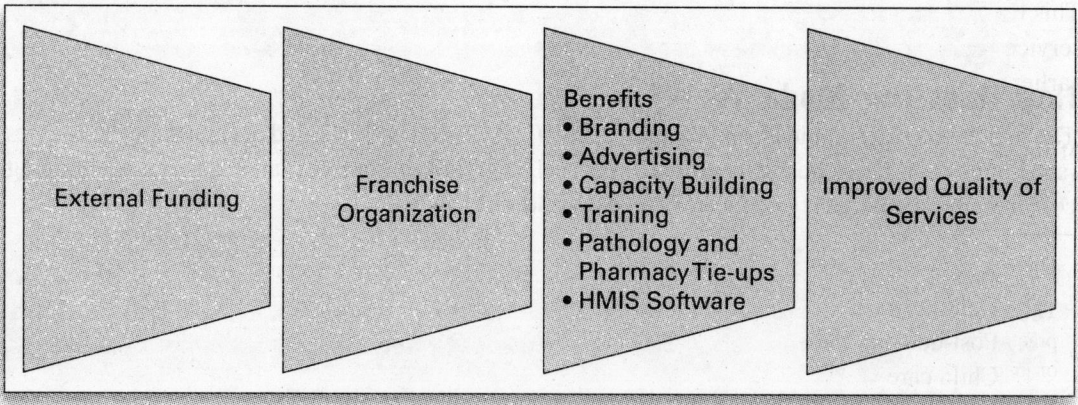

Source: Adapted from organization documents and information received from the organization.

[2]http://merrygold.org.in/, accessed on 2 August 2013.

Besides this, Merrygold is also responsible for providing the L1 and L2-tier franchises with the following benefits:

1. Capacity building and training of medical and paramedical staff. ·
2. Development of vendors and procurement at competitive prices.
3. Regulating quality assurance systems (medical audits).
4. Marketing of the network.
5. Helping the network avail various government schemes by putting the franchises in touch with the relevant district health authorities.
6. Branding support to franchises by giving them a brand name including installation of standard signage, glow sign boards, clinical posters, branding of hospital premises and providing hospital stationery.

Other benefits to the franchisees are:

1. The franchisee receives the Health Managment Information Systems (HMIS) software and training in it.
2. Pathology assistance by Metropolis Laboratories.
3. Pharmacy assistance by Guardians Pharmacy.
4. Training and orientation of Merrysilver and Merrytarang partners.
5. Facilitating corporate tie-ups (if possible).
6. Management development programmes.

Other Benefits to Merrygold Health Network Franchisees

According to Birendra Kumar, team leader of MGHN in Lucknow, 'The franchise usually opts for this arrangement because the MGHN mobilizes more footfalls in the hospitals with the help of Merrytarang workers. More institutional deliveries and family planning services in the hospital means more turnover and more revenue generated.'

Source: Interview transcripts of Birendra Kumar.

The social franchising network created by HLFPPT provides all the services listed in Figure 6.4. This results in an improvement in the array of services and enhances their quality. The bouquet of services provided to the franchisee helps in setting up protocols and systems for the hospital which earlier might not have had the benefit of these.

The business model of MGHN rests on the principle of 'increased volume and specialization of the health care facility to drive costs down and result in better patient outcome'. The services

Quality Assurance at MGHN

The MGHN system has a team of gynaecologists. HLFPPT has developed 13 protocols mainly for clinical practices at the hospital level. The HLFPPT team does quality audits and visits the hospitals routinely. One-on-one meetings with doctors and paramedical staff are held to discuss how the quality may be improved. An analysis of quality assurance scores for all L1 hospitals was done as per Figure 6.5 and as per quarter eight, nearly 100% of the checklist was completed on the quality assurance scale.

Source: Interview transcripts of Birendra Kumar.

Figure 6.4
Services Provided by the Network

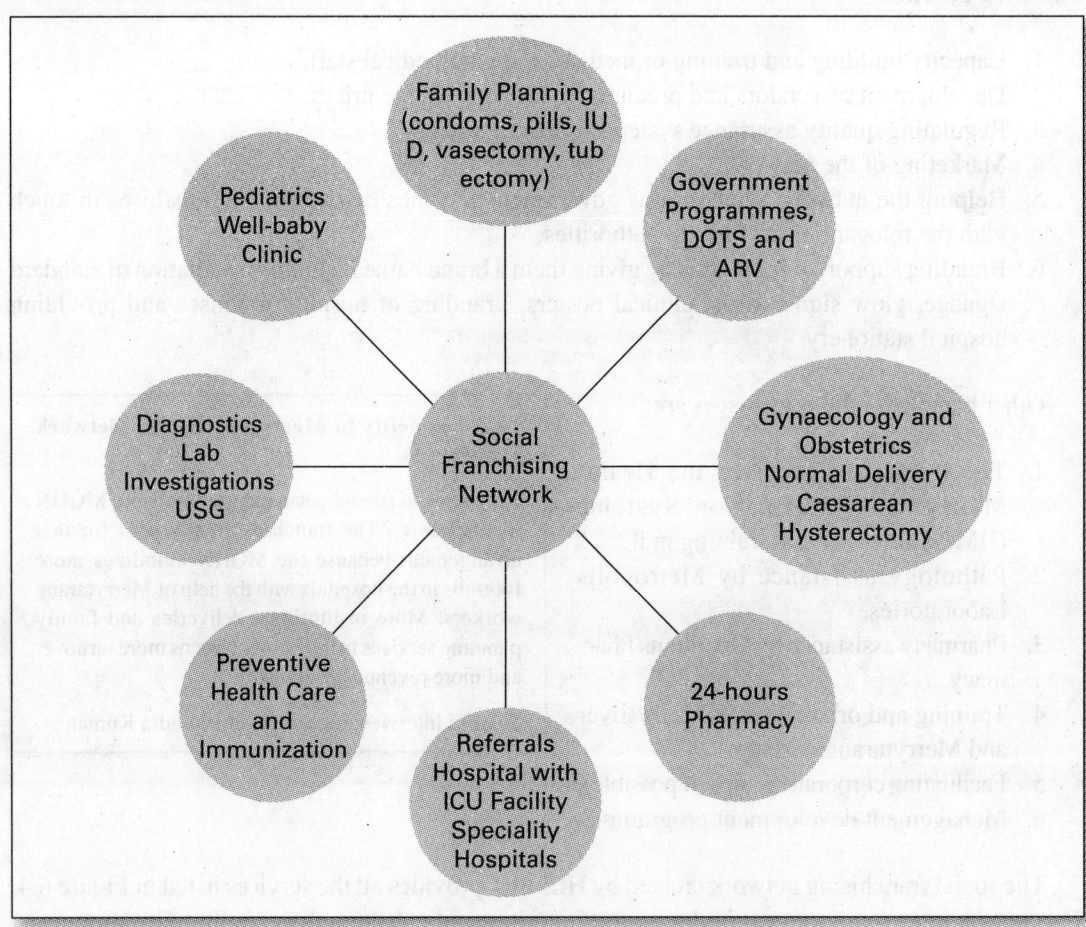

Source: Adapted from organization documents and information received from the organization.

franchised out are priced at 50–60% less than market price. The franchise is usually a 15–20-bedded facility spread over a 6,000 sq. ft area.

The franchise at each level is required to have a particular level of infrastructure and for L1 and L2, a licensing fee is required. No revenue share is required for L2 and L3. This is described in Table 6.1.

Cost Structure of Merrygold Health Network

In 2007, the cost of services had been fixed at modest rates when Merrygold was initiated. Over the years, the cost of services has gradually increased. For instance, as per Table 6.2, the cost of normal delivery for general-ward patients has gone up by approximately 66% over five years. Similarly, the

Figure 6.5
Comparative Analysis of Quality Assurance Scores of All L1 Health Facilities

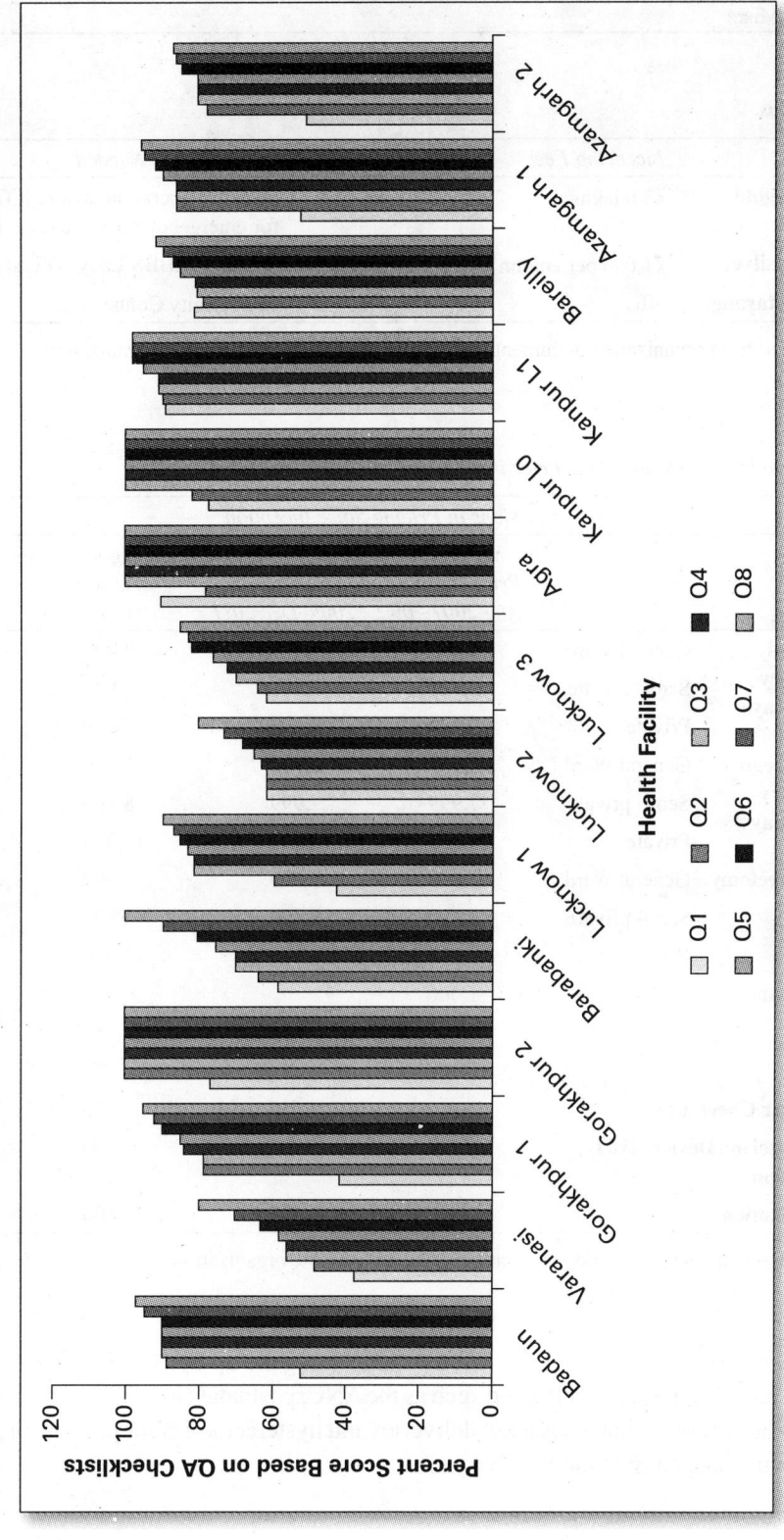

Source: Report by Futures Group.

Table 6.1

Franchise Terms

Level	Licencing Fee	Revenue Share	Infrastructure Needed
L1-tier Merrygold	₹3.0 lakhs	3%	20 bed + operation theatre (OT) + Personnel for emergency obstetric care (EmOC)
L2-tier Merrysilver	₹1,000 per annum	NIL	5 beds + MBBS/Lady AYUSH +Asst
L3-tier Merrytarang	NIL	NIL	Community Connections

Source: Adapted from organization documents and information received from the organization.

Table 6.2

Services Offered by MGHN and Their Price in Comparison to Market Price

			Revisions in Pricing Since Inception			
S.No.	Service		Merrygold Price (in INR) Aug 2007– 09	Merrygold Price (in INR) Aug 2009–Dec 2011	Merrygold Price (in INR) Dec 2011– till date	Market Price (non-metro range) in INR
1.	**Normal Delivery (Two days)**	General Ward	1,499	1,999	2,499	3,450–11,050
		Semi- private	2,499	2,499	2,999	
		Private	3,999	3,999	3,999	
2.	**Caesarean Delivery (Five days)**	General Ward	4,999	6,999	7,999	9,500–22,000
		Semi- private	7,999	7,999	8,999	
		Private	11,999	11,999	11,999	
3.	**Hysterectomy**	General Ward	5,999	5,999	7,999	3,500–22,000
		Semi- private	8,199	8,199	8999	
		Private	12,999	12,999	12,999	
4.	**Day Care**		1,000			Varied
5.	**ANC**		50	50	50	100–300
6.	**PNC**		50	50	50	100–300
7.	**Regular Check-ups**		50	50	50	Varied
8.	**Intrauterine Device (IUD) Insertion**		99	99	100	250–400
9.	**Sterilization**		999	999	1,500	1,000–3,000

Source: Organization documents and information received from the organization.

cost for a caesarean section for general-ward patients has gone up by 60% in the same time period. Many costs, however, remain unchanged such as the ANC, postnatal care (PNC) and costs for regular check-ups. The cost of normal/caesarean deliveries and hysterectomies for patients in private rooms also remains unchanged over the last five years.

The reason for the increase in some costs could be attributed to two reasons:

1. Increased cost of services incurred by the franchises.
2. These services are more utilised than the others so increasing their costs will increase profits for the franchises.

All services offered are significantly lower than the market price for them in other private facilities. For example, the cost of a normal delivery in a private facility can go as high as ₹11,050 while it is 2.7 times lower at MGHN and priced at ₹3,999.

Evidence of Impact

Utilization of Services

Table 6.3
Evidence of Impact from 2007 Onwards till May 2012

Services	2007–08	2008–09	2009–10	2010–11	2011–12 (till May)	Total
ANC Check-ups	25,066	44,874	192,955	467,971	35,984	766,850
Institutional Deliveries	5,785	9,669	36,028	75,928	9,319	136,729
Sterilization	355	734	1,921	7,499	158	10,667
IUD	1,284	1,973	11,191	23,109	1,050	38,607

Source: MGHN figures received in June 2012.

From Table 6.3, it is evident that institutional deliveries have gone up significantly, nearly 23.6 times from 2007 to 2012. Similarly, sterilization went up 30 times in the same time frame in the MGHN. Utilization of ANC check-ups went up 30 times as well from 2007 to 2012. Thus, impact, in terms of uptake of services has had a steep incline.

Discussion

The MGHN initiative is a laudable one. In a short span of time, small nursing homes and clinics providing maternal care and family planning services have been branded, their quality upgraded and patient load increased as a result of the initiative across UP. Social franchising initiatives as can be seen in MGHN seem to provide better quality of patient care and have the clinical protocols streamlined for better output and improved quality of services.

Social franchising models also do well economically because they result in covering large areas of population which might or might not be underserved by the existing government system. The reason why MGHN is hailed as a success is because it provides maternal health services at an affordable price with quality assured.

At regular intervals, HLFPPT has been revising the costs of services, in order to cover the expenses of the franchises as well as looking to profit margin. There is concern in some quarters that the footfall at the MGHN facilities might reduce because of schemes such as Janani Suraksha Yojana (JSY) being provided at the government facilities. If the MGHN network is accredited by the government as institutions where schemes such as JSY may be implemented as well, the issue of reducing footfalls will not arise. This linkage with the government system might be useful for the future.

The initial idea while setting-up the three-tier system was also for referral between L2 and L1. However, since the L2 facilities have MBBS doctors, complicated cases are taken up by L2 and not usually referred. For greater economic efficiency, the L1 and L2 facilities could be consolidated and all these facilities could be given L1 status.

Way Forward

MGHN has been scaled-up throughout UP covering 36 districts. Expanding the network in difficult areas within UP will help strengthen the fact that social franchising as a model can be replicated in different social settings. The challenge also lies in replicating MGHN across the different states of India. There is a move towards this and hopefully states such as Rajasthan might take this up in the future.

References

IFPS Technical Assistance Project (ITAP). 2012. Social Franchising as a Public-Private Partnership Model—Lessons Learned from the Merrygold Health Network of Uttar Pradesh, India. Gurgaon, Haryana: Futures Group, ITAP. Available at http://futuresgroup.com/index.php/resources/publications/social_franchising_as_a_public_private_partnership_model, accessed on 2 August 2013.

Government of India (GoI). 2011. Family Welfare Statistics. Statistics Division, Ministry of Health and Family Welfare, Government of India.

Lafontaine, F. 1992. 'Agency Theory and Franchising: Some Empirical Results'. RAND *Journal of Economics*, 23: 263–83.

Monatgu, D. 2002. 'Franchising of Health Services in Low-income Countries'. *Health Policy and Planning*, 17(2): 121–30.

National Family Health Welfare 2005–06. 2007. International Institute for Population Sciences (IIPS) and Macro International. Volume I. Mumbai, India: IIPS.

Ravindran et al. 2011. 'Are Social Franchises Contributing to Universal Access to Reproductive Health Services in Low-income Countries?' *Reproductive Health Matters*, 19(38): 85–101.

Sample Registration System (SRS). 2007–09. Planning Commission, Government of India. Available at http://censusindia.gov.in/vital_statistics/SRS_Bulletins/Bulletins.html, accessed on 2 August 2013.

Human Resources

7. Addressing Issues of Human Resources and Quality of Care:
The Yashoda

7

Addressing Issues of Human Resources and Quality of Care: The Yashoda

Radhika Arora

Across India, initiatives to encourage institutional deliveries to improve maternal and child health are being rolled out. Government schemes, such as the Janani Suraksha Yojna (JSY) under the National Rural Health Mission (NRHM), have contributed to the increase in institutional deliveries from 7.39 lakhs per year in 2005–06 to about 1 crore in 2009–10 (GoI 2012). Over 50% of women who previously had home deliveries chose to deliver their babies at a health-care facility according to recent evaluations of the JSY (2011). The increase in institutional deliveries has implications on infrastructure, human resources, availability of drugs and equipment and supplies, all of which impact quality of care, ultimately affecting maternal and newborn mortality and morbidity (JSY 2011). These would also have

> **Interview Byte: Dr Kaliprasad Pappu**
>
> '…[B]ecause birth is not only an obstetrical event. It has to do with social and physical security. Family and community support has always been there, so when we are getting the mothers to come to deliver in the facility we were looking around to see who could do this in the current system and what we saw were the nurses. The clinicians were so busy delivering babies that no one had the time to really counsel them. We felt an acute need for someone who could be a counsellor to the mother, who could engage with the system on behalf of the mother to get the best for the mother and the newborn … That was the basic need, more so when we looked around in our states which are high-focussed states …'
>
> *Source:* Dr Kaliprasad Pappu, Director, Programmes, Norway India Partnership Initiative, © PHFI, 2011.

an effect on the services a woman and her family receive at the institutional level, which may influence decisions regarding choice of place of delivery in the long run.

In 2008, under the umbrella of the NRHM, the state governments with support of the Norway India Partnership Initiative (NIPI) launched the Yashoda Programme in Madhya Pradesh, Bihar, Odisha and Rajasthan. The Yashodas, as they are known in Madhya Pradesh, Rajasthan and Odisha and Mamta as they are called in Bihar, are a new cadre of volunteer health workers, brought into the system to improve the quality of maternal and newborn care, at public health-care institutions that have a high rate of institutional deliveries (Ramani 2010). Their role as facilitator, counsellor and link between the medical staff and the mother is primarily to improve the quality of care for a mother and her newborn, supporting the work being done already to generate demand and provide quality services with respect to institutional deliveries. The Yashoda Programme is now being implemented in several districts of four states—Rajasthan, Bihar, Madhya Pradesh and Odisha. This case study describes the work being done under the Yashoda Programme in the Alwar District of Rajasthan.

The Yashoda Programme

As the number of deliveries at public health facilities increases, human resources available at the facilities are often stretched thin to provide basic, essential clinical care. This leaves little scope for the provision of important, but seemingly less-than-critical aspects of maternal care, such as psychological support during deliveries, initiating breastfeeding and counselling on newborn care. The Yashoda programme presents an innovative cadre of voluntary health workers introduced in select government health facilities to support, counsel and assist a new mother from the time she comes into the facility to deliver to the time she leaves with her newborn. Pradeep Choudhry, State Programme Officer, NIPI–United Nations Office for Project Services (UNOPS), explained to the research team visiting the intervention area in Alwar District, Rajasthan:

> The aim of the Yashoda Programme is to focus on institutional deliveries… The Yashoda came in as the link between women—mothers—being brought to the hospital towards helping her in the delivery, learning about newborn care—washing the baby, breastfeeding, bonding with the baby. (Interview: 17 June 2011)

Role of a Yashoda

The Yashoda worker's role fits into UNOPS–NIPI's larger Continuum of Care approach towards improving maternal and newborn health in India (PHFI 2011). Her role is designed so that she fits into the existing human resource structure of a medical establishment (see Box 7.1). While the Yashoda is the link between the medical staff and the patient, her duties are strictly non-clinical in nature.

From the time a pregnant woman enters the health-care facility to deliver her child, till the

---

Interview Byte: Leena

'My first baby was a male child. Unfortunately, after five days he passed away. I had no knowledge about how I should have taken care of him. When I was chosen to be a part of Yashoda and I had to teach other mothers about child care, I felt I got an opportunity to ensure that I could teach the other mothers from my mistakes, they will know how to look after their baby or what are the symptoms that indicate that the child is unwell. All the things that I didn't know, which is why I lost my baby, being a Yashoda I want to ensure that no mother makes the same mistakes that I made.'

Source: Leena, Yashoda Worker, Zanana Hospital, Alwar District, © PHFI, 2011.

Box 7.1: Key Role and Features of a Yashoda

- Focus on postnatal and newborn care and encourage retention of women in the facility for 48 hours after delivery.
- Immunization and all other mandated services for mother and child to be ensured
- Helping the woman register as JSY beneficiary
- Weighing of babies
- Ensuring cleanliness of bed, ward & toilets at the hospital
- Honorarium as payment
- Over 400,000 women were assisted by the Yashoda till 2010

Source: Information shared by NIPI-UNOPS 2011.

time she leaves, the Yashoda's role is to support the new mother. She begins by assisting the mother with the paperwork and registration process (see Figure 7.1). She handholds the patient through the labour processes and also assists nurses with the non-medical aspects of the actual delivery. On the birth of a baby, the Yashoda supports the mother in early initiation of breastfeeding. She ensures immunization of the child (through prior counselling and support after birth of child). She counsels the mother on looking after herself post delivery and on newborn care—from how to swaddle a newborn to breastfeeding (focussing on correct feeding practices) and nutrition for the mother as well. This is also when the Yashoda provides information and counselling on family planning.

The first 24 to 48 hours after delivery are the most crucial for the newborn baby and mother. During this period, the Yashoda will support the mother for immediate and exclusive breast feeding; orient the mother about basic newborn care and immunization and assist the nurse in various postnatal care (PNC) activities for making the newborn and the mother comfortable.

Features of a Yashoda

The Yashoda is a female volunteer worker with a minimum level of education; she is usually a member of the community, familiar with the local language and customs of the people. Often she lives less than five kilometeres from the facility to which she is assigned. This makes her commute to the facility easy and she can also be reached easily. It is also advantageous because the Yashoda worker is familiar to the mothers who come into the facility to deliver and she can interact with them even after they leave the facility—keeping an informal track of both the mother and her newborn (Interview: Pradeep Choudhry, 17 June 2011).

Recruitment

The post of a Yashoda was open to women from the community with a minimum education level of Class VIII. Applications were received on the basis of advertisements for the position placed in newspapers.

Remuneration

As a volunteer worker, a Yashoda is given an incentive amount of ₹100 per delivery, with a ceiling amount of ₹3500 per Yashoda worker per month. This limit was imposed to prevent professional discord between the Yashoda and nurses who had higher levels of education and professional qualifications, even though the mention of a ceiling indicates that the amount a Yashoda earns every month varies, with no minimum guaranteed income.

Figure 7.1
Time Allocation by Yashoda

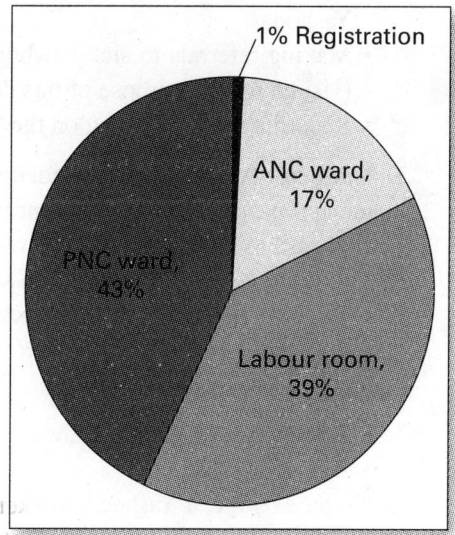

Source: Presentation on Assessing and Supporting NIPI Interventions (ASNI) PHFI, University of Oslo and the Royal Norwegian Embassy.

Training

Each recruit undergoes a three-day training session on the roles and responsibilities she has to undertake before starting work as a Yashoda worker. Training is required to enable the Yashoda worker to develop skills that will help her execute her role as a carer, counsellor and facilitator. At the same time, developing capacity of supervisors to monitor and support the Yashoda is essential towards ensuring better quality of services and motivation levels of the Yashoda.

The Programme

Yashoda workers were posted at the community health centre (CHC) and district hospital (DH) level, though the low-case load at the CHC level led to a lower utilization; their services were better utilized at the DH level (Ramani 2010).

Details of Yashodas at a Health Care Facility

1. Each establishment is assigned up to 24 Yashoda workers, numbers calculated on the basis of the load of deliveries.
2. Supervising the Yashodas are two retired nurses [Grade-I]. In the intervention area we visited, there was one retired nurse supervising the volunteer workers. The supervisor's role is:

   - Typically an eight-hour shift from 12 noon to 8 in the evening.
   - Tasks include tracking the activities of the Yashodas, supervision, checking on babies for signs of sickness and general well-being, working on rosters and duty-schedules of the Yashodas.
   - Making referrals to sick newborn care unit (SNCU) in the intervention district of Alwar (visited for the purpose of this documentation).
   - Recording and reporting on the Yashoda's work.

3. **Uniform:** A Yashoda is provided with a pink shirt-apron with her name embroidered on it; the apron makes it easy to identify a Yashoda worker. She is also given space to sit and a cupboard to keep her things, as well as, store registers/notebooks used for record keeping.[1]
4. The Yashodas work in batches of six, over three-day shifts. Every fourth day—the day after a night shift—is the day off. Each batch of volunteer workers has a time-bound shift to complete:

   - Day 1: 7.30 AM to 2 PM
   - Day 2: 2.30 PM to 7.30 PM
   - Day 3: 7.30 PM to 7.30 AM
   - Day 4: Off day

5. On an average, a Yashoda worker handles 20–30 cases (deliveries) monthly. The absolute numbers would vary monthly (Interview: Pradeep Choudhry, 17 June 2011).

---

[1]Early days of Yashoda indicated that a space for a Yashoda to sit during her shift and access to a toilet were important to a Yashoda worker.

Impact of the Yashoda Programme

Often health care facilities have overstretched health care resources, leaving a gap in aspects of care—such as PNC and counselling. The Yashoda worker was brought in to address this gap in services, her role being a blend of a counsellor, guide and facilitator to the women delivering at hospitals.

Results from a recent PHFI-University of Oslo (2011) study indicate that 81% of women at the Alwar District Hospital reported being attended by a Yashoda in the PNC ward. Essential PNC check-ups such as temperature and blood pressure monitoring were received by 30–40% of women in the intervention areas compared to less than 20% in the control areas (see Figure 7.2). Interviews with new mothers indicated that services had improved after the introduction of the Yashoda workers at the facility. For many, this was the first delivery at the facility level—which meant unfamiliar surroundings and being away from family members. Interviews with mothers delivering in the facility for the second time (after the introduction of the Yashodas) indicate a great improvement in the delivery of services in terms of easing hospital procedures for the mother, supporting the mother and newborn through counselling and helping her seek medical support for herself and her child should the need arise. PNC was reported to have increased after the introduction of the Yashodas who made a difference by undertaking simple tasks such as making the mother more comfortable after delivery, especially for those who underwent caesarean section deliveries, providing information on nutrition for the new mother and advice on family planning (Interview: Pradeep Choudhry 2011). The young mothers reported an increase in their awareness of newborn care on issues such as cord care, breastfeeding, preventing hypothermia and identifying symptoms of distress/illness in

Figure 7.2
PNC Check-up Indicators

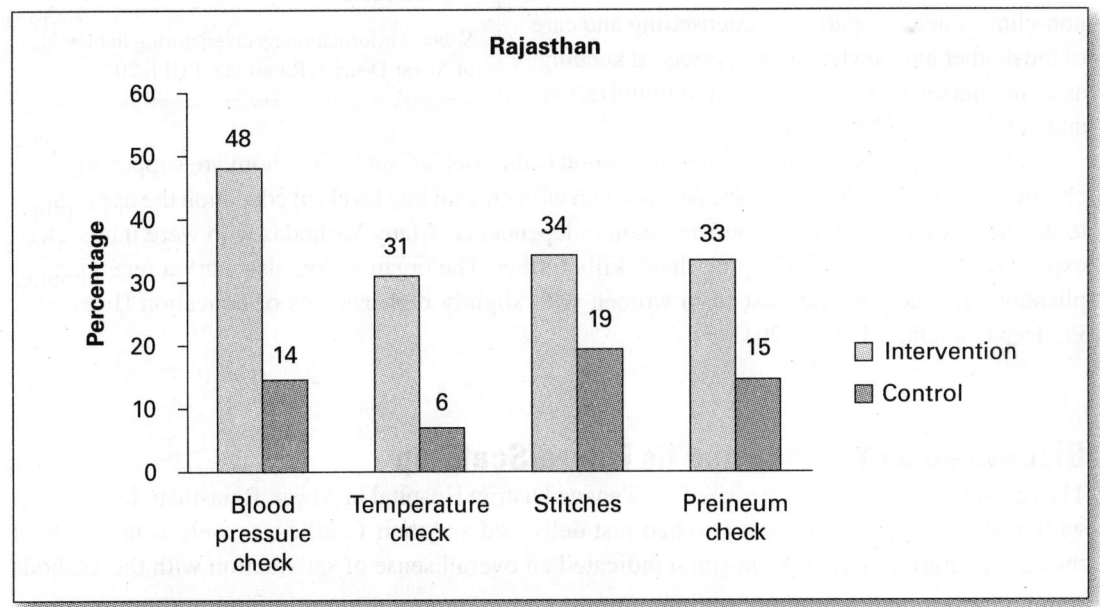

Source: Presentation on Assessing and Supporting NIPI Interventions (ASNI) PHFI, University of Oslo and the Royal Norwegian Embassy.

the newborn, after information sharing by the Yashodas. For a woman in labour, the Yashoda can provide important psychological comfort in an unfamiliar setting.

Studies on the impact of the Yashoda Programme indicated improvements in two important aspects of newborn care in the intervention districts, immunization and initiation of breastfeeding (see Box 7.2). The improvement in immunization, however, was also seen in the control districts, probably due to the impact of the NRHM. Ninety percent of the mothers in both the intervention and control districts reported initiation of breastfeeding, keeping baby warm and immunized. Immunization at the Alwar District Hospital went up to 90% (BCG and oral polio vaccine [OPV]). The impact of the Yashodas on breastfeeding was more evident as 76% of women initiated breastfeeding five hours after delivering through caesarean section in the intervention areas, compared to 44% in the control areas.

The Assessing and Supporting NIPI Interventions study (ASNI) also reports improved newborn indicators (counselling and practice) in the intervention areas where both the Yashoda and the ASHA worker were present. For example, mothers in Alwar were almost four times more likely to have received counselling on keeping babies warm compared to mothers in the control district. Birth registration was also 2.5 times higher in the intervention district (PHFI 2011).

Interviews with nurses and hospital staff indicate that the introduction of the Yashodas provided them much needed support, crucial as the numbers of institutional deliveries increase. Yashodas ease the workload of the hospital staff by assisting with non-clinical duties (apart from counselling and care of the mother and newborn) such as record keeping, assisting nurses in the labour room, immunizations and helping with PNC care.

> **Box 7.2: Impact of Yashoda Programme**
>
> - Breastfeeding Intervention: 76% women initiated breastfeeding five hours after delivery through caesarean section as compared to 44% in control areas.
> - Better information on PNC, newborn care (cord care, breastfeeding, keeping babies warm, looking for signs of distress in newborn).
> - 90% immunization (BCG and OPV) in Alwar District.
> - Additional support to nursing staff in non-clinical care.
>
> *Source:* Information received during field work in Alwar District, Rajasthan, PHFI, 2011.

There has also been an impact on the Yashodas themselves, many of whom are supporting their children and families. The programme has given women with low levels of education the opportunity to develop skills, earn a livelihood and gain independence. Many Yashodas who were interviewed expressed an interest in developing their skills further. The organization also started receiving applications for the Yashoda post from women with slightly higher levels of education (Interview: Pradeep Choudhry, 17 June 2011).[2]

Discussion on Yashoda and Its Future/Scale-up

The research and filming team visited the Zanana District Hospital in Alwar, Rajasthan. Interactions with Yashodas, nurses, women who had just delivered and their families, as well as members of the administrative staff at the hospital indicated an overall sense of satisfaction with the Yashoda

[2]Interview with Pradeep Choudhry, State Programme Officer, NIPI–UNOPS held on 17 June 2011 at the Zanana District Hospital, Alwar, Rajasthan. © PHFI, 2011.

Programme, while also acknowledging the gaps and challenges present in the programme. This section outlines some of the challenges and discusses issues of scale-up in the context of the benefits and drawbacks of the Yashoda Programme.

Challenges

The Yashoda Programme has clearly contributed towards improving information dissemination and awareness generation amongst new mothers in the intervention areas. Data shows improvement in immunization levels, weighing of newborns and PNC. Staff members of the health facility interviewed during field visits also acknowledge the support received by them as a result of the implementation of the Yashoda Programme—especially in the counselling of new mothers and keeping track of PNC indicators such as blood pressure and temperature, weighing of baby and initiating breastfeeding. The Yashoda's role was also found to ease record keeping and housekeeping duties of the nursing staff. However, the programme presents its own set of challenges.

1. **Integration:** Integrating the Yashoda worker within the existing human resources structure of health care facilities without the Yashoda challenging the role of the nurses was one of the first challenges of the programme. Initial problems faced by the Yashoda included not having a space for her to sit in the ward or keep her belongings while on duty. This was tackled at various levels:
   - **Role:** Clearly defining the role of the Yashoda. Restricting her role to that of a non-clinical nature, thereby ensuring that the role of the Yashoda was distinct from that of a trained nurse.
   - **Remuneration:** Imposing an upper limit on the honorarium that the volunteer Yashoda would earn per month. This way she would not earn more than her nursing colleagues who would have typically invested more time and money in their education and training.

2. **Challenges from the Yashodas' Perspective**
   - **Role:** Restricting the role of a Yashoda might help integrating her more easily with the nursing staff, but over time a person who has had exposure to such a programme, would like to develop her education and work skills and grow in her career. The Yashodas expressed a desire for skill-building and additional capacity building to expand the scope of their work.
   - **Capacity Building:** Additional skill building of a Yashoda would also help institutions use this cadre more efficiently within their systems.
   - **Remuneration:** If there are fewer than expected births in a particular month, the amount a Yashoda earns in that month leads to very low levels of income, making livelihood especially difficult for those who are widowed and/or have children to support.

3. **Challenges for the Programme**
   - Funds for sustaining the programme in the long term: who will pay the Yashoda worker on a long-term basis?
   - How does the Yashoda worker complement and enhance the newer cadres of health workers that have been brought in under the NRHM?
   - Increased training capacity for skill building of new and older generations of Yashoda workers for more effective utilization of the Yashoda's role.

Scale-up

The Yashoda Programme is part of the Norway India Partnership Initiative's larger Continuum of Care approach towards maternal and child health. Along with the this programme, UNOPS–NIPI also supports the state governments to run home-based newborn care programmes in Rajasthan, Bihar and Odisha, which provide a more comprehensive frame within which to initiate interventions on counselling, awareness and services on basic maternal and newborn care.

The programme in Rajasthan was initiated with pilot interventions in three districts. Within a year, the government expanded the implementation of the Yashoda Programme in all the districts of Rajasthan with the continuing support of UNOPS–NIPI.

The need for careful preparations for scale-up and sustainability of a programme such as this is acknowledged. The need for adequate training and supervisory mechanisms to ensure effective replication and quality of services was emphasized during our interactions with the UNOPS–NIPI team (Interview: Kaliprasad Pappu, PHFI, 2011).[3] Long-term growth and career plans of a Yashoda worker to keep her motivated, dedicated and efficient, as well as the finances required for the incentives would need a long-term financial commitment. A commitment would also be required to support the administrative expenses and training and recruitment needs of a large-scale programme of this nature.

After demonstrated success, complete ownership by the government and its willingness to support the Yashoda Programme is crucial. Thus, sustainability of the programme and scaling-up the Yashoda concept would depend on the impact of the programme and the subsequent support by the government partners.

'The process of scaling-up (of programmes) requires very careful preparation and the need (for the Yashoda Programme) is very obvious to the states those who have implemented it in three districts… There is a need to look at them (Yashodas) as a cadre and see to where it would be going in a few years' time. We are working trying to understand from the system what the different possibilities are (for scale up). It's good to have this career progression in mind but this we are firming up from within the health system because it's basically the health system (which will absorb the Yashoda). Everyone feels the need for a kind of career progression.'

Source: Dr Kaliprasad Pappu, Director Programmes, NIPI (in-person interview, PHFI 2011, New Delhi).

References

Public Health Foundation of India (PHFI) and Centre for Development and the Environment Institute of Health and Society. 2011. 'Assessing and Supporting NIPI Interventions'. Public Health Foundation of India and Centre for Development and the Environment Institute of Health and Society. University of Oslo, Norway.

Government of India (GoI). 2012. First Annual Report on Health. Ministry of Health and Family Welfare, GoI.

National Health Systems Resource Centre (NHSRC). 2011. Programme Evaluation of the Janani Suraksha Yojna. New Delhi. Available at http://nhsrcindia.org/pdf_files/resources_thematic/Public_Health_Planning/NHSRC_Contribution/Programme_Evaluation_of_Janani_Suraksha_Yojana_-Sep2011.pdf, accessed on 5 August 2013.

Ramani, S. 2010. Notes Parallel Session II. Paper presented at Maternal Health Task Force Conference. New Delhi. 31 August.

Suggested Reading

NIPI. 2010. Operational Guidelines for Yashoda/Mamata: An Enabling Intervention for Quality Maternal and Newborn Care at the Facility Level. Available at http://www.nipi.org.in/Items/Resources_ManualsAndGuidelines_YashodaOperationalGuidelines_New.pdf, accessed on 6 August 2013.

[3]In-person interview with Dr Kaliprasad Pappu at New Delhi. © PHFI, 2011.

Quality Initiatives in Health Care Services

8. Quality Assurance Programmes (QAPs) in Public Health Facilities

8

Quality Assurance Programmes (QAPs) in Public Health Facilities

Sanghita Bhattacharya and Radhika Arora

Quality Assurance Programmes (QAPs) address different aspects of how quality of care can be embedded into the health system. In the context of maternal and newborn care, the issue of quality is particularly important as the enormous increase in institutional deliveries due to the Janani Suraksha Yojna (JSY) scheme and other initiatives by the government, has resulted in overcrowding and compromised quality of care. The potential gains, in terms of lives saved for mothers and babies by providing quality of care during pregnancy and delivery, are enormous. Across less-developed countries, an estimated half of all maternal deaths could be prevented with 95% coverage of quality facility births, around 150,000 women saved each year and for newborns, just over one-third of all neonatal deaths could be avoided (WHO, UNICEF, UNFPA and The World Bank 2007).

> Quality means clinical effectiveness, safety, and a good experience for the patient. (Godlee 2009)

> Quality…. Doing the right thing, at the right time, in the right way, for the right person, and having the best possible results.

> (Institute of Medicine 2001)

With rapid expansion in access to maternal care and institutional deliveries under the Reproductive and Child Health Programme Phase II (RCH-II), especially due to JSY, the conditional cash transfer (CCT) scheme for institutional deliveries implemented since 2005, institutional deliveries in India have increased from 40.7% in 2005–06 to 72.9% in 2009–10 (UNICEF 2009). The scale and rapid rate of uptake of institutional births has, however, brought a number of challenges to the public health sector. The high demand for care at selected hospitals has resulted in massive overcrowding and an inevitable decline in the quality of care that women receive. The most serious consequence is the avoidable mortality of mothers and newborn babies, which undermines the goals of RCH-II and the National Rural Health Mission (NRHM). Moreover, poor quality may act as an obstacle to further increases in institutional births as women and communities recognize the shortfall in safe and respectful care, thus preventing the Government of India from achieving universal coverage.

Institutional births have gone up due to JSY as people from remote areas are also coming to the facility, so it is very important for us to ensure that the newborn and mother are well taken care of ... [T]his we can do by improving the quality of the services. (Interview with Medical Officer, District Hospital, West Bengal, PHFI, 2001)

What Is Quality of Care in Health?

As per the quality of care framework, Tables 8.1 and 8.2 highlight the key areas in which the quality improvement process can be undertaken (detailed concept note on Quality of Care is provided in Appendix 1).

Table 8.1

Elements of Quality of Care

Structure	Description
1. Physical Resources	The resources required to enable the provision of quality care **infrastructure, equipment, drugs and supplies**.
2. Human Resources	Care provided by appropriately **trained and supervised** providers; numbers of staff **adequate** to meet the demand for care.
Process	
3. Competent and Efficient Care	Care consistent with scientific knowledge, internationally recognized **good practice**. Care is **safe** (**clean** birth practices, avoidance of iatrogenic harm); **timely** and **responsive** (respectful, promoting autonomy, equitable). Care documented adequately.
Outcome	
4. Clinical Effectiveness	Good clinical **outcomes** achieved (e.g., mortality reduction)
5. Satisfaction with Care	Patient/provider satisfaction high.

Source: Based on Donabedian (1966; 1997), Hulton et al. (2000) and Institute of Medicine (1990).

Table 8.2

Aspects of Quality Improvement

	Aspects of Quality Improvement
Equity	Services are provided to all people who require them.
Accessibility	Ready access to services is provided.
Acceptability	Care meets the expectations of the people who use the services.
Appropriateness	Required care is provided and unnecessary or harmful care is avoided.
Comprehensiveness	Care provision covers all aspects of disease management from prevention to remediation psycho-social aspects of care are considered.
Effectiveness	Care produces positive change in the health status or quality of life of the patient.
Efficiency	High-quality care is provided at the lowest possible cost.

Source: World Health Organization (2000).

Quality Assurance Programme under National Rural Health Mission

Quality assessment is an integral part of the NRHM. In order to establish and institutionalize quality assurance and improvement in RCH services, district quality assurance cells (DQACs) are being set-up. The Family Planning Division of the Ministry of Health and Family Welfare (MoHFW), Government of India has formalized quality assurance cells (QAC) and by now all the states in the country have constituted a state and district quality assurance committee.

In October 2005, a working group on quality assurance (QA) in RCH-II was set-up, consisting of programme divisions and development partners, to design an internal and independent quality monitoring mechanism at the institutional level on a sample basis. The activities were conducted in three phases.

First, an operational manual was developed by United Nations Population Fund (UNFPA) (the identified technical assistance agency) for assessing service quality covering core programmatic elements of maternal health, immunization, family planning services, availability of essential infrastructural facilities and RCH outreach services. The draft tools and the manual were finalized in August 2006 (National Institute of Health and Family Welfare 2008).

Second, the QA process was piloted in six states (Assam, West Bengal Karnataka, Maharashtra, Uttar Pradesh and Uttaranchal—one district each in five states and two districts in Uttar Pradesh) with technical as well as financial support from development partners, continued support of research agencies and participation from medical colleges. The reports of the state quality assessments carried out on sample facilities by the designated field agencies were shared with the respective district QA units. After incorporating their recommendations, the reports were shared with the District Health Societies to initiate action on recommendations with support and oversight by each State Mission Director (National Institute of Health and Family Welfare 2008).

Third, pilot activities were scaled-up to cover the entire state. Elements for which quality is assessed include access to services, equipment and supplies, professional standards, technical competence and continuity of care. With respect to safe motherhood and newborn care, aspects assessed include facility infrastructure, transport arrangements, communications, equipment functionality, service equipment, supplies inventory, staff training and knowledge/skills and availability of protocols (National Institute of Health and Family Welfare 2008). The QA procedure involves a series of visits to health facilities by the district quality assurance group (QAG), a team of three district-level health officials. This team uses QA checklists to review the readiness of the facility to offer services and the measures the quality of services provided. The QAG team then communicates the gaps in readiness or quality identified by them to the medical officer in charge and suggests actions for improvement, before leaving the facility. Follow-up visits are made to the facility every four months, during which progress in addressing the gaps identified previously is assessed. The QA checklists provide easy procedures to

> **Benefit of QAP**
>
> 'If you have a QAP in a hospital, the efficacy of treatment in the hospital improves and so does the efficiency of the utilization of the different assets such as infrastructure, manpower and equipment. Quality does not come along with a lot of expenditure; it only requires a lot of motivation from the staff right from the top to the bottom levels, including the state level and the district level. It is doable and government or public institutions should be motivated enough to be able to take up this challenge and do it.'
>
> *Source:* Senior Official, Department of Health, Government of West Bengal.

Figure 8.1
Accreditation Oriented Quality Improvement Framework in India

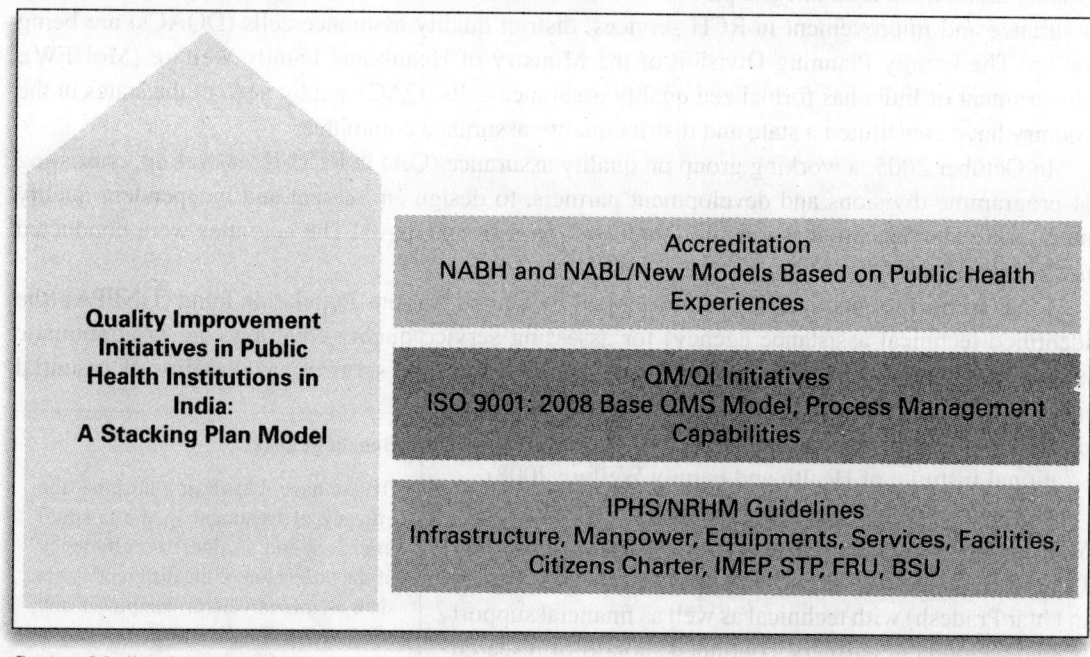

Source: Medica Synergy (2010).

provide an aggregated score for each individual facility with respect to input (readiness), process (how the service is delivered) and outcome (performance) (Khan et al. 2008).

NRHM follows a step-wise approach in attaining quality standards and Figure 8.1 represents that approach.

STEP I

The Indian Public Health Standards (IPHS), one of the core strategies of NRHM, lay down the minimum norms for services to be provided and the infrastructure and human resources that each facility should have in place. IPHS are based on the recommendations of the task group under the Director General of Health Services which was set-up for the purpose. The standards presently developed are for: (a) primary level health facilities, i.e., subcentres (SCs) and primary health centres (PHCs) and (b) secondary level health facilities, i.e., community health centres (CHCs) constituting the first referral units (FRUs) and district hospitals (DHs). They prescribe minimum standards, less resource intensive than those used for larger institutions and easily applicable in rural/resource poor settings. IPHS provide a yardstick to measure the services being provided in the public health facilities. With these standards, it will be possible to objectively grade the different facilities and take up remedial action accordingly. IPHS is a novel concept to fix benchmarks of infrastructure including buildings, manpower, equipment, drugs, and quality assurance through the introduction of treatment protocols.

The IPHS guidelines pertain to:

1. Services to be assured at each level.
2. Human resources structure with essential qualifications for each post.
3. List of essential drugs, kits and other equipment.
4. Accountability mechanisms including participatory management structures (such as patient welfare committees, their constitution and functions).
5. Quality assurance in service delivery (cleanliness, hygiene, blood storage, waste management).
6. Physical infrastructure—location of the centre, building layout.
7. Display of charter of patient rights.
8. Quality control (internal and external monitoring instruments).
9. Record maintenance.

NRHM provides concrete service guarantees including skilled attendance at all births, emergency obstetric care and basic newborn care. At all health centres it is mandatory to display (a) agreed service guarantees and details of human and financial resources at the facility, (b) a Charter of Citizen's Health Rights highlighting the services to be given to the citizens and their rights in that regard and (c) outcomes of various monitoring mechanisms in simple language for widespread understanding. IPHS, Citizen's Charter of Health Rights and PHC/block health plans are intended to serve as monitoring yardsticks of health facilities at the PHC/block levels (Government of India, Ministry of Health and Family Welfare 2005).

STEP II

Quality management systems (QMS) certificate by Bureau of Indian Standards (BIS), BIS is the official national government body for standardization and accreditation of products and systems, originally catering to industrial goods and processes. In recent years, growing focus on management systems has spurred BIS to develop accreditation norms for quality management systems. Currently, BIS provides International Organization for Standardization (ISO) certification in quality management systems to health centres. The Indian Standard (IS) 15551:2003 provides guidelines for process improvements in health service organizations, while the IS 15784:2007 certificate was developed by BIS for health care facilities which follow a sound management system, adhere to medical ethics and provide quality health care services to consumers in a transparent manner. The IS defines the requirements from secondary and tertiary level health care facilities, speciality and super-speciality hospitals. It was formulated to regulate the mushrooming of substandard hospitals and nursing homes playing with the health of consumers. This standard covers areas such as access to facilities, assessment and continuity of care, patients' rights and education, care of patients, management of medication, hospital infection control, continuous quality improvement and responsibility of the management, etc. The process of applying for an IS certificate involves first setting-up a documented quality management system in the facility and then applying for the certificate. The facility is then subjected to a series of audits on various aspects of quality management. Corrective actions need to be taken and verified on the audit observations. The certificate is granted when all systems have been put in place as per the standard. ISO facilities are subject to periodic audits by BIS to ensure maintenance of quality processes as per standards (BIS 2010).

STEP III

National Aaccreditation Board for Hospitals and Health Care Providers

The National Accreditation Board for Hospitals and Health Care Providers (NABH) was set-up in 2005 as a constituent board of the Quality Council of India (QCI).[1] It was set-up to establish and operate an accreditation programme for health care organizations. It is also an institutional member of the International Society for Quality in Health Care (ISQua).[2] NABH works as an autonomous body and offers accreditation for hospitals, blood banks, medical testing labs, small health centres, centres of other systems of medicine (Ayurveda, Yunani, Unani, Siddha and Homeopathy—collectively known as AYUSH), wellness centres, etc., (NABH 2009).

The NABH is structured to include an accreditation committee for recommending or denying grant of accreditation, changing the scope of accreditation or launching new initiatives; a technical committee responsible for drafting and periodically reviewing accreditation standards and guidelines; an appeals committee deals with hearing appeals made against adverse decisions by applicants. It has a panel of assessors and experts for conducting facility assessments on compliance with accreditation standards. NABH also conducts training of health administration officials in implementing quality management systems in their institutions and undertaking quality improvement measures in order to obtain accreditation certification (NABH 2009).

NABH standards for hospitals have 10 chapters incorporating 100 standards and 514 objective elements. These include patient care, management of medication, hospital infection control, continuous quality improvement, facility management and safety, human resources and information management systems. Health care institutions must attain the relevant standards before applying for accreditation. Subsequently, NABH makes a series of assessment visits to the facility and recommends corrective action as required. The final assessment report (by independent assessors) determines the grant of the accreditation certificate to the institution. The certification is for three years, with one surveillance visit during the period. Certification can be renewed on the basis of reassessment reports on request from the certified institutions (NABH 2009).

[1] QCI was set up in 1997 as an autonomous body by the Government of India jointly with the Indian industry (represented by industrial associations on the QCI Board) to establish and operate the National Accreditation Structure for conformity assessment bodies.

[2] International Society for Quality in Health Care (ISQua) is an international body which grants approval to accreditation bodies in the area of health care as mark of equivalence of accreditation programme of member countries.

Quality Assessment Programme under the National Health Systems Resource Centre

The National Health Systems Resource Centre (NHSRC) was set-up to serve as an apex body for technical assistance, dissemination and for functioning as a centre of excellence for facilitating the centre and the states in the quality assessment programme (QAP). Its specific objectives include developing capacities in a network of institutions and individuals to improve the efficiency, effectiveness and quality of health systems through interventions at the national, state, district and sub-district level and facilitating the process of developing decentralized and accountable service delivery systems with community ownership and public participation in governance mechanisms (NHSRC 2010).

Quality improvement is one of the seven thematic areas of NHSRC's functioning. NHSRC explicitly states, 'Availability of health services and the necessary inputs does not directly equate to improved utilization, unless efforts are made to improve the quality and comprehensiveness of the services provided at the public establishments across the country.' One thrust area of NHSRC's work is on improving the quality of health care facilities leading to a system of accreditation within the public health system which could be linked to flexible financing to meet and maintain these standards (NHSRC 2010).

Based on the international standard (ISO 9001:2008), NHSRC initiated a programme to bring health facilities (district hospitals) up to the required standards for certification and piloted this model programme in eight states, Uttaranchal, Rajasthan, Uttar Pradesh, Madhya Pradesh, Chhattisgarh, Bihar, Jharkhand and Odisha, in 2007–08.

The objectives of the programme were (see Figure 8.2):

Figure 8.2
Steps of QAP Project

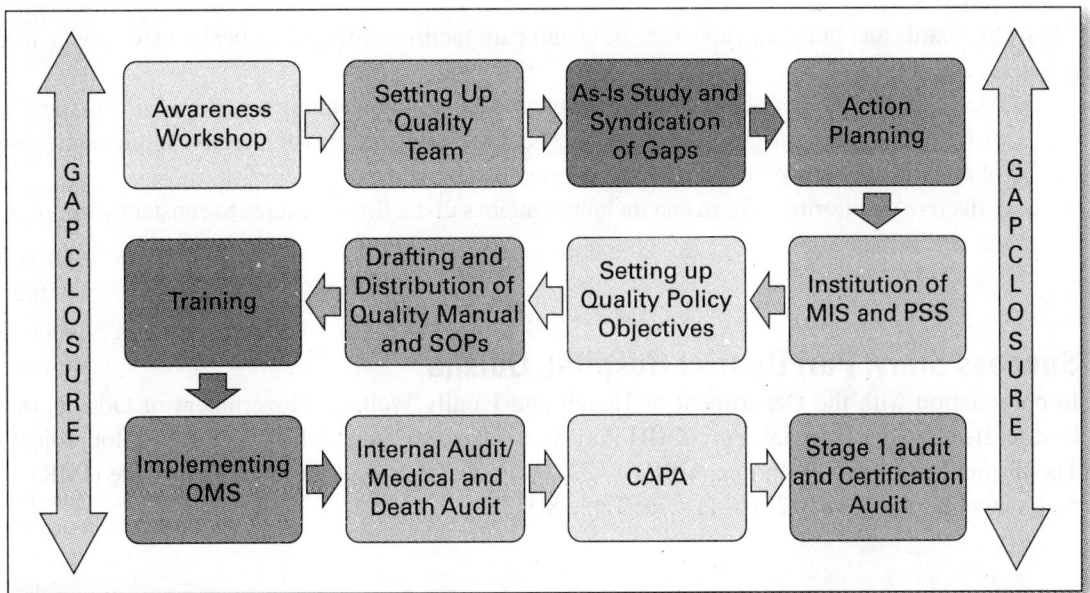

Source: Medica Synergy (2010).

1. Helping in identifying existing gaps and their root causes and formulating strategies and action plans to bridge these identified gaps.
2. Developing a methodology of quality improvement applicable to particular health facilities, based on rational utilization of available funds and participatory management structures, to reach the desired standards. Such a methodology should also factor in patient perception, equity and access and identify measures to monitor them.
3. Facilitating the improvement of systems and processes of service delivery in the health care facilities to meet the stipulated standards.
4. Handholding the health care facility by the provision of competent personnel, aimed at the achievement of prevailing ISO 9001 standards and also making efforts for continual improvement.
5. Developing process documents including a quality manual, work instructions and protocols which are required to achieve improvement in health care delivery and ISO certification.
6. Assisting the facility in its internal audit process, carrying out corrective and preventive action, conducting customer perception surveys/employee satisfaction surveys and facilitating development of action plans, etc.

The QAP led to the development of:

1. Quality manuals, procedures and work instructions to institute quality improvement and maintenance processes.
2. Standard treatment protocols (STPs) for ensuring delivery of uniform and standardized services.
3. Benchmarks based on local needs and sensitivities, focussed at improving the quality of services.
4. Standards and building capacities of health care facilities for quality health care service delivery.
5. Mechanisms for interfacing with the hospital management committees (*Rogi Kalyan Samitis* [RKS]), hospital managers and the district health administration for effective implementation of documented processes for quality improvement.
6. Effective monitoring system that includes patient satisfaction measures to constantly improve on performance.

Success Story: Puri District Hospital, Odisha

In consultation with the Department of Health and Family Welfare, Government of Odisha, the District Headquarter Hospital, Puri (DHH Puri) was selected as one of the sites for the pilot project. The district has a crude birth rate (CBR) 17.5/1,000 population and infant mortality rate (IMR) is 80 (Annual Health Survey 2010–11) (see Table 8.3).[3]

[3]http://www.censusindia.gov.in/vital_statistics/AHSBulletins/AHS_Baseline_Factsheets/Odisha1.pdf, accessed in January 2012.

Table 8.3

Profile of Health Facilities in Puri District

Type of Institutions	Number
District Hospital	1
District Post-partum Centre	2
Community Health Centres	7
Primary Health Centres (Upgraded)	2
Primary Health Centres (BPHCs)	3
Primary Health Centres (PHCs[N])	40
First Referral Unit (FRU)	3
Rural Family Welfare Centre	11
Urban Family Welfare Centre	1
No. of Post-partum Centre	2
Mobile Health Units (MHU)	6
No. of Subcentres	221

Source: Medica Synergy (2010).

The Puri District Hospital has a capacity of 260 beds and caters to a population of 1,697,983 (Census 2011). This hospital functions as a secondary-level referral centre for the public health institutions below the district level, such as subdivisional hospitals, CHCs, PHCs and SCs (see Table 8.3).

NHSRC, along with the technical support agency (TSA), undertook the QAP programme here. Medica Synergy Pvt. Ltd, a health care services and consultancy firm headquartered in Kolkata was appointed as the TSA for the state of Odisha and throughout the implementation of the programme, a technical assistant from the firm was placed at the hospital.

The primary objectives of the pilot were:

1. Attaining the IPHS in terms of services delivered with available inputs.
2. Attaining IPHS in terms of infrastructure, manpower, equipment and supplies within availability of resources and prevailing governance constraints.
3. Developing process documents including a quality manual, work instructions and protocols adequate to achieve ISO certification.
4. Keeping focus on requirements for NABH certification/accreditation standards while developing the processes and the system for certification to ISO 9001 standards.

The following section describes the various steps that were taken by NHSRC to ensure quality:

1. **As-is Process**: Conduct a detailed organizational audit of the structure and process of delivery care at the facility. This involved a survey which reviewed manpower, equipment, infrastructure, processes including training and capacity building activities, services and facilities provided, along with legal compliance. This also included all support processes including nursing, housekeeping and laundry services, etc.

2. **Mapping the to-be Processes and Gap Filling**: To develop 'to-be' process, identifying and incorporating the existing gaps based on the survey and work on developing recommendations to overcome these gaps. This involved:

- Development of documents including a quality manual, procedures and work instructions to institute processes, maintain and improve the functions.
- Development of a handy broad framework of standard treatment protocols for ensuring delivery of uniform and standardized services.
- Development of benchmarks, based on local needs and sensitivities, focussed at improving the quality of services provided.
- Development of an effective management information system to elicit actionable feedback.
- Building the capacity of the respective health care facilities for service delivery. This includes basic orientation and training to hospital managers or the resource group meant to help this process and providing capacity building training to the existing staff at the health care facilities. It also includes active handholding and guidance as they test out and put new processes into place.
- Orienting RKS about their roles in quality improvement of health care facilities and how to budget for needs and how to raise and utilize resources.

3. **Implementation**: Facilitate the process of implementation.

- To liaison with the RKS, hospital managers and district health administration for effective implementation of documented processes.
- To handhold the health care facility for achievement of the prevailing ISO 9001 standards.

4. **Auditing and Certification**: Coordinating with ISO authorities, getting the district health facility audited and enabling the facility to get certified.

Implementation Process
Table 8.4 details the implementation process that was followed at Puri District Hospital.

Table 8.4
Reports for Implementation of the QAP in Puri District Hospital

Process	Activity
Phase 1	
1. Kick off meeting at the state level	• Key in demonstrating the commitment of the state to the process.
2. Kick off meeting at the hospital level	• Introduction to technical assistance agencies and initial buy–in of the key operational team of the facility.
3. Gap analysis study/As-is mapping	• Facility and process assessment and mapping at each department.
4. Capacity building of all staff members on ISO 9001 and key QI principles	• Capacity building of hospital staff.

(Table 8.4 Continued)

(Table 8.4 Continued)

Process	Activity
4. Gap analysis/process mapping dissemination meetings with the various departments/functional areas	• Creating awareness about the various lacunae existing in their areas and creating buy-in for the suggested improvement measures.
Phase 2	
1. Development of to-be process	• Standardized Manuals and Protocols 1. Hospital operations manual (details in Annexure 2). 2. Quality manual, SOPs/STPs for better functioning and service delivery. 3. Quality management handbook
2. Two-three rounds of dissemination workshops with each department/ functional area	• Increasing the understanding of staff on new processes. Also, acts as a key forum for incorporating suggestions and changes recommended by team in order to increase the ownership of the documents.
3. Capacity building sessions	• Increasing capacity building on allied areas. 　◦ Biomedical Waste Management 　◦ Infection Control 　◦ Materials Management 　◦ Customer/Patient Interfacing 　◦ Medical Records Maintenance 　◦ Equipment Management 　◦ Health and Safety 　◦ Fire Fighting 　◦ Disaster and Emergency Management 　◦ RKS—Role in Quality Management
Phase 3	
Internal auditors training	• Creation of a cadre of staff with capability to audit the quality management system (QMS).
Internal audits	• Developing a system of internal audits as a process and system monitoring mechanism.
Management review meetings	• Developing an apex process forum for review of the processes and the quality management system. • Developing suitable corrective and preventive action for continual improvement and overall monitoring of the achievement of quality policy and objectives of the hospital.
External audit (certification and surveillance)	• Development of a process for external checks and validations of the established QMS.

Source: Medica Synergy (2010).

Effect of the Quality Assurance Programme at the Puri District Hospital

Over time, there have been manifold improvements and upgradation in the quality of services being provided at the hospital. The Outpatient Department (OPD) patient turnover showed a steep increase; there has been an increase of 8,936 patients (4%) in the year 2007–08 and 30,597 (13%)

in the year 2008–09, resulting in an overall increase of 39,533 (17.2%) patients in the last two years (see Figure 8.3). The in-patient department (IPD) has seen an increase from 25,119 in 2007–08 to 37,456 in 2008–09, a jump of 49% (see Figure 8.4). This is primarily due to improvements in terms of expansion of infrastructure, manpower and the delivery process in the hospital, based on the QMSs.

However, the manpower status of the hospital shows there has not been a significant increase in manpower, in line with the increase in patient load.

Considering the non-availability of major surgery and super-speciality services at the hospital, the average length of stay (ALOS) is four days. The bed occupancy rate of the hospital is more than 100% and the average bed occupancy rate of the hospital is 121%.

As per the Patients' Satisfaction Survey Report for OPD patients, it is found that the Satisfaction Index for patients has increased remarkably by 20%. Similarly, the Satisfaction Index of the hospital employees improved by 6%, i.e., from 37% to 43%. All this is reflected in an increase in the volume of in-patients, which is attributed to the improved quality of health services. Figures 8.5 and 8.6 show attributes of the Satisfaction Indices for inpatient department (IPD) patients and

Figure 8.3
OPD Patients Turnover

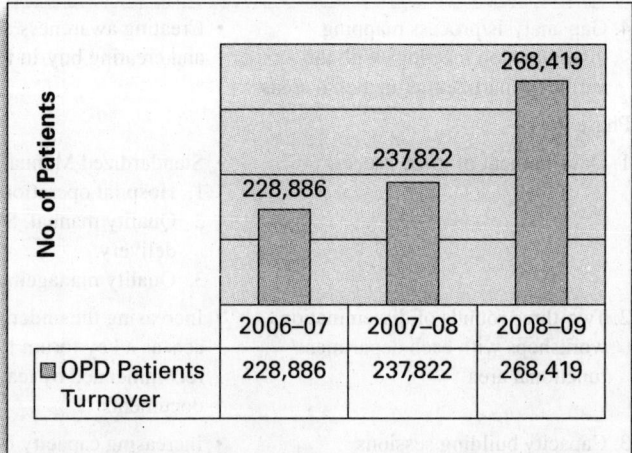

Source: Medica Synergy (2010).

Figure 8.4
IPD Patients Admission

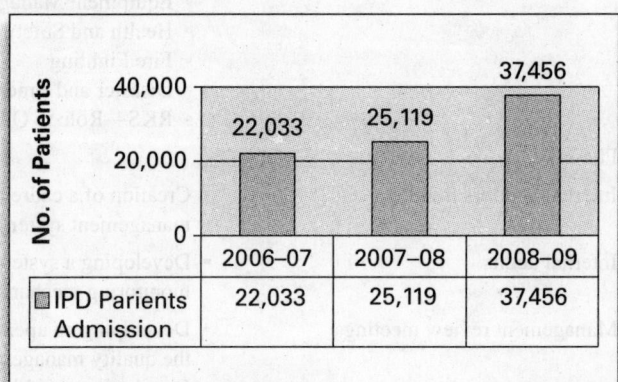

Source: Medica Synergy (2010).

employees. The data compares results from Phase 1, 2008 and Phase 2, 2009.

There was an increase in institutional deliveries due to improvements in infrastructure and manpower (auxiliary nurse midwives (ANMs) and staff nurses), equipment, maintenance of privacy and cleanliness. The hospital also provided essential facilitates in terms of availability of a blood bank, anaesthetist and gynaecologist, which have resulted in an increase in caesarean deliveries (see Figure 8.7).

Maternal deaths have shown a sharp decline, mainly due to the training received by all the staff nurses and ANMs in skilled birth attendance, early detection of complicated cases and improved referral systems.

Figure 8.5

Patient Satisfaction Index

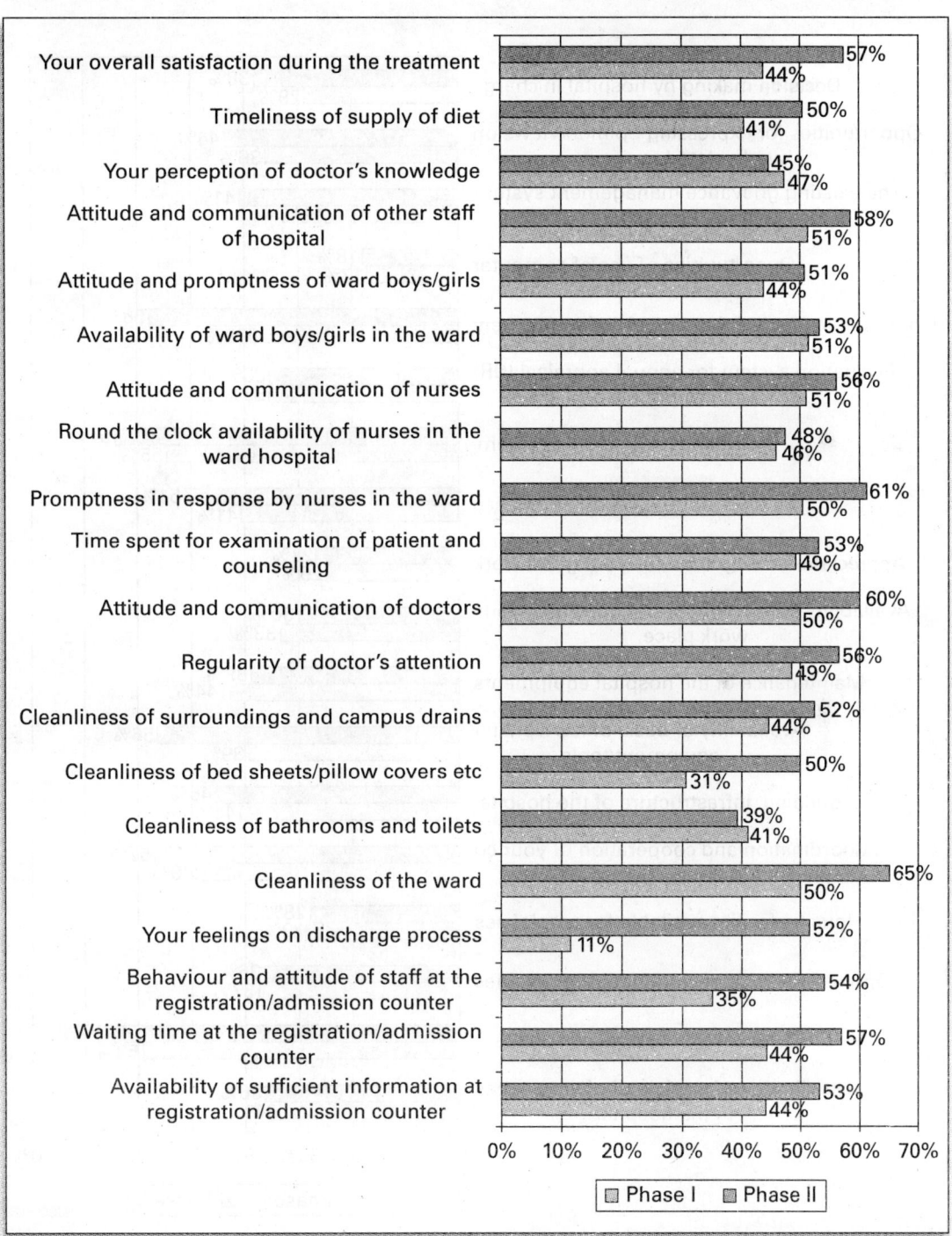

Source: Medica Synergy (2010).

Figure 8.6

Employee Satisfaction Index

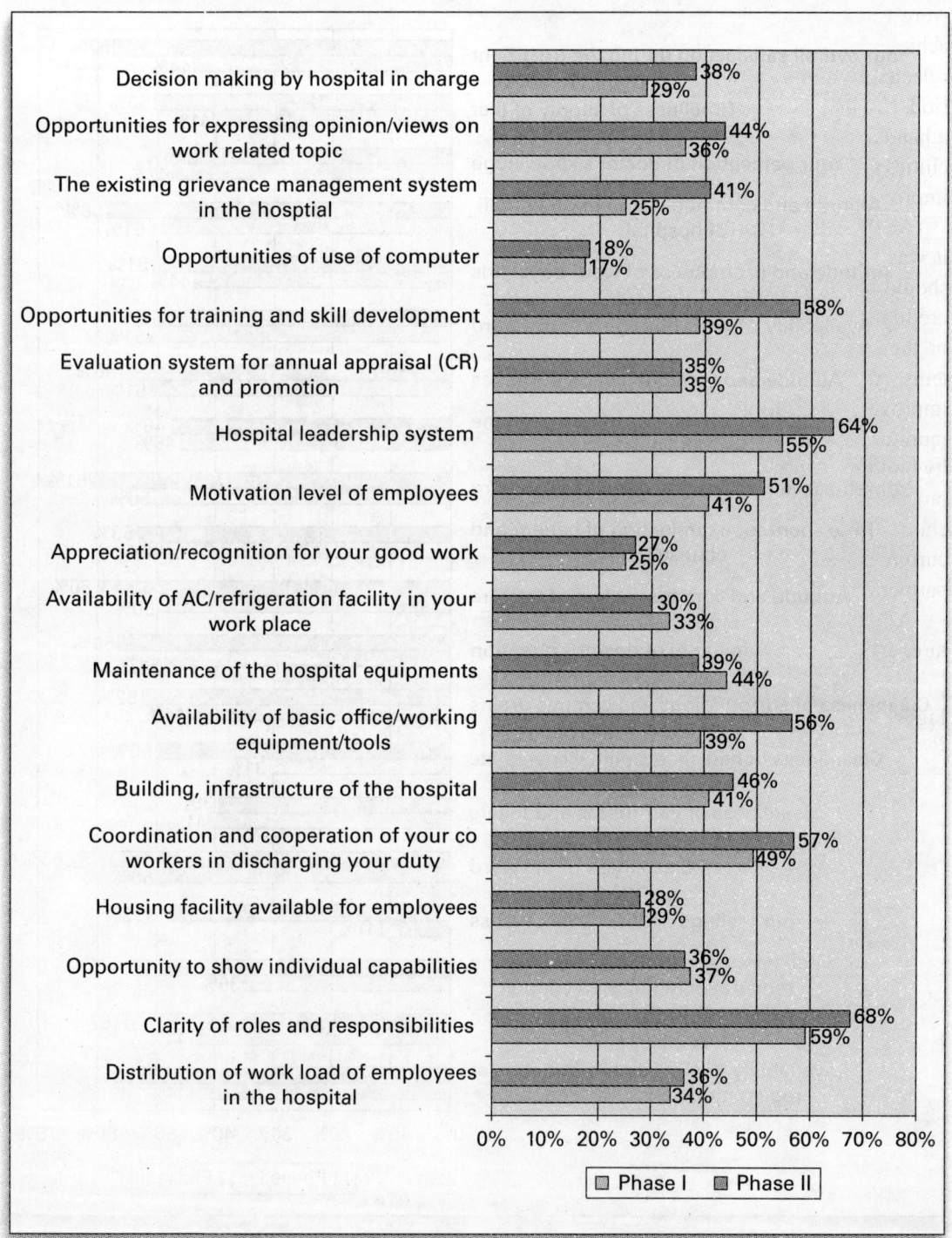

Continuous Quality Improvement

The objectives of the pilot initiatives were to establish a QMS system and achieve ISO 9001 certification for the selected facilities. During the project period, NSHRC extended support through a handholding process in which the facilities focussed on striving for continual improvement.

At the end of the pilot initiatives, it was recommended that the hospital should strive towards the target of accreditation under the existing NABH or the state/national accreditation systems. An accreditation targeted quality improvement (QI) system will bring in a target-oriented approach and will provide milestones to monitor the continual improvement process. One of the key elements of the QI process is the capacity building of hospital staff on the various aspects of quality management and also on key hospital processes and allied areas. However, the continuous improvement process faces the threat of constant churn in the hospital team which takes place due to transfers and retirements. Another problem in current capacity building process is that each of these projects is dependent on technical assistance partners (see Figure 8.8).

A QAP which aims to improve the overall functioning of the health facility in terms of infrastructure, equipment and human resources and ensures that care is provided as per the standard norms,

Figure 8.7

Deliveries (Normal and Caesarean)

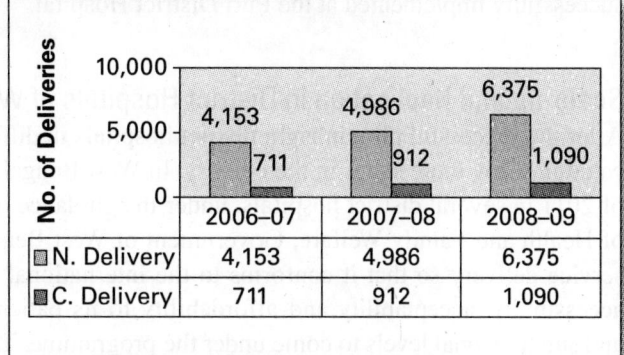

	2006–07	2007–08	2008–09
▣ N. Delivery	4,153	4,986	6,375
▣ C. Delivery	711	912	1,090

Source: Medica Synergy (2010).

Figure 8.8

Total Births versus Maternal Deaths

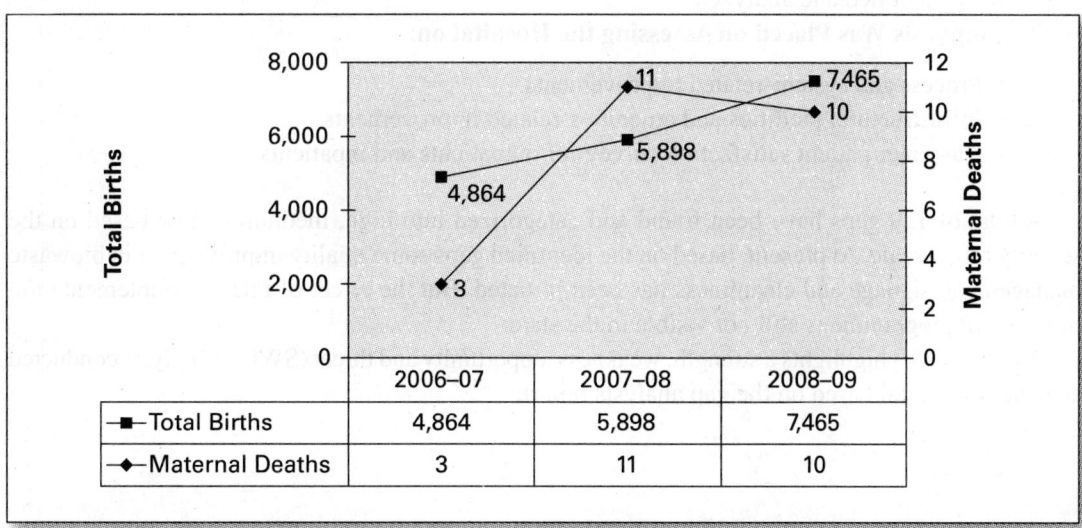

	2006–07	2007–08	2008–09
■ Total Births	4,864	5,898	7,465
◆ Maternal Deaths	3	11	10

Source: Medica Synergy (2010).

if implemented well, can lead to good clinical outcomes (e.g., mortality reduction) and satisfaction with care (e.g., patient and provider satisfaction). This was apparent after the QAP programme was successfully implemented at the Puri District Hospital.

Scale-up and Replication in District Hospitals of West Bengal

After the successful pilot in eight district hospitals in different states in India, the model was replicated in a few more states in the country. In West Bengal, it is being scaled-up since the beginning of 2011 in several district hospitals, under the guidance of the MoHFW/NHSRC. The Department of Health and Family Welfare, Government of West Bengal, in its bid to strengthen the quality of service delivery so that it conforms to the international standard (ISO 9001:2008) and enhances accessibility, acceptability and affordability to its patients, has identified 12 hospitals at district and subdivisional levels to come under the programme. The NHSRC is coordinating and providing technical assistance for this.

The present programme is at the formative phase. Some actions have been initiated, the gap analysis has been conducted and accordingly the action plan is being developed. The following steps have been completed in one of the selected facilities (Bangur Hospital):

> **Interview Byte of a Health Official**
>
> 'When we started, we did not have any accreditation programme, it was just a QAP, now we are aiming for ISO certification. We started with three hospitals, now we are replicating 12 more and we are thinking of scaling-up the programme.'
>
> *Source:* Senior Official, Department of Health, Government of West Bengal.

1. **As-is and Gap Analysis**: The various processes of the hospital were analyzed based on clustering of various services/issues into management, clinical services, support services and cross-departmental issues. The four clusters were further divided into thematic (management and cross departmental issues) and services (clinical and support) groups. Along with the As–is process mapping, key gaps in each area were identified and analyzed.

2. **Emphasis Was Placed on Assessing the Hospital on**:

   • Process and system-related improvements.
   • Infrastructure, facilities and amenities-related improvements.
   • Customer/patient satisfaction survey for outpatients and inpatients.

A total of 129 gaps have been found and categorized into high, medium or low based on the severity rating scale. At present, based on the identified gaps some quality improvement in biowaste management, signage and cleanliness has been initiated. But the effect of Phase 2 implementation of the QAP programme is still not visible in the state.

The Figure 8.9 highlights a strength, weakness, opportunity and threat (SWOT) analysis conducted at Bangur Hospital based on the gap analysis report.

Figure 8.9
SWOT Analysis

STRENGTHS
- Proactive leadership and Competent Staffs
- Model public health facility hospital of the state with most advanced technology
- Having capacity to cater 45,000 IP and 400,000 OP patients with various diagnostics facilities at affordable rates
- Availability and Easy access to local vendors
- Locational advantage for getting sanctioned manpower specially doctors and nurses

OPPORTUNITIES
- Commitment of State Health Department to pump in the required fund for development/improvement of hospital
- Initiation of West Bengal Facilitated Quality Assurance Programme (FQAP) to implement QMS and creation of brand
- Implementation of Health Insurance schemes after ISO Certification
- Implementation of IPHS guidelines that are in line with the need of District Hospitals

WEAKNESS
- Basic needs of patient like toilet facilities, safe drinking water, patient relatives' waiting area are lacking
- Shortages of Manpower and equipments as per the sanctioned bed
- Undecided Vision, Mission and Goals for the hospital and lack of accountability at various functional levels.
- Absence of individual key performance indicators, departmental quality objectives/indicators
- Lack of analysis of operational statistics

CHALLENGES
- Meeting the increasing expectations of the patients with medical advancements
- Shortage of human resource considering the rise of patient load every year (eg. There have been 9% increase in IP patient load without any increase in IP beds)
- After ISO certification, there may be significant increase in patient load with higher expectations
- Less scope for expansion of infrastructure in the available space and old buildings

Source: Medica synergy, 2010, report submitted to National Health System Resource Centre, unpublished.

Annexure 1

Table 8A.1
Key Findings Based on Gap Analysis—Puri District Hospital

Areas Identified for Improvement	Planned Interventions	State-level Support Required
A. Infrastructure, Facilities and Amenities		
1. Casualty facilities—resuscitation area and equipment, emergency crash cart, etc.	The various infrastructure, facility and amenities-related requirements	Funding for improvements through RKS/ mission funds.
2. Amenities for patients at OPD—help desk, waiting chairs, toilets.		
3. Signages at all locations.		

(Table 8A.1 Continued)

(Table 8A.1 Continued)

Areas Identified for Improvement	Planned Interventions	State-level Support Required
4. Clinical Laboratory—space and facilities.	are detailed in the following:	
5. Radiology unit—infrastructure as per requirements.		
6. Stores—facilities and improvement of storage conditions.	– Infrastructure Improvement plan.	
7. Beds/Bed-side lockers in various wards.	– Signage plan and specification.	
8. Paediatric beds/bassinets in paediatric wards.		
9. Toilets in various wards (non-working/broken condition).	Both these reports will also have indicative budgets for implementation.	
10. Operationalizing the recovery area in the operation theatre (OT).		
11. Operationalise the new kitchen building.		
12. Repairing the mortuary cold storage unit.	The reports shall be submitted to state/ district authorities for implementation.	
13. Space and facilities for medical record storage.		
14. Medical equipment needs repairing at various locations.		
15. Proper zoning and space utilization in OT and labour room.		
B. Process/System Improvements		
1. Standard Operating Protocols/Standard Treatment Protocols (SOPs/STPs) for better functioning and service delivery.	NHSRC will provide technical support for: – Development of STPs.	The mission directorate/ RKS required to support the training/capacity building sessions by means of funds for conducting the sessions such as refreshment costs for the participants, cost of producing handouts (photo copying).
2. Effective system for management of outsourced services.		
3. Patient rights—feedback forms, complaints boxes, patient/ citizens charter.	– Development of STPs with guidance of NSHRC.	
4. Mass casualty handling plan.	– Implementation support of protocols through one to one site meetings with various department units.	
5. Waiting time improvement and queuing system at OPD.		
6. Lab quality and safety plan.		
7. Patient and operator safety in radiology unit.		
8. Inventory control system for stores.		
9. Availability of emergency life saving drugs at various wards/ units and their monitoring.	– Training and capacity building sessions on various issues such as BMW, medical documentation, infection control, etc.	
10. Death audits on a monthly basis.		
11. Improving medical documentation system—history and assessment, doctors/nurses notes, temperature, pulse and respiration chart (TPR) Chart, I/O charting, orders sheet, discharge summaries.		
12. Improving infection control—infection control manual, environmental surveillance in OT and labour room, instrument sterilization system in OT.	– Capacity building of RKS. – QMS based on ISO covering objective-oriented planning, internal audits, management review	
13. Effective linen and laundry system.		
14. Improvement of cleaning and sanitation levels.		

(Table 8A.1 Continued)

(Table 8A.1 Continued)

Areas Identified for Improvement	Planned Interventions	State-level Support Required
15. Improving fire safety—firefighting plan, ideal location for extinguishers, firefighting training for all staff members.	process, corrective and preventive actions leading to continuous quality improvement.	
16. Improving biomedical waste management—segregation, timely collection and proper disposal.		
17. Improving equipment management—inventory, preventive maintenance planning and user level checks and verifications.		

Source: Medica Synergy (2010).

Annexure 2

Table 8A.2
Hospital Operation Manuals

Manual Name	Formats
Casualty and Minor Injuries Department	Casualty register
	Medico legal case register
	Brought dead register
	Emergency On-call visits register
	Emergency drugs indent register
	Duty list of casualty medical officers
Ward Management including Admissions and Discharge	Bed head ticket
	Money receipt (for air-conditioning (AC) ward)
	Ward admission and discharge register
	Death register
	Bed vacancy register
	Emergency medical officer (EMO) specialist call register
	Referral register
	Oxygen indent register
	Diet register
	Regular medicine indent register (D/E/N)
	Emergency medicine indent register
	Daily round register
	OT call register
	Day, evening and night instruction register

(Table 8A.2 Continued)

(Table 8A.2 Continued)

Manual Name	Formats
	AC ward advance register (wherever AC wards are available)
	AC ward admission register (wherever AC wards are available)
	AC ward discharge register (wherever AC wards are available)
	Discharge certificate
	Blood bank officer (bbo) call register
	Intake output chart
	Discharge summary
	Discharge against medical advice
	Patient incident form
	Employee incident form
	Blood transfusion flow sheet
	TPR chart
OPD	OPD register (male)
	OPD register (female)
	OPD ticket
	Laboratory investigation requisition-cum-reporting slip
	X-ray requisition slip
	Ultra sonography (USG) requisition slip
	Injection registers
	Anti-rabies vaccination register (new cases)
	Anti-rabies vaccination register (old cases)
	Medico legal case register (male and female)
Operation Theatres and Recovery Rooms	OT booking register
	OT call register
	Operating list
	Consent for procedure, treatment, anaesthesia, high-risk consent
	Fumigation register
	Anaesthesia register
	Surgery register—general surgery
	Surgery register—obstetrics and gynaecology
	Surgery register—orthopaedics
	Narcotics and psychotropic drugs register
	Dead inventory register
	Consent for surgery
	Patient incident form

(Table 8A.2 Continued)

(Table 8A.2 Continued)

Manual Name	Formats
	Employee incident form
	Blood transfusion flow sheet
	High-risk consent
Radiology, Imaging and Other Investigations	Radiology OPD register
	MLC issue register
	Paid issue register
	Unpaid issue register
	USG register
	Electrocardiogram (ECG) register
	Audiometry register
Laboratory Services	Pathology investigations register
	Master list of equipment requiring calibration
	Laboratory calibration schedule
	Laboratory investigation-cum-report format
Blood Bank	Request for blood transfusion
	Donor register/form
	Master blood stock register
	Blood issue register
	Blood cross matching register
	Blood grouping form
	Blood testing register
	Thalassemia patient free blood register
	Blood reaction register
Physical Medicine and Rehabilitation	Daily patient attendance register
Mortuary and Autopsy Services	Information on medico legal cases (MLC)
	Post-mortem information register
	Post-mortem report
Enquiry, Patient Registration and User Fee Collection	Help/information desk register
	Casualty ticket register (paid)
	Casualty ticket register (unpaid/bpl)
	Daily money collection and deposit register
	X-ray Slip
	Electrocardiogram (ECG) Slip
	Pathology OPD and IPD

(Table 8A.2 Continued)

(Table 8A.2 Continued)

Manual Name	Formats
	Dental
	Ear, nose and throat (ENT)
	Ambulance and mortuary van
	Free slip
	IPD slip (also available at pharmacy counter/admission counter)
Stores and Inventory Management	Annual medicine and consumables requirement plan
	Approved drugs and consumables list
	Main stock book
	Date of expiry register
	Local purchase indent format
	Minimum inventory for drugs
	Medicine indent register
	Emergency medicine indent register
	Oxygen issue register
Procurement and Outsourcing Management	Annual medicine and medical consumables requirement plan
	Approved drugs and consumables list
	Main stock book
	Purchase indent
	Minimum inventory for drugs and consumables
	Supplier's evaluation
Hospital Security Management	Security incidents report
	Security attendance register
Training and Development	Competence matrix
	Training attendance sheet
	Post training feedback
	Annual post training evaluation
Ambulance and Transport Services	Ambulance log book
	Ambulance moving order book
	Mortuary van moving order book
Dietary Services	Diet feedback register
	Food quality register
	Diet register
Laundry and Linen Services	Laundry register
Housekeeping	Housekeeping and cleaning schedule
	Housekeeping checklist-cum-report

(Table 8A.2 Continued)

(Table 8A.2 Continued)

Manual Name	Formats
Infrastructure Maintenance `Management	Master list of equipment
	Master list of approved agencies
	Preventive maintenance checklist
	Breakdown servicing register
	Annual civil maintenance checklist and report
	Plumbing maintenance schedule and report
	Master list of fire extinguishers
	Fire extinguisher maintenance card
Biomedical Waste Management	Biomedical waste management plan
	Employee incident form
Document and Data Control	Master list of control formats and manuals
	Master list of external standards
	Internal document distribution and issue acknowledgement sheet
	Document/format change request
Control of Records	Master list of records and retention plan
Control of Non-conforming Hospital Services	Hospital services non-conformity register
Corrective and Preventive Actions Management	Corrective/preventive action log
Internal Quality Audits	List of internal quality auditors
	Audit plan
	Audit checklist
	Non-conformity summary report
Management Review	Minutes of the meeting

Source: Medica Synergy (2010).

References

Bureau of Indian Standards. 2009. Annual Report 2008–09. New Delhi: Bureau of Indian Standards. Available at http://www.bis.org.in/org/AnnualReport0809.pdf.

Census of India. 2011. Registrar General of India. New Delhi: Government of India.

Godlee, F. 2009. 'Effective, Safe and a Good Patient Experience'. *BMJ*, 339: 4346.

Government of India (GoI). 2005. 'National Rural Health Mission—Framework for Implementation'. New Delhi: Ministry of Health and Family Welfare, Government of India.

Institute of Medicine (IOM). 2001. Crossing the Quality Chasm: A New Health System for the 21st Century. Washington, DC: Healthcare Quality: Institute of Medicine.

Khan, M.E., Mishra, A., Sharma, V. and Varkey, L.C. 2008. 'Development of a Quality Assurance Procedure for Reproductive Health Services for District Public Health Systems: Implementation and Scale-up in the State of Gujarat'. New Delhi: Population Council.

Medica Synergy. 2010. 'Reports for Implementation of the QAP in Puri District Hospital'. (unpublished). Report submitted to National Health System Resource Centre, Delhi.

National Accreditation Board for Hospitals and Health Care Providers. 2009. General Information Brochure 2009. New Delhi: National Accreditation Board for Hospitals and Health Care Providers.

National Health Systems Resource Centre (NHSRC). 2010. Note on Quality Processes. Available at http://nhsrcindia.org/index. php?option=com_content&view=article&id=68:quality-process&catid=49:quality-processes&Itemid=74, accessed in February 2012.

National Health Systems Resource Centre (NHSRC). 2010. Quality Improvement. Thematic Area http://nhsrcindia.org/index. php?option=com_content&view=article&id=54:quality-improvement&catid=36:thematic-areas&Itemid=58, accessed in February 2012.

National Institute of Health and Family Welfare. 2008. Guidelines and Manuals. Available at: http://nihfw.org/nchrc/ GuidelinesAndManuals.html, accessed in January 2012.

UNICEF. 2009. Coverage Evaluation Survey. National Fact Sheet. New Delhi: UNICEF India Country Office.

WHO, UNICEF, UNFPA and the World Bank. 2007. 'Maternal Mortality in 2005'. Estimates Developed by WHO, UNICEF, UNFPA and The World Bank. Geneva: WHO.

WHO. 2000. 'Strategies for Assisting Health Workers to Modify and Improve Skills: Developing Quality Health Care—A Process of Change'. Geneva.

Suggested Readings

Ministry of Health and Family Welfare, Government of India. 2008. The Indian Public Health Standards. Available at http://mohfw. nic.in/NRHM/iphs.htm, accessed in January 2012.

National Institute of Health and Family Welfare (NIHFW). 2008. 'Quality Assurance in RCH-II Services'. Presentation made at the Workshop for Senior and Mid-level Managers on Improving Quality of Care in Health Sector. Shimla, 4–8 June.

Quality Council of India. 2009. 'Role of QCI/NABH in Health Care Improvement'. Presentation made at the Workshop on Quality, Equity and Accountability under NRHM. Bhubaneshwar, 4–6 September.

Woodward, A.C. 2000. Issues in Health Services Delivery, Discussion Paper 1. Improving Provider Skills. Strategies for Assisting Health Workers to Modify and Improve Skills: Developing Quality Health Care—A Process of Change. Evidence and Information for Policy. Department of Organization of Health Services Delivery. Geneva: WHO. Available at http://www. who.int/hrh/documents/en/improve_skills.pdf.

Appendix 1

Concept Note: Quality of Care

Quality means clinical effectiveness, safety, and a good experience for the patient. (Godlee 2009)

Interest in the quality of health services in developing countries is on the rise, with increasing efforts towards maintaining acceptable quality standards (Thomason and Edwards 1991). In order to focus on quality care there is a need for an understanding of what constitutes quality. In a health system, quality broadly encompasses clinical effectiveness, safety and a good experience for the patient and implies care which is effective, patient-centered, timely, efficient and equitable (IOM 1990, Murray 1999).

Quality of care (QOC) is a substantive field of policy, programming and research in public health and many definitions and conceptualizations exist. QOC draws upon two widely accepted frameworks: the Institute of Medicine (IOM) Framework of QOC (IOM 1990 and 2001) and the Hulton Framework (Hulton et al. 2000).

Why Quality of Care?
• Client satisfaction
• Provider motivation
• Quality costs less
• Improved health outcomes

IOM QOC framework asserts that 'quality of care is the degree to which health services for individuals and populations increase the likelihood of desired health outcomes and are consistent with current professional knowledge' (IOM, 1990). Developed in 1990, the IOM QOC framework is widely used as the basis of a great deal of research activity to improve health care organization and delivery. Developed primarily for the purposes of measurement of quality as part of routine quality improvement, IOM set out six priorities for quality improvement addressing the six key dimensions of health care system functioning. These are:

1. Safe—avoiding injuries to patients from the care that is intended to help them.
2. Effective—providing services based on scientific knowledge to all who could benefit.
3. Patient-centered—providing care that is respectful/responsive to individual patient preferences, needs and values, ensuring that patient-values guide all clinical decisions.
4. Timely—reducing waits and harmful delays for those who receive and give care.
5. Efficient—avoiding waste, including waste of equipment, supplies, ideas and energy.
6. Equitable—providing care that does not vary in quality due to characteristics such as gender, ethnicity, geographic location and socio-economic status.

The Hulton framework sets out that 'quality of care is the degree to which maternal health services for individuals and populations increase the likelihood of timely and appropriate treatment for the purpose of achieving desired outcomes that are both consistent with current professional knowledge and uphold basic reproductive rights' (Hulton et al. 2000). The Hulton framework tries to look at quality of maternity care and measuring quality within an institutional context. Ten key elements are defined to represent the provision and the experience of care and for each element; standards, criteria and selected indicators are put forward (see Figure 8A.1).

Figure 8A.1
Quality of Institutional Delivery Services—10 Elements of Care

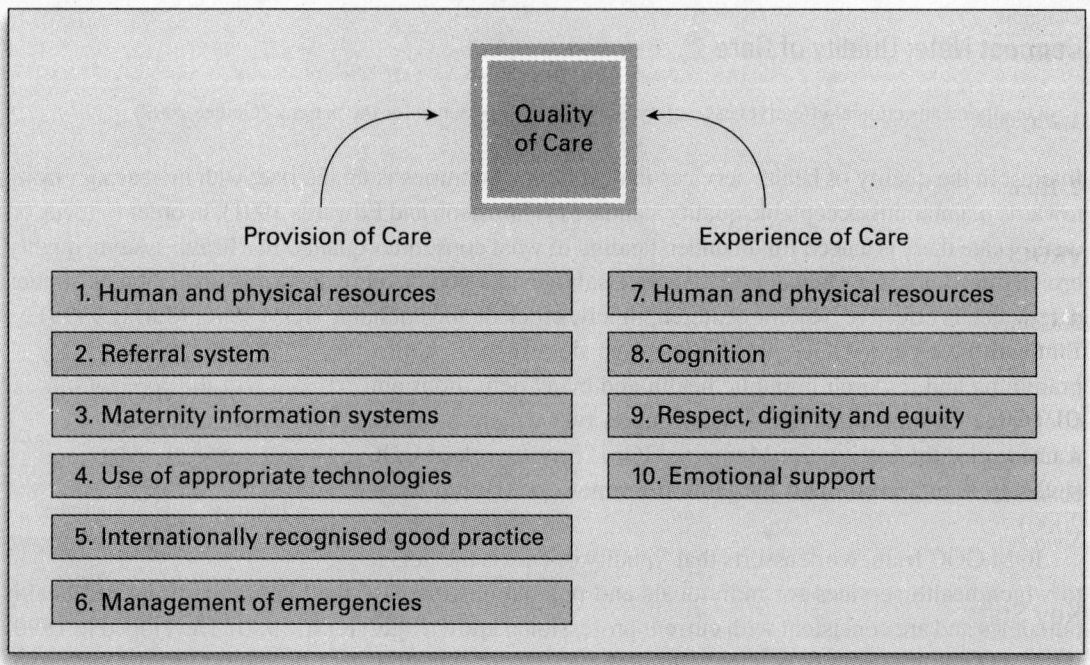

Source: Hulton et al. (2000).

In terms of the provision of maternity care, the six elements are:

1. Human and physical resources
2. The referral system
3. Management information systems
4. Use of appropriate technologies
5. Internationally-recognized good practice
6. Management of emergencies

With reference to the experience of care, the four elements are:

1. Human and physical resources
2. Cognition
3. Respect, dignity and equity
4. Emotional support

The domains to comprehensively capture all elements of quality of care are listed in Table 8A.3 (Bell and Avan 2010).

Table 8A.3

Elements of Quality of Care

Domains	Description
STRUCTURE	**Organizational factors that define the health system under which care is provided**
1. Physical Resources	The resources required to enable the provision of quality care **infrastructure, equipment, drugs and supplies.**
2. Human Resources	Care provided by appropriately **trained and supervised** providers; number of staff **adequate** to meet the demand for care.
PROCESS	**The interactions between users and health care providers; it can be thought of as the actual delivery and receipt of care**
3. Competent and Efficient Care	Care consistent with scientific knowledge, internationally recognised **good practice**. Care is **safe** (**clean** birth practices, avoidance of iatrogenic harm); **timely** and **responsive** (respectful, promoting autonomy, equitable). Care documented adequately.
OUTCOME	**The consequences of care**
4. Clinical Effectiveness	Good clinical **outcomes** achieved (e.g., mortality reduction).
5. Satisfaction with Care	Patient/provider satisfaction high.

Source: Donabedian (1966; 1997), Hulton et al. (2000) and Institute of Medicine (1990).

Key Stakeholders in Quality Improvement Process

- Policy and decision-makers
- Health providers
- Communities and service users (see Figure 8A.2)

Figure 8A.2

Stakeholders in Quality Improvement Process

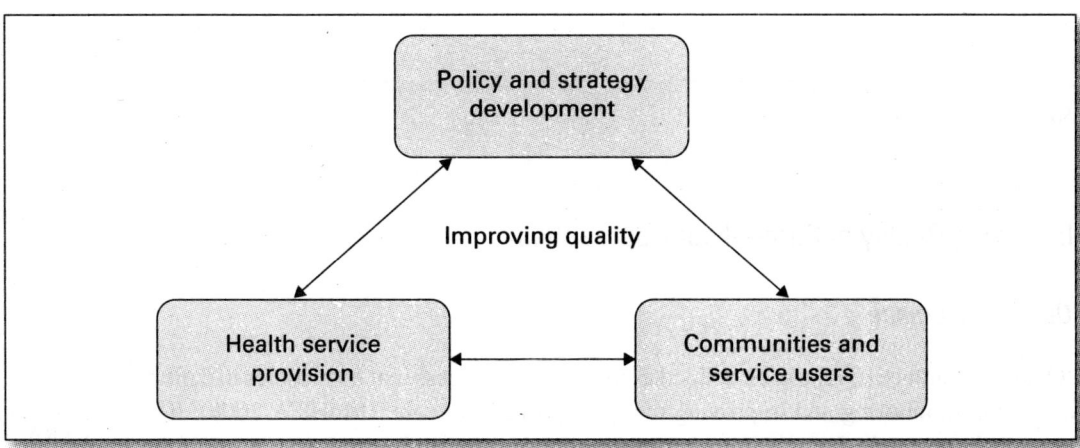

Source: WHO (2006).

A Process for Building a Strategy for Quality Improvement

There are seven activities (elements) within the three categories of analysis, strategy and implementation: understand the problem, plan, take action, study the results and plan new actions in response (see Figure 8A.3). One of the key elements of this approach is that it is very dynamic as it's based on results. The strategy needs to be modified as the approach of implementation (WHO 2006).

Figure 8A.3

Process for Building a Strategy for Quality Improvement

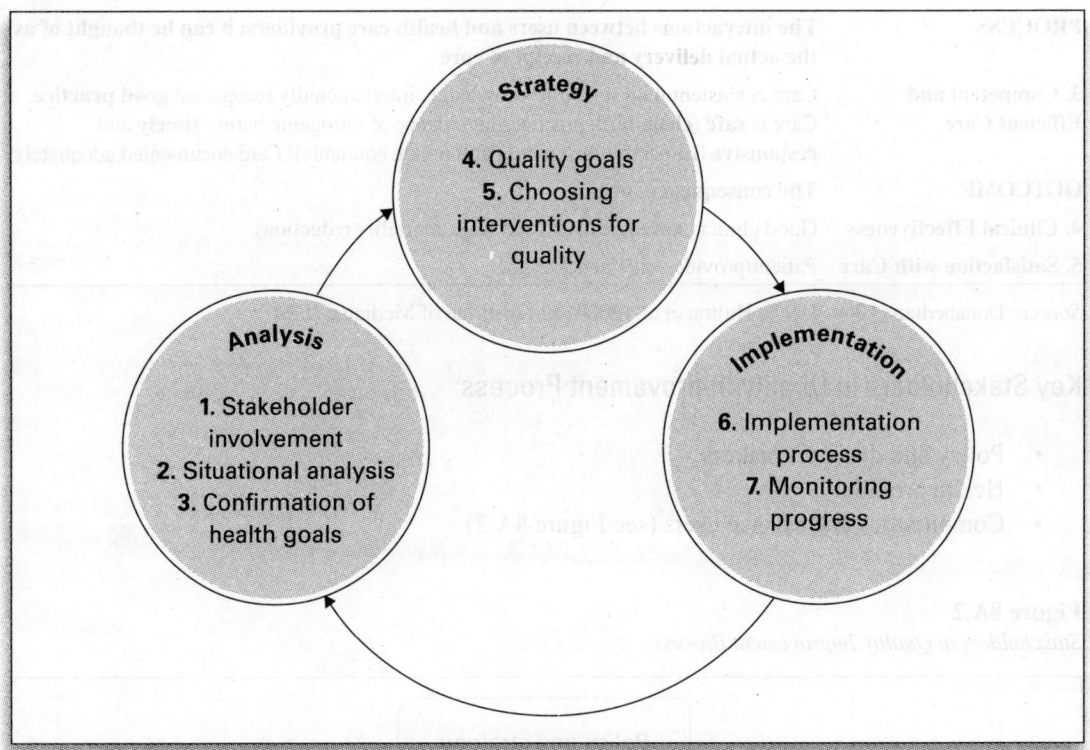

Source: WHO (2006).

Improving Quality of Care—Four Approaches

Quality Assurance

'Quality assurance (QA) can be defined as mechanism/process that contributes to defining, designing, assessing, monitoring and improving the quality of health care' (MoHFW 2008). It sets standards, assesses how standards are met and accordingly takes corrective action.

Continuous Quality Improvement (CQI)

The approach most commonly used for rapid cycle improvement in health care is the plan-do-study-act method in which four repetitive steps are carried out over the course of small cycles (see Figure 8A.4) (Varkey 2007).

Figure 8A.4
Plan-Do-Study-Act Cycle

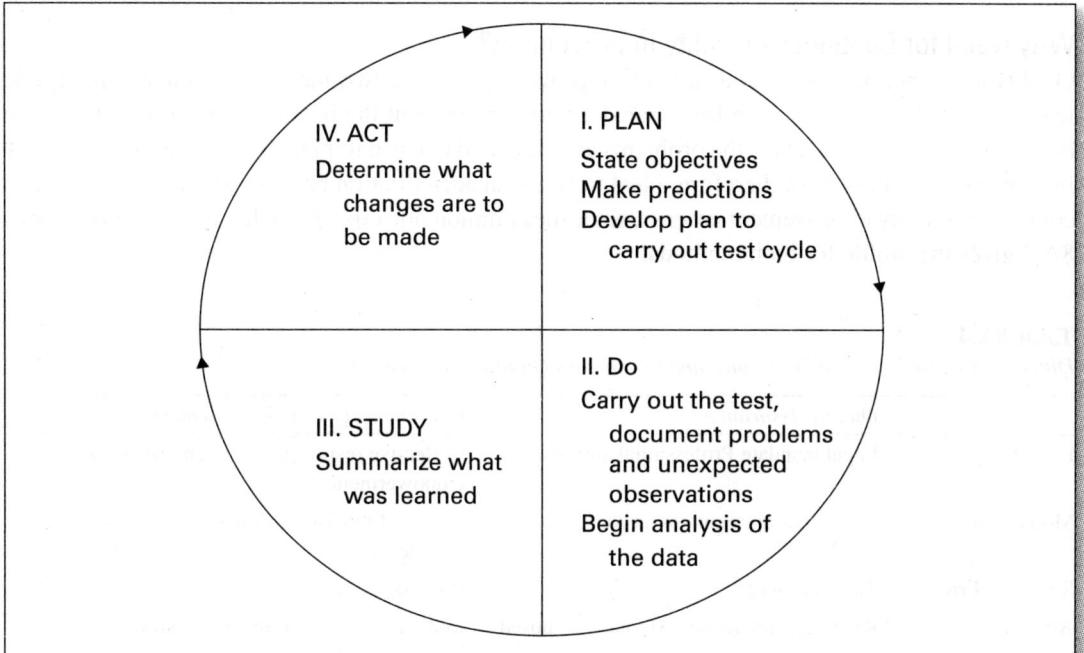

Source: Langley et al. (2009).

System Improvement

Identified systems to be improved, i.e., supply of drugs; assess how well standards are met and take corrective action.

Total Quality Management (TQM)

It encompasses

- Building an organizational culture
- Focus on clients

- Development of human resources
- Creating an enabling environment
- Quality assurance
- Continuous quality improvement

Perfect care may be a long way off, but much better care is within our grasp. (IOM 2001)

Why Need for Continuous Quality Improvement?

Quality assurance and continuous quality improvement are the two faces of the same coin, as one leads to the other. The first step for a transformation process at the health service institutions is to begin with accreditation. Once the problems are identified one can implement the continuous quality improvement process. It is, therefore, ideal to begin an accreditation process simultaneously with a continuous quality improvement process, since the common objective is quality improvement. Table 8A.4 gives the profile for both methods.

Table 8A.4

Differences between Quality Assurance and Continuous Quality Improvement

	Quality Assurance	*Continuous Quality Improvement*
Legitimacy	Legal mandate Professional authority	Collective responsibility client satisfaction staff empowerment
Motivation	Accreditation regulator as consumer	A way of thinking that fosters competition and excellence
Source of Error	The employee	Process, system
Attitude	Reserved, defensive, externally imposed	Internal orientation, self-motivation
Approach	Primarily focus on clinical result	Focus on process
Spectrum	May focus on special departments	Whole organization and all process

Source: Modified from Leebov and Ersov (1991).

References

Bell, J. and Avan, B. 2010. 'Developing a Framework and Instrument to Assess the Quality of Delivery Care: A Work in Progress. Executive Summary No. 5. Immpact, University of Aberdeen.

Godlee, F. 2009. 'Effective, Safe and a Good Patient Experience'. *BMJ*, 339: 4346.

Donabedian, A. 1966. 'Evaluating the Quality of Medical Care'. *Milbank Q* 2005, 83(4): 691–729.

Donabedian, A. 1997. 'The Quality of Care. How Can It Be Assessed?' *Archives of Pathology and Laboratory Medicine,* 121(11), 1145–115.

Hulton, L.A., Matthews, Z., Stones, R.W. 2000. 'A Framework for the Evaluation of Quality of Care in Maternity Services'. Southampton: University of Southampton.

Institute of Medicine (IOM). 1990. 'Medicare—A Strategy for Quality Assurance'. Volume I. Washington DC: National Academy Press.

IOM. 2001. 'Crossing the Quality Chasm: A New Health System for the 21st Century'. Washington, DC: Healthcare Quality, Institute of Medicine.

Langley, G.J., Nolan, K.M., Nolan, T.W., Norman, C.L. and Provost, L.P. 2009. *The Improvement Guide: Practical Guide to Enhancing Organizational Performance*. San Francisco, CA: Jossey-Bass.

Leebov, Wendy, Ersoz, Clara Jean. 1991. *Health Care Manager's Guide to Continuous Quality Improvement*. Chicago: American Hospital Publishing.

Murray, C.J.L. and Frenk, J. 1999. 'A WHO Framework for Health System Performance Assessment. Global Programme on Evidence and Information for Policy'. Washington DC: World Bank.

Ministry of Health and Family Welfare (MoHFW). 2008. 'Quality Assurance for District Reproductive and Child Health Services in Public Health System: An Operational Manual'. Ministry of Health and Family Welfare, Government of India.

Thomason, J. and Edwards, K. 1991. 'Using Indicators to Assess Quality of Hospital Services in Papua New Guinea'. *International Journal of Health Planning Management*, 1991(6):309–11.

Varkey, P. et al. 2007. 'Basics of Quality Improvement in Health Care'. Available at: http://www.med.unc.edu/cce/files/education-training/QI%20methods.pdf, accessed in April 2012.

World Health Organization (WHO). 2006. 'Quality of Care: A Process for Making Strategic Choices in Health Systems'. Geneva. Available at http://www.who.int/management/quality/assurance/QualityCare_B.Def.pdf, accessed in January 2012.

Referral Transport

9

Emergency Referral Transport: The GVK-EMRI Model

Raj Mohan Panda and Sourav Neogi

Background

The current estimated maternal mortality ratio (MMR) in India is 212 per 100,000 live births (SRS 2007–09). This translates into about 63,000 pregnant women or new mothers dying annually, often from preventable causes (UNICEF 2008). Almost 59% of maternal deaths in India are due to obstetric complications (SRS 2003). Most maternal deaths are due to five direct causes: haemorrhage, obstructed labour, eclampsia, sepsis and unsafe abortion. These complications can occur without forewarning and can rapidly become life threatening (Babinard and Roberts 2006). Access to appropriate, affordable and timely transport affects women's chance to receive preventative and emergency obstetric care that is essential for their survival. It is widely accepted that reduction of the MMR needs easy accessibility to emergency obstetric care (EmOC) facilities for all women having obstetric complications, which requires a well-functioning referral transport system. The World Health Organization (WHO) estimates that 75% of maternal deaths can be prevented through timely access to childbirth related care (Babinard and Roberts 2006). Evidence suggests that most obstetric emergencies can be managed if comprehensive emergency obstetric care (CeEmOC) is reached within 12 hours, with the exception of obstetric haemorrhage which requires attention within two hours. Timely access to care also helps reduce other long-term maternal health problems including obstetric fistula caused by obstructed labour (Porter 2007). Emergency transport referral mechanisms, thus, play an important role in achieving Millennium Development Goal (MDG) 5—to reduce maternal mortality by 75% by 2015 from 1990—as well as improving maternal health in general.

The Role of Transport in Accessing Maternal Health Services

The most commonly reported problem is distance to a health facility, reported to be a big problem by a quarter of the women who didn't seek service to a health facility. Expectedly, distance is a greater challenge for rural than urban women. One-third of rural women cite distance as being a big obstacle to obtaining medical care. Delay in reaching a health facility is one of 'the three delays'. Referral transportation (RT) also indirectly affects the other two 'delays', that is, the decision to seek care and delay in receiving adequate care (Thaddeus and Maine 1994). Several factors hinder the decision to seek care on the part of the individual, the family or both. The lack of a systemic and functional inter-institutional referral transport facility is a major factor for the delay in receiving adequate and appropriate care for complicated referral cases. In the Indian context, the referral system assumes much more importance because tribal and remote areas are poorly served by health care facilities. This is compounded by the lack of a proper public transport facility and corresponding relative high cost for private transport—which can add to delay in reaching the facility, increasing risk in case of obstetric emergencies. Interventions such as referrals are complex in nature, work best as an integral part of the health system and have to be designed so. Referral systems have been recognized as crucial component of the health system since the Alma Ata Declaration. Studies using modelling techniques have predicted that maternal mortality decline will reach a threshold of 35% if access to emergency obstetric care is not provided and that referral and transport strategies, alongside other interventions, could contribute to as much as an 80% reduction in maternal mortality (Goldie et al. 2010). Although delay has been recognized as an important contributing factor to maternal mortality and morbidity, case studies on these interventions to prevent delay and their subsequent effects on maternal health care are rare in the developing world. There are very few studies which have focussed exclusively on the transport mechanism for referral (for maternal health) and its impact on EmOC in India. This case study was designed to bridge the gap and focus on the issue of referral transport for maternal health care as well as highlight the determinants of an efficient transport/referral system and its importance in lowering maternal mortality and morbidity.

Objectives of the Case Study

- To study the determinants of an efficient referral transport for EmOC and prevent neonatal complications.
- To understand how existing referral transport (through the study of two models) functions at three different levels (state, district and block levels).
- To discuss these case studies and their relevance for policy and programmes concerning the role of referral transport in the reduction of maternal mortality.

Methodology

To understand the present situation with regard to the referral system, an in-depth desk review of literature was carried out to identify the different RT systems operating in the country (with specific focus on maternal care and EmOC in the country). Apart from published studies and reports, the review also examined various programme implementation plans (PIPs), evaluation reports, best practices (*Directory of Innovations Implemented in the Health Sector*, 2008, Solution Exchange e-discussions), Popline, newsletters, journals, etc. The team also met as well as communicated over email and phone with a number of government officials, development agencies and non-governmental organizations (NGOs) within India. Interviews with stakeholders (in-depth interviews with key personnel of the emergency referral transport services in both the models) and interactions with beneficiaries also greatly informed the process. Field trips were also undertaken to gather relevant information that was not available from existing sources. Access to grey literature and project reports and documents provided by the agencies administering these models also helped shape the case study.

Features of a Referral Transport System

A referral transport system is an integral part of an effective referral system. This has been summarized by Murray et al. from various studies.

Requirements of an Effective Referral System

Establishing a responsive emergency referral system—and the transportation mechanisms supporting these referrals—demands tightly interlocking components that can quickly interact and safely transfer a woman from the site of complication onset to a definitive level of care (see Box 9.1). The window period to make this transfer and receive emergency care is small, and if exceeded, debilitating and life-threatening. For example, in the case of the post-partum haemorrhage (PPH), women may have a window of only two hours between the onset of PPH and death. In this short period of time, the components of the referral system that need to be tightly interlocked include clinical judgement, stabilization and transfer protocols, communications technology, transportation and cost arrangements. This highly time-sensitive referral process is even further challenged in the case of neonatal complications which, in some cases, such as asphyxia, would require immediate treatment. Where referral mechanisms have been implemented they are frequently designed for obstetric emergencies; further work on referral is clearly needed to bridge the methods in place to bring emergency care to both mothers and newborns.

> **Box 9.1 Effective Referral System**
>
> - An adequately resourced referral centre (adequate staff, equipments, supplies, budget, managers).
> - Communications and feedback systems.
> - Designated transport.
> - Agreed setting–specific protocols for the identification of complications.
> - Personnel trained in their use.
> - Teamwork between referral levels.
> - Unified records system.
> - Mechanism to ensure that patients do not bypass a level of the referral system.
>
> *Source:* Murray and Pearson 2005.

The GVK-Emergency Management and Research Institute Model

This referral transport system was started by GVK Emergency Management and Research Institute (GVK-EMRI) in August 2005 with a modest beginning of 30 ambulances to cater to the population across 50 towns of Andhra Pradesh. Later in the same year, the organization signed a contract with the Government of Andhra Pradesh to expand their service to cover the entire population of the state with a fleet size of 802 ambulances. From this humble beginning in one state in India, the initiative has spread to 12 states and two union territories. GVK-EMRI's vision is to respond to 30 million emergencies and save one million lives annually by delivering quality services through a combination of leadership, innovation, technology and research and training. The model invested in these critical elements in the early years. Once they had the right combination of people, resources and leadership, they started expanding rapidly into many states in India.

Public–Private Partnership

Emergency medical systems (EMS) can only be put in place with careful planning and implementation and the various components should be linked to ensure that the system functions as one unit (Kobusingye et al. 2005). An EMS must be sensitive to and meet the needs of the poor. Issues of access to the system, hinder use by a lot of people who need these services. There are different means of achieving access to EMS. One such mechanism is through the means of a public–private partnership (PPP). GVK-EMRI is one of the public–private models that the state and central governments have supported to strengthen the health system towards improving access to health care. Gov-

> **Addressing Emergency Delivery**
>
> According a senior partner, Emergency and Medical Learning Centre in GVK-EMRI, out of nearly 3,500 patients who are picked up every day, some of them deliver in the ambulance itself. He said, 'Our personnel (emergency medical technicians [EMTs]) who are working in the ambulance are trained to conduct a normal delivery as well as a complicated delivery. We train them and organize some workshops on "how to conduct deliveries". We have obstetric mannequins and use them to train EMTs.
>
> The best advice we give to the EMT is, take the patient to the nearby hospital. Institutional delivery is the best. But sometimes, if it is unavoidable they will conduct the delivery. They park the ambulance on one side of the road and they conduct the delivery in the ambulance itself. And every day, almost about seven–eight deliveries are taking place in the ambulance itself, almost 1 to 1.5% of pregnant women are transported by ambulance in the state of Andhra Pradesh.'
>
> *Source:* Interview with senior partner at GVK-EMRI.

ernment provides funds for operational expenses (expenses for fuel, salary of the ambulance staff, emergency response centre (ERC) staff, phone bill expenses, maintenance of ambulance, etc.) and capital expenses (ambulance cost). The private partner (GVK-EMRI) complements the hardware by providing management skills, innovation, execution and technological capabilities to improve service delivery. The model which initially started in Andhra Pradesh has been scaled-up across many states in India. In Andhra Pradesh, ERC, training infrastructure, etc., are owned by GVK-EMRI.

Processes

How the GVK-EMRI Model Enables Access to Health

'Access' is the ability to reach, obtain or afford entrance to services (Parker 1974). Around four million deaths per year (cardiac, road accidents, maternal, suicide attempts, neonatal/infant/pediatric, diabetic related, etc.) occur due to the absence of the 4As[1]:

- Access to a universal toll-free number.
- Availability of a life-saving ambulance to quickly reach the nearest and appropriate health facility.

[1]Leadership in non-profit organization Making a difference in saving lives since April 05. Available at http://tidescoimbatore.com/presentations/venkat_changavalli.pdf, accessed on 4 May 2012.

Figure 9.1
GVK-EMRI and Access to Health Care

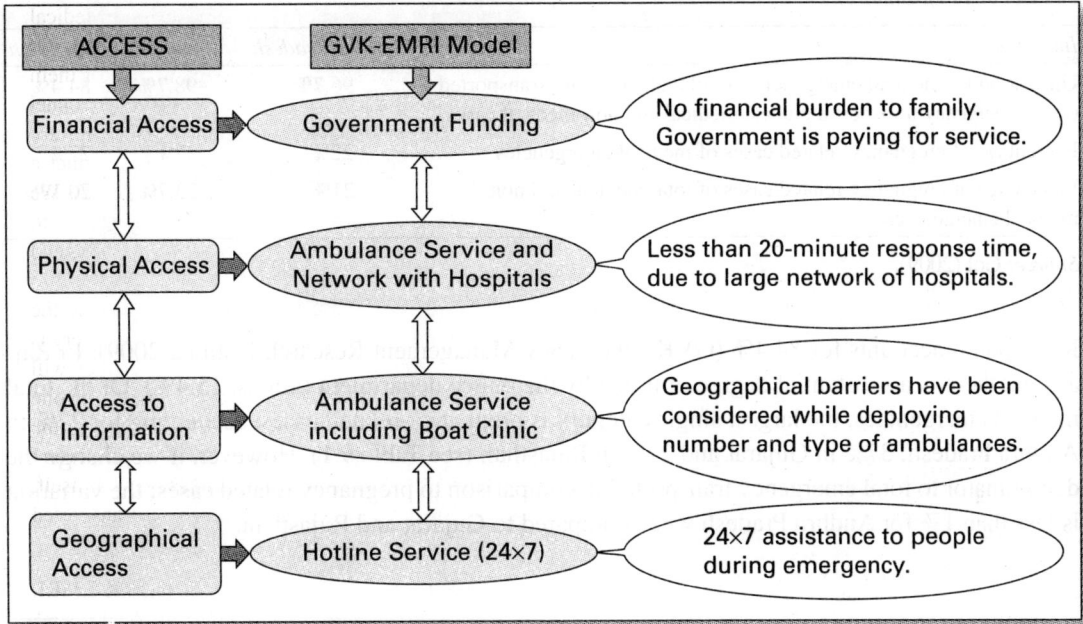

Source: Authors' own.

- **A**ffectionate care by trained paramedics (compassion, ability, resourcefulness and energy).
- **A**ffordability by every citizen.

Figure 9.1 illustrates how the GVK-EMRI model has been addressing different access factors.

Coverage of the Intervention: GVK-EMRI in Various States of India

GVK-EMRI is functioning in various states in India; however, it is important to note that the intervention was started in Andhra Pradesh and then replicated in other parts of the country (GVK Emergency Management Research Institute 2009).

Presently, EMRI services are available in Andhra Pradesh, Gujarat, Uttarakhand, Tamil Nadu, Rajasthan, Goa, Karnataka, Assam, Meghalaya, Chhattisgarh and Himachal Pradesh (specific details provided in Annexure 1 and description provided in Annexure 2).

Percentage of Pregnant Women of the Total Medical Emergencies with Access to GVK-EMRI Services

While the GVK-EMRI may be used as a general emergency service, it is largely used for medical emergencies. In Andhra Pradesh this accounts for 96.7%, in Gujarat it accounts for 98.7% and in

Table 9.1

Pregnancy-related Cases as Percentage of Emergencies Transported under GVK-EMRI from Andhra Pradesh, Gujarat and Rajasthan

Indicator	Andhra Pradesh	Gujarat	Rajasthan
Utilization for medical emergencies of total emergencies transported (total emergency transport includes: medical and non-medical cases)	96.7%	98.7%	84.4%
Percentage of pregnancy-related cases of medical emergencies	22%	37%	27%
Percentage of pregnancy-related cases of total medical and non-medical emergencies	21%	33.7%	20.13%

Source: GoI (2009).

Rajasthan it accounts for 84.4% (GVK Emergency Management Research Institute 2009). In Rajasthan, there is a substantial degree of usage by the police department (almost 15.4%). Of the total medical emergencies, the largest single category is pregnancy-related cases, accounting for 22% in Andhra Pradesh, 37% in Gujarat and 27% in Rajasthan (see Table 9.1). However, if we change the denominator to total emergency transported in comparison to pregnancy related cases; the variation is less than 1% for Andhra Pradesh when compared to Gujarat and Rajasthan.

Salient Features of the Model

Resources

Ambulance

Two versions of ambulances are available under the EMRI model, which are described as follows:

- **Basic Life Support (BLS)**: The ambulances are equipped with bigger oxygen tanks, as they often head into rural areas where they cannot rely on quick refills. It has a washbasin with a foot operated tap. They have three types of stretchers for different situations, each of which is designed to make it easy to lift and transport a patient in and out of the ambulance. It has a public address system.
- **Advanced Life Support (ALS)**: An ALS version is available with cardiac monitor and defibrillator in addition to all the provisions of the BLS ambulance.

Infrastructure

The physical infrastructure includes the administrative campus with ERC training facilities, hostel for students, ambulance parking lot, etc. In Andhra Pradesh, GVK-EMRI has its own campus and initial investment has been made. Investment towards infrastructure is a one-time expenditure, which could be upgraded and modified based on need and volume.

Cost of Services (No Cost to Citizen)

The services offered by GVK-EMRI are free for the beneficiaries/patients. The services are subsided by the government. Majority of the state governments are paying from the National Rural Health Mission (NRHM) budget and some states are paying from their own budgets for the expenses incurred for providing these services. The beneficiaries/patients also get cashless service for primary stabilization at the receiving hospitals.

Training and Capacity Building

Training in lifesaving obstetrics skills was found to contribute towards reducing maternal deaths in Nigeria and other settings (Ijadunola et al. 2010). Emergency triage assessment and treatment, a part of WHO integrated management of childhood illness strategy, has been used in many countries to improve paediatric emergency care (WHO 2000). There are also protocol based emergency care procedures in ALS in obstetrics laid down by the American Academy of Family Physicians. EMRI conducts a course for science graduates on basic life support skills during the foundation (EMT) programme. EMTs are trained to conduct normal and complicated deliveries. Training has been imparted to them by using mannequins during the institutional phase followed by hospital phase for hands-on clinical training and ambulance phase for real-time pre-hospital care orientation.

Conducting Research and Building Capability in Emergency Medical Systems

EMSs are a neglected topic and part of 10/90 gap in health research, whereby less than 10% of global research investment is spent on problems affecting 90% of the world's population (Murray and Pearson 2005). It is noteworthy to mention that EMRI continually invested in research activities in three categories, i.e., operations research, systems research and medical research so that the services can be upgraded based on the research results. Under operations research, there is focus on predicting the future state of health care, disease incidence, better utilization of resources and redefining processes. Systems research mainly addresses capturing best practices in EMS/prevention of emergency. Effectiveness of intervention in specific emergency conditions, integration with hospital care come under the medical research category. The research system at EMRI

Research and EMRI

The global standard in getting a call and reaching the patient is around eight minutes and EMRI is trying its best to meet those standards. The senior partner of the research division at EMRI opined that providing emergency transport services in different regions in a large country like India was a huge challenge. He said that it was a challenge to achieve the global standard in different terrains such as hills, mountains desert and in places which had no proper roads. He says, 'We do research on such issues to understand what should be the standard for that specific region. We analyze all these issues and then we come up with our own understanding on the issue.'

Another example cited is research on ERC. According to the senior partner, earlier they had the communication officers (COs) and dispatch officers (DOs) responding to calls at ERC. Then through their research they found that sometimes because of these two agents the call taking time was two to three times more as compared to a single-channel communication (which they have implemented recently). Thus, one component of delay was reduced.

Source: Interview with senior partner at GVK-EMRI.

designs and conducts locally appropriate studies that establish effectiveness of certain processes by studying outcomes. They also conduct economic analysis of their processes which helps them choose appropriate sub-systems.

Communications Systems

An emergency referral system has both linked and independent components and all components should work together to operate in an efficient manner. This would differ from model to model. The role of communication systems cannot be overstated. The best of referral systems would fail if they do not reach their patients in time and they have no contact with hospitals as they help transport patients to the hospitals (Murray and Pearson 2005). Innovations are needed to provide efficient referral communication in different settings in the country to gain access to the emergency care interventions that already exist. Equipping primary health care centres with appropriate numbers (emergency toll-free numbers or numbers of ambulances) will help clients to reach out at short notices.

Emergency Response Centre (ERC) in EMRI

In the ERC, communication takes place with multiple stakeholders. It is open 24×7. All ERC staff is trained in communication skills. Attention has been given to the response time. At the EMRI ERC, the employee has a strong understanding about the region and using software application support ambulances will be dispatched. The ERC software has local maps of the region where the services are rendered.

- **Communication with Client (toll-free number, etc.):** Integrated Emergency Response Service for medical, police and fire emergencies with single universal toll-free number '108', is a 24×7 emergency service. Toll-free number is accessible from landline or mobile. Emergency help reaches in an average of 18 minutes.
- **Communication with Ambulances (transporter):** Once the emergency has been identified by the ERC staff, they obtain the address of the patient along with their mobile number and other relevant information. After that the ERC operator contacts the pilot (driver) of the selected ambulance. EMTs are also being informed about the nature of the patient. The pilot also communicates with the patient to find the location of the house. The EMTs communicate with the family members of the patient to find out the condition of the patient and provide basic support for actions (pre-arrival instructions) which could be followed by the family members.
- **Communication with Caregiver (while transporting to nearest health facility):** While the patient is being transported in a state-of-the-art EMRI ambulance to a nearby hospital, communication with caregivers at the hospital is maintained to prep are the facility to receive the patient. Vital data about the patient is recorded and relayed to the hospital so that the facility has adequate time to receive the patient as well as be informed about what procedures should be in place to save/treat the patient. The Emergency Response Services has signed memorandums of understanding (MoUs) with over 6,800 hospitals throughout the country and these hospitals provide primary stabilization free of cost for the first-24 hours.

Service Delivery

- **Pre-hospital Care:** Pre-hospital care is that which is provided on-scene and en route and through online medical support by the ERC physician until the patient arrives at a formal health facility capable of providing definitive care. It should comprise basic strategies with proven effectiveness such as the deployment of trained paramedics/personnel with basic life support skills. Triage by paramedics is important to screen which patient goes where. The level of training of paramedics in basic lifesaving skills improves a patient's outcomes (Murray and Pearson 2005)·

- **Emergency Care during Transportation en Route**

  An emergency medical technician (EMT), who is essentially a paramedic working in the ambulance, provides care at scene and en route to hospital with the ambulance driver (called pilot who as well is trained in simple skills). This is established as a cardinal piece in pre-hospital care. At GVK EMRI, emergency response centre physicians (ERCP) stationed at the ERC are available 24×7, provide advice to these EMTs and support in all cases, thus, ensuring that all patients receive due care. Therefore, EMRI helps in reduction of maternal and infant deaths across operational states by expeditious transport of pregnant ladies and safe assisted delivery option while en route, whenever there is an impending delivery situation.

- **Emergency Care at Health Facilities**

  The capabilities of formal health facilities for providing emergency maternal health care vary immensely between states and districts in India. Ideally appropriate facilities which can provide such kind of care for maternal health emergencies such as obstructed labour should be mapped out well in advance in all areas and patients should be transferred within appropriate time so that lives can be saved. To do these an effective triage system is important so that appropriate cases can be transferred to the appropriate facilities. Very often precious time and lives are lost because patients are taken to facilities where the desired and definitive care is not provided. The emphasis on appropriate 'systems' engagement ensures that proper communication is given to first responders, so that they know where and when to refer patients and can receive feedback about cases that they have managed (Murray and Pearson 2005). The WHO guidelines for essential trauma care list comprehensively the most appropriate resources for various levels of health care facilities.[2]

Discussion: Barriers and Facilitators of the GVK-EMRI Model

Quality Management System

The aim of quality care would be that it is effective, safe, timely, efficient, community-centered and equitable. When we discuss the quality components of a referral transport model, it has many

---

[2] See Importance of Effective Emergency Medical Transport in Addressing Maternal Complications: Case Study, EMRI 108 EMS Service in Andhra Pradesh. Available at http://www.emri.in/images/stories/EMRI_Journel_Round%20 10.pdf, accessed on 13 April 2012.

dimensions; however, the two most important dimensions are promptness of the service and the care provided en route.

Promptness of the Service

The popular perception of every urban call being reached within 20 minutes and every rural call within 40 minutes is being achieved. However, at times delays do occur. What is worth noting is that there is an objective, documented and verifiable system in place for measuring the time taken from the moment of receiving the call to the moment of reaching the patient and the time taken to deliver the patient to the facility.

Once the ambulance carries out an average of eight trips per day, delays become almost inevitable—necessitating the addition of another ambulance in the same area. The last mile in terms of geographic coverage requires a disproportionately high increase in number of ambulances. The number of ambulances would also have to rise in areas with increased utilization so as to guarantee quality in terms of promptness.

Care Provided en Route

In order to provide care en route there should be investment in training a cadre of paramedical staff and equipping the ambulances with all the necessary equipment and consumables.

Training of Drivers and other Support Staff

EMRI Hyderabad has a state-of-the-art training facility. There are classrooms for training, hostels for the trainees, training equipment and training protocols and processes in place for testing and certifying skills.

Coordination—Hospital Linkages

One of the key functions that EMRI performs is to engage private hospitals who would participate in the emergency response service and provide cashless service primary stabilization for the patient. For this purpose, EMRI has met with large numbers of private hospitals and signed MoUs with them. The percentage of referrals to private health facilities is 35% in Andhra Pradesh. The choice of the hospital is based on patient's choice, condition of the patient and facilities at the receiving hospital.

Annexure 1: Coverage of the EMRI Model till May 2012

- Andhra Pradesh—April 2012: 752 ambulances covering the entire state with 100% population coverage.
- Gujarat—August 2007: 506 ambulances throughout the state with 100% coverage.
- Uttarakhand—May 2008: 140 ambulances covering entire state with 100% coverage.
- Tamil Nadu—September 2008: 436 ambulances covering 100% of the population.

- Goa—September 2008: 33 ambulances covering 100% of the state.
- Karnataka—November 2008: 517 ambulances covering 100% of the population.
- Assam—November 2008: 283 ambulances covering 100%of the population. One boat ambulance is also functioning.
- Meghalaya—February 2009: 44 ambulances.
- Himachal Pradesh—July 2010: 112 ambulances.
- Madhya Pradesh: 102 ambulances.
- Chhattisgarh—January 2011: 172 ambulances.
- Union Territories (Daman and Diu/Dadra Nagar Haveli): 13 ambulances.

Annexure 2: Experiences of Two States: Andhra Pradesh and Gujarat

Andhra Pradesh

EMRI began operations in Andhra Pradesh on August 2005, with a fleet of 30 ambulances. Later R. Raju (Satyam) donated another 40 ambulances to EMRI in the year 2006–07, making a total of 70 ambulances run by EMRI on its own. In the third year of operations (2007–08), EMRI expanded the ERS to the entire state of Andhra Pradesh under PPP mode, with the Government of Andhra Pradesh contributing an additional 432 ambulances, bringing the total ambulances in operations to 502. GVK-EMRI—Andhra Pradesh launched an additional set of 150 ambulances on 16 February 2009. Today, GVK-EMRI operates with 752 ambulances covering the entire state, handling over 5,000 emergencies per day. In Andhra Pradesh, the operating cost for each ambulance per month is ₹95,000 and as operations stabilized in Andhra Pradesh, the Government of Andhra Pradesh took over 95% of the operating cost.

The emergency transportation provided in a state-of-the-art ambulance is free. It has been co-ordinated by state-of-the-art emergency ERC with 24×7 services. In addition to that, the call to the number 108 is a toll-free service accessible from both landline and mobile. Currently, in Andhra Pradesh GVK-EMRI is receiving around 30,000 calls and responding to 3,500 emergencies per day. EMRI has tie-ups with 3,331 private hospitals in Andhra Pradesh, apart from the government hospitals that can handle emergencies. These hospitals provide free stabilization services for the first-24 hours to the patient. Initially, the cost of Indian-built ambulances was ₹21 lakhs approximately for an ALS version and about ₹15 lakhs for the BLS version of ambulance. However, with the increase in the numbers, the cost has come down to ₹15 lakhs for an ALS ambulance and ₹11 lakhs for the BLS ambulance. According to daily reports of ambulance usage, each ambulance is averaging four–five trips per day. Operating cost per ambulance per month is ₹95,000 as per the current MoU with Government of Andhra Pradesh.

Gujarat

EMRI started operating in Gujarat in August 2007 with a fleet of total 61 ambulances across nine districts of the state. Currently, EMRI's 108 services are available across entire Gujarat covering all 26 districts with a fleet of over 403 ambulances. The capital cost for purchase and equipping the ambulances as well as for land and building of the ERC was provided by the Government of Gujarat (GoG) under NRHM. As per the daily report of 31 December 2008, ambulances were dispatched in case of 8.24% of all the calls received since the operations began in Gujarat (NHSRC 2008). Of these dispatches, medical emergencies were almost 99%. Out of the total medical emergencies, 33.7% were pregnancy related. EMRI has tie-ups with 2,050 private hospitals in Gujarat, apart from 1,381 government hospitals that can handle emergencies. These hospitals provide free stabilization services for the first-24 hours to the patient. As per the MoU signed between GoG and EMRI, the procurement of these ambulances is done by EMRI with funds from GoG (₹15.75 lakhs for ALS and ₹9.75 lakhs for BLS ambulances).

In Gujarat, the state government is contributing 95% of the operating cost and 100% of the capital cost. After analysis of the audited expense statements of the Gujarat model for 2007–08 and 2008–09, the operating expenses came down by approximately 22% (cost reduced from ₹2,871 in first year to ₹634.85 in second year).

All direct costs for 108 GVK-EMRI are being borne by the respective state governments.

References

Babinard, J. and Roberts, P. 2006. Maternal and Child Mortality Development Goals: What Can the Transport Sector Do? Washington, DC: World Bank. Available at http://www.eldis.org/go/topics/resource-guides/health&id=33302&type=Document, accessed on 2 March 2012.

Government of India (GoI). 2009. 'Study of Emergency Response Service—EMRI Model'. NHSRC, Ministry of Health and Family Welfare, Government of India.

Goldie, S.J., Sweet. S., Carvalho, N., Natchu, U.C.M. and Hu, D. 2010. 'Alternative Strategies to Reduce Maternal Mortality in India: A Cost-effectiveness Analysis'. PLOS Med, 7(4): e1000264. DOI: 10.1371/journal.pmed.1000264. Available at http://www.plosmedicine.org/article/info%3Adoi%2F10.1371%2Fjournal.pmed.1000264, accessed on 2 April 2012.

GVK Emergency Management Research Institute. 2009. EMRI Documents Annexure-A-16: National Performance Report.

Ijadunola, K., Ijadunola, M., Esimai, O. and Abiona, T. 2010. 'New Paradigm Old Thinking: The Case for Emergency Obstetric Care in the Prevention of Maternal Mortality in Nigeria'. BMC Women's Health, 10(6). Available at http://www.biomedcentral.com/1472-6874/10/6, accessed on 13 April 2012.

Kobusingye, O., Hyder, A., Bishai, D., Hicks, E.R., Mock, C. and Joshipura, M. 2005. 'Emergency Medical Systems in Low and Middle-income Countries: Recommendations for Action'. Bulletin of the World Health Organization, (83): 626–31. Available at http://www.who.int/bulletin/volumes/83/8/626.pdf, accessed on 3 May 2012.

Ministry of Health and Family Welfare. 2008. Directory of Innovations Implemented in the Health Sector. Department for International Development. Ministry of Health and Family Welfare, Government of India. Available at http://planningcommission.nic.in/reports/genrep/health/Directory_of_innovations_march.pdf, accessed on 15 May 2012.

Murray, S.F. and Pearson, S.C. 2005. 'Maternity Referral Systems in Developing Countries: Current Knowledge and Future Research Needs'. Social Science & Medicine, 62(2006): 2205–15. Available at http://www.amddprogram.org/d/sites/default/files/Murray%20and%20Pearson_2006_Maternity%20referral%20systems%20in%20developing%20countries.pdf, accessed on 29 March 2012.

National Health Systems Resource Centre (NHSRC). 2008. Study of Emergency Response Service (EMRI Scheme). Ministry of Health and Family Welfare, Government of India.

Parker, A.W. 1974. 'Primary Care: Where Medicine Fails'. In S. Andreopoulos (ed.), The Dimensions of Primary Care: Blueprints for Change, pp. 15–77. New York: Wiley.

Porter, G. 2007. 'Transport, (Im) Mobility and Spatial Poverty Traps: Issues for Rural Women and Girl Children in Sub-Saharan Africa'. A paper prepared for the international workshop Understanding and Addressing Spatial Poverty Traps: An International Workshop, Spier Estate, Stellenbosch, South Africa. Available at http://www.odi.org.uk/resources/docs/3536.pdf, accessed on 2 March 2012.

Sample Registration System (SRS). 2006. Maternal Mortality in India: 1997–2003. Trends, Causes and Risk Factors. New Delhi: Registrar General, Government of India.

SRS. 2007–09. 'Special Bulletin on Maternal Mortality in India 2007–09'. Office of Registrar General, India.

Thaddeus, S. and Maine, D. 1994. 'Too Far to Walk: Maternal Mortality in Context'. *Social Science and Medicine*, 38(8): 1091–10.

UNICEF. 2008. 'Maternal and Perinatal Death Inquiry and Response—Empowering Communities to Avert Maternal Deaths in India'. UNICEF, New Delhi, India. Available at http://www.unicef.org/india/MAPEDIR-Maternal_and_Perinatal_Death_Inquiry_and_Response-India.pdf, accessed on 5 May 2012.

World Health Organization (WHO). 2000. 'Management of the Child with a Serious Infection or Severe Malnutrition: Guidelines for Care at the First-referral Level in Developing Countries'. Department of Child and Adolescent Health and Development, World Health Organization, Geneva. Available at http://whqlibdoc.who.int/hq/2000/WHO_FCH_CAH_00.1.pdf, accessed on 28 March 2012.

10

Low-cost Referral Transport: The Janani Express

Sourav Neogi

Background and Overview

High maternal mortality remains an issue of concern for India. As per UN estimates, nearly 63,000 Indian women, accounting for almost 18% of estimated global maternal deaths, die every year due to causes related to pregnancy and childbirth.

One of the predominant causes of maternal mortality is the delay incurred in providing pregnant mothers with appropriate and adequate medical care on time. A key necessity in ensuring that rural women opt for institutional deliveries and leverage the benefits of Janani Suraksha Yojana (JSY) is the availability of emergency transport facilities to transfer pregnant women on time to the nearest hospital for delivery. Access to appropriate, affordable and timely transport affects women's ability to receive preventive and emergency obstetric care (EmOC) that is essential for their survival. It is widely accepted that reduction of the MMR needs easy accessibility to EmOC facilities for all women having obstetric complications which, in turn, require a well-functioning referral transport system.

World Bank Transport Strategy estimates that 75% of maternal deaths can be prevented through timely access to childbirth-related care, facilitated by transport. As per evidence suggests that most of the obstetric emergencies can be managed if Comprehensive Emergency Obstetric Care (CeEmOC) is reached within 12 hours, with the exception of obstetric haemorrhage which requires attention within two hours (Forster et al. 2009). Timely access to care also helps reduce other long-term maternal health problems including obstetric fistula caused by obstructed labour. Emergency transport referral mechanisms, thus, play an important role in achieving Millennium Development Goal 5—to reduce maternal mortality by 75% by 2015 from 1990—as well as in improving maternal health in other ways.

Statement of the Problem

Distance to a health facility is one of the most commonly reported problems by a quarter of the women; who didn't seek service to a health facility. Covering the distance to health care facilities is a greater challenge in rural areas as compared to urban areas. One-third of rural women cite distance as being a big obstacle to obtaining medical care (VikasSamvad 2008). Delay in reaching a health facility is one of 'the three delays'. Referral transportation also indirectly affects the other 'two delays', which are delay in the decision to seek care and in receiving adequate care (Thaddeus and Maine 1994). Several factors hinder the decision to seek care on the part of the individual, the family or both. Some prominent ones are lack of money, poor roads and cost of transportation. Social factors such as gender, social norms and culture also create hindrance.

The lack of a systemic and functional inter-institutional referral transport facility is also a major factor for the delay in receiving adequate and appropriate care for complicated referral cases. Studies throughout low-middle income countries on EmOC have stressed the importance of referral transport and how distance proves to be significant factor in delay in seeking medical care. However, there are very few studies which have focussed exclusively on referral transport for medical health care/EmOC in India. This case study will concentrate on the issue of referral transport for maternal health care.

Madhya Pradesh—Where Are We?

Madhya Pradesh, located in the middle of the country, is one of the biggest states in India in terms of land area. A large part of the state is still underdeveloped and faces extreme climatic situations. Key health indicators for the state are not encouraging. The terrain, poor road conditions and lack of public transport make it difficult for locals to reach nearby health facilities, especially during an emergency. Even until recently, unavailability of emergency transport coupled with poor road connectivity was identified as major reasons for delay in pregnant women reaching delivery centres (Government of Madhya Pradesh 2008).

The coverage by public health facilities in Madhya Pradesh is poor as compared to Government of India (GoI) norms and other states in India. As of October 2001, Madhya Pradesh had established only 53% of community health centres (CHCs) required in accordance with GoI norms. For sub-health centres (SHCs), primary health centres (PHCs) and district hospitals, the corresponding figures was 84%, 71% and 80% respectively.

The average number of villages and the extent of the rural area covered by a SHC in MP are 5.99 and 36.46 km^2 respectively, compared to the all India average of 4.27 villages and 22.81 km^2 (GoI 2000).

In 1993, only 16% rural households needed to travel less than half a km to access a PHC, whereas 29% needed to travel between 2–5 km and 40% had to travel 5–10 km (Government of Madhya Pradesh 2008).

Data from National Family Health Survey-3 (NFHS-3 2007) suggests that the situation has not improved much. Among those who do not use government health facilities, the lack of accessibility is clearly a major deterrent as among the main reasons for their non-use are poor quality of care (63%), lack of a nearby facility (51%) and long waiting time (26%).

Clearly, access to a functional government health facility during an emergency is a challenge in Madhya Pradesh. Hence, the state government decided to establish a referral transport system, but the concept of a transport system linked to 24×7 call centres for coordinated operation of this system was initiated at a later stage.

Janani Express

Janani Express was launched on 15 August 2006 to increase institutional deliveries by ensuring a transport facility round-the-clock for pregnant women, particularly in rural areas, to take them to the nearest health facility. It was decided that the scheme would be implemented in two blocks of each of the 10 selected districts in the first stage. However, the scheme was launched across all the 38 districts in at least one block of the district. In the first phase, the 'Janani Express Scheme' was launched by the government under a public–private partnership (PPP). It is now operational in 308 blocks of the state and nearly 40% of the beneficiaries of JSY are availing the scheme.

Essential Features of the Janani Express Model

Janani Express Yojana is offering a 24-hour referral transport facility to urban and rural beneficiaries for both above poverty line (APL) and below poverty line (BPL) families. Vehicles used under this scheme are hired from the private sector. Tenders are invited at the district level and further agreements are made on pre-fixed criteria. On an average, two vehicles are available in each block at ₹15,000 to ₹20,000 per month. The costs are fixed at ₹150 for a distance up to 25 km and ₹250 beyond this. Services are free for BPL and chargeable for APL. The vehicle is also utilized to transport sick and malnourished children who need to be referred. The vehicles are stationed at block headquarters with 24×7 services. These vehicles are strategically placed at 24×7 institutional delivery points located across the district in such a way that no village takes more than 30 minutes to reach.

Figure 10.1
Janani Ambulance

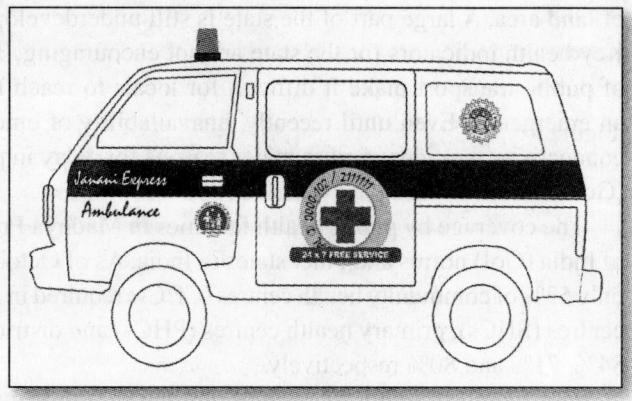

Source: PPT by UNICEF in Bhopal, Madhya Pradesh.

Centrally Located 24×7 Call Centre

Initially mobile numbers of the Janani Express drivers were distributed in the community. The community members used to call directly to the driver for the Janani Express vehicle. However, this system didn't work that well for various reasons. Later on, the concept of a call centre was introduced to the system. The entire call centre part was conceptualized, developed and implemented by United Nations Children's Fund (UNICEF). UNICEF also prepared a software for the call centre which captures data regarding the performance of the Janani Express service.

A call centre is located in all the district hospital campuses and has four dedicated operators working for eight-hour shifts. During the day shift, two operators work in the call centre; however, in the evening and at night one operator operates the centre. The call centre is provided with two dedicated telephone lines one of which is a toll-free number 102. Both the numbers are publicized in the community through radio, posters, banners and the Accredited Social Health Activist (ASHA). The call centre is also equipped with a computer in which all information about the caller and patient is gathered. On receiving the call, the operator diverts the nearest vehicle to the village and also informs the nearby delivery centre to be prepared for incoming patient. This is required to control the fleet of vehicles and to ensure coordinated contact. The monthly report is generated through the software and submitted to the District Health Society.

Training

Training is a very important component of any programme. However, no trained paramedical/medical personnel accompany the pregnant woman in the Janani Express and she is only accompanied by family members. The Janani Express drivers are trained in first aid. In the vehicles oxygen cylinders are available.

Communication and Coordination

As shown in the Figure 10.2, the patient's family calls the call centre directly to inform about the patient's condition and location. Based on preliminary enquiry, the call-centre employee writes down

Figure 10.2

Coordination between the Agency and Beneficiaries/Service Providers: A Graphical Depiction

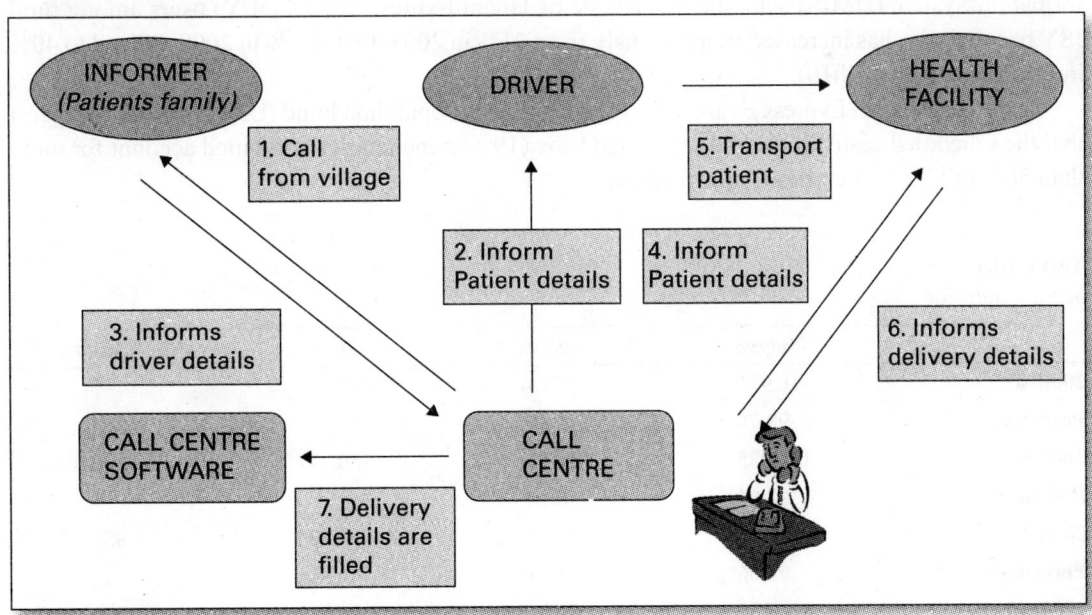

Source: UNICEF.

all the necessary details, calls the Janani Express driver and provides him with information regarding the location of the pregnant women. After that, the call centre calls the patient's family and gives details of the driver including his number. The call-centre employee meanwhile also informs the health facility regarding the patient's arrival to avail delivery services in the facility. All information is recorded in the call-centre software by the call-centre employee.

Achievements

Call centre software developed by UNICEF captures service statistics on a daily basis. The service statistics have been analyzed by UNICEF periodically.

Since its introduction the Janani Express Scheme has shown encouraging results as per service statistics. Fifty percent of all beneficiaries are BPL cardholders for whom the service is free. Although Janani Express is primarily meant for pregnant women it has also been used for other health emergencies. Table 10.1 provides the service statistics for Janani Express over the years, showing more than 95% use of the vehicle by pregnant women.

As per the May 2010 presentation of Ministry of Health and Family Welfare, 79% of community leaders are aware of the Janani Express which results in higher usage of the service. At present, there are a total of 625 vehicles in 308 blocks across the state (Agnani 2010).

The average number of beneficiaries availing services per day has increased tremendously since its inauguration. The average number of emergencies transported per day has increased from 47 in 2006 to 904 in 2010 and of which pregnancy-related cases are reported to be 882 per day.

The scheme has increased its coverage over the years. As per the state Health Management Information System (HMIS) data, the percentage of Janani Express Yojana (JEY) users among rural JSY beneficiaries has increased tremendously from 21% in 2007–08 to 36% in 2008–09 and to 40% in 2009–10 (Agnani 2010).

Findings of Janani Express Evaluation, United Nations Population Fund (UNFPA) (2007) suggest that the scheduled caste (36%) and scheduled tribe (19%) beneficiaries combined account for more than 50% of all beneficiaries (Agnani 2010).

Table 10.1
Service Statistics

	Pregnant	Others	Total	Daily Case Load
2006–07	16,971	213	17,184	47
Percentage	98.76%	1.24%		
2007–08	146,025	4,452	150,477	412
Percentage	97.04%	2.96%		
2008–09	303,220	7,269	310,489	851
Percentage	97.66%	2.34%		
2009–10	322,255	7,429	329,684	904
Percentage	97.75%	2.25%		

Source: www.mohfw.nic.in/.../M.P.%20Janani%20Express-04.07.10.ppt, accessed in April 2011.

Costing

Vehicles used under this scheme are hired from private sector. Tenders are invited at district level and further agreements are made on pre-fixed criteria. On an average, two vehicles are available in each block. Rate of contract varied from ₹8,700 per month to ₹17,500 per month. The costs are fixed at ₹150 for a distance up to 25 km and ₹250 beyond that.

As per UNFPA, the average cost per client was ₹377 and average cost per km was ₹9 in 2007. However, due to the increase in number of patients/pregnant women using the services there is a greater utilization of the vehicles and per client trip, cost reduced to ₹248 in 2009–10.

The call centre is part of a model in which the state government has made direct investment. As per state government data, the establishment cost of a call centre is a one-time expenditure of approximately ₹2 lakhs. The running cost is ₹30,000 per month (Agnani 2010).

References

Agnani, M. 2010. 'Janani Express—Low Cost Referral Transport in Madhya Pradesh'. Presentation shared by UNICEF, Madhya Pradesh.

Forster, G., Simfukwe, V. and Barber, C. 2009. 'Use of Intermediate Modes of Transport for Patient Transport: A Literature Review Contrasted with the Findings of the Transaid Bicycle Ambulance Project in Eastern Zambia'. London: Transaid.

Government of India (GoI). 2000. Bulletin on Rural Health Statistics in India, Rural Health Division, MOHFW, GoI.

Government of Madhya Pradesh. 2008. 'Medium Term Health Sector Strategy Madhya Pradesh'. Department of Public Health and Family Welfare, Government of Madhya Pradesh. Available at http://www.health.mp.gov.in/archives/mths.pdf, accessed in April 2011.

National Family Health Survey (NFHS-3) 2005–06. 2007. 'International Institute for Population Sciences (IIPS) and Macro International'. Volume I. Mumbai, India: IIPS.

Thaddeus, S. and Maine, D. 1994. Too Far to Walk: Maternal Mortality in Context. *Social Science and Medicine*, 38(8): 1091–10.

UNICEF. 2010. 'Toolkit—Operating Perinatal Referral Transport Services in Rural India'. UNICEF, India. Available at http://www.unicef.org/india/Referral_Transport_book-Final_PDF.pdf, accessed in 2011.

VikasSamvad. 2008. Status of Child and Maternal Health in Madhya Pradesh and India; A comparative analysis from NFHS-3 report VXZIZ. Available at http://www.righttofoodindia.org/data/status_of_child_and_maternal_health_in_mp_and_india_analysis_from_nhfsIIIreport.pdf, accessed in 2011.

Section B
Addressing Direct Causes of Mortality

Sub-themes

Newborn Care (Hypothermia)
Post-partum Haemorrhage (PPH)

Section B
Addressing Direct Causes of Mortality

Direct causes of maternal and newborn mortality for the purpose of this book have been defined as causes (and innovations to address them) that directly impact the health of a mother and her newborn. The causes—mostly clinical—include haemorrhage, sepsis, pre-eclampsia and eclampsia, unsafe abortion and obstructed labour (WHO 2013). The larger directory of innovations found innovations such as home-based care for newborns, emergency transport, government programmes such as the Janani Suraksha Yojana, delivery huts for women, new technology for baby warmers and emergency obstetric care training (EmOC) which address the direct causes of maternal and newborn mortality.

This section presents two case studies of innovations which respectively address the issue of post-partum haemorrhage (PPH) in women and newborn hypothermia in neonates. Both innovations demonstrate the use of simple technologies and programmes developed around the use of these low-cost technologies towards the management of PPH and newborn hypothermia separately.

The case study on RAKSHA Project illustrates the use of the non-pneumatic anti-shock garment (NASG) in the management of PPH. In 2007, Pathfinder International, a non-government organization (NGO) with support from the MacArthur Foundation implemented the RAKSHA Project towards the management of PPH. The programme used a continuum of care approach towards the management of PPH. It began with strengthening the community's capacity for prevention and management of PPH to developing the skills of health workers towards the identification and management of PPH through the active management of the third stage of labour. The programme included administration of an appropriate drug (uterotonic), use of a Kelly's Pad and the innovative non-pneumatic anti-shock garment (NASG).

The second case study in this section is addressing newborn hypothermia. Newborn hypothermia affects approximately 1.8 million babies born in India. Hypothermia in newborns can lead to death, low IQ, diabetes and heart diseases. Hypothermia can affect any newborn irrespective of the climate in the region of their births. Preterm babies are especially vulnerable to hypothermia. The Embrace infant warmer is a low-cost infant warmer which has been piloted in parts of India. This case study discusses the use and potential scale-up of the Embrace infant warmer at the facility and community level as well as at the level of emergency transportation.

Reference

World Health Organization. 2013. Available at http://www.who.int/mediacentre/factsheets/fs348/en/index.html, accessed on 5 August 2013.

Newborn Care (Hypothermia)

11. Warmth for Newborns: The Embrace Infant Warmer

11

Warmth for Newborns: The Embrace Infant Warmer

Madhavi Misra

Genesis

Embrace started as a classroom exercise for four Stanford University students who were given an assignment to design an incubator that costs less than 1% of the traditional incubators for low birth weight (LBW) babies. The students researched and travelled around India and Nepal and found that even if the traditional incubator is made with low-cost technology, it would require a constant supply of electricity. The need to make cheaper incubators was certainly a worthwhile enterprise, but more importantly this was the crying need to save the lives of babies, especially in developing and underdeveloped countries.

Need

Every year globally, 20 million premature and LBW babies are born; four million of them die and many that survive grow up to have low IQ, diabetes and heart diseases. 1.2 million of these deaths occur in India alone. Some of these health problems could be avoided by providing these babies with warmth. To reduce mortality, clinicians often supplement the infant's innate heat production with an external supply of heat such as an incubator, a radiant warmer, a hot water bottle or a warming blanket (Sherman et al. 2006). By maintaining a stable thermal environment, the infant is given an optimal chance of physical development, thus providing a favourable chance of survival (Sherman et al. 2006). Neonatal hypothermia after birth is a worldwide issue (Costeloe et al. 2000) across all climates (Christensson et al. 1988, Johanson et al. 1992, Tafari and Olsson 1973) and prolonged exposure can lead to harm and in severe cases, death. It is important to keep preterm infants warm immediately after birth, especially during resuscitation. This is problematic even when routine thermal care guidelines are followed. The newborn cannot shiver (Scopes and Tizard 1963) and relies on interventions to protect it against exposure to cold. The ability to maintain equilibrium between heat loss and heat gain (Buczkowski-Bickmann 1992) despite variation in environmental temperatures is restricted during the first-12 hours of life (Smales and Kime 1978). While within the uterus, a constant heat supply from utero-placental circulation provides the foetus with a relatively stable thermal environment, upon birth the infant's transition from a warm, wet uterine environment to a relatively cold, dry extra-uterine environment exacerbates heat loss. Successful adaptation, therefore, requires rapidly elevating heat production immediately after delivery (Gunn and Gluckman 1995). While adaptation is ongoing, the infant is readily susceptible to a net heat loss resulting in a drop in body temperature.

As Rahul Panicker, the founder of Embrace explains,

> Imagine being flung into ice cold water, that is the same level of thermal shock a new born baby feels at a room temperature and these are babies, therefore, struggling for survival soon after birth and these are the babies that we are trying to help through our infant warmer.

After birth, deep body and skin temperature of the preterm newborn can drop at a rate of approximately 0.1°C and 0.3°C per minute respectively unless immediate action is taken. Silverman et al. (1958) showed that reducing heat losses in preterm infants in the first few days after birth increased survival rates. The infant attempts to compensate for heat loss by diverting energy from metabolism for growth into heat production, but this process is usually neither sufficient nor sustainable for ongoing thermal regulation. As such, many infants suffer from hypothermia. Mortality rates of newborn infants are directly correlated with the duration and degree of hypothermia. In particular, LBW infants subjected to periods of hypothermia during neonatal transport have significantly higher mortality rates than those not subjected to hypothermia. Early intervention in the delivery suite is, therefore, of high priority if hypothermia is to be prevented.

Standard Care for Preterm and Low Birth Weight Babies to Prevent Hypothermia

Standard care to prevent hypothermia includes providing a warm delivery room at a minimum of 25°C (although rarely achieved in practice), drying the infant thoroughly, especially the head, immediately after birth, removing any wet blankets, wrapping in a pre-warmed blanket, pre-warming any contact surfaces, eliminating drafts and close proximity to outside walls. Radiant warmers (if available for resuscitation and stabilization) allow easy access and are effective in preventing heat losses, provided that the infant is immediately dried and placed under the pre-warmed heater. Although the infant gains heat by radiation, there are increased potential losses through convection and evaporation and these are exacerbated if the infant is inadequately dried. Servocontrol is advantageous for the avoidance of overheating or under heating if absorption of heat is being obstructed by coverings.

The measures to prevent hypothermia fall into two groups: first are the measures to ensure barriers to heat loss and second is the provision of external heat sources. The first group mainly focusses on reducing evaporative heat losses and includes wraps and head coverings made from a variety of materials such as bubble wraps made of plastic or single layer gowns. These are used alone or in conjunction with radiant warmers or incubators (the second category). The second category also includes the use of heated blankets (where the infant is thoroughly dried and placed on the mother's chest and abdomen with a light blanket around them). These can reduce radiant and conductive heat loss and promote temperature stabilization.

All of these interventions have potential disadvantages, for example, Newton and Watkinson (2003) reported that significantly more infants (with gestational ages less than 30 completed weeks), wrapped in polythene bags were hyperthermic (greater than 37°C) when compared to unwrapped historical controls. Brun et al. (1997) noted that a chemical hot pack during resuscitation of a newborn infant resulted in third-degree burns and recommended that these should not be used unless the peak temperature of the pack is less than 44°C.

Kangaroo mother care (KMC) or skin-to-skin care is a World Health Organization (WHO) recommended practice for preterm or LBW babies. It is a powerful, effective and easy-to-use method to promote the health and well-being of infants born preterm as well as full-term. KMC is given by a mother to her child by placing the child on her bare chest to give warmth from skin to skin, exclusive breastfeeding and giving all necessary care (physical and psychological) to the child without removing the child from the mother's chest.

KMC's key features are:

- Early, continuous and prolonged skin-to-skin contact between the mother and the baby.
- Exclusive breastfeeding (ideally).
- It is initiated in hospital and can be continued at home.
- Small babies can be discharged early.
- Mothers at home require adequate support and follow-up.
- It is a gentle and effective method that avoids the agitation routinely experienced in a busy ward with preterm infants.

History of Incubators

An incubator is an enclosed device with a mechanism underneath, to keep the enclosed space heated. The enclosed space is created by using a transparent material (acrylic/plexiglass/fibreglass) to enclose the space above the baby tray. Air or oxygen is passed through a filter; a humidifier is used as well. Low-noise levels are maintained to avoid harming the baby's hearing. The enclosed space may have provision for armholes, lined with plastic/latex to allow handling and touching the infant, without removing him/her from the heated space (AIIMS 2006).

The incubator was invented in 1891 and innovations in improving the technology continued well into the first half of the 20th century, making a difference to infant care (O'Donnell 1990). Annexure 1 has Table 11A.1 comparing the recent innovations in baby warmers/incubators. These should be seen in the context of providing alternatives to the Embrace infant warmers. Comparison should be made in terms of price, ease of usage and effectiveness.

The group at Stanford University realized that most babies born in the developing word do not have the benefit of using the traditional incubators. A number of reasons are responsible for this, such as the high cost of keeping babies in the incubators, need of constant supply of electricity, large demand for incubators against the short supply of incubators, etc.

Embrace is trying to bridge this gap by innovating to meet the needs of those that live in developing countries, especially in the rural areas. Embrace acknowledges that KMC is one of the best social innovations to have happened in the recent past. It is, however, reported by doctors that compliance is an issue, especially in rural areas, due to issues of cultural sensitivity—having the mother exposed in a setting where privacy is difficult to ensure and convenience—especially when the mother has other chores and multiple children to take care of. Embrace is trying to make mothers feel successful in caring for their babies by enabling KMC for as long as possible and completing the warm chain when KMC is not possible, all while continuing to have the baby close to the mother.

Development of the Embrace Baby Warmer

The Embrace infant warmer is constructed to be similar to a heated water mattress, a device that has proven to be both safe and efficacious (Gray et al. 2004). It looks like a miniature sleeping bag and uses an innovative application of existing phase-changing technology (see Image 11.1). It is expected to be effective, inexpensive, durable, portable and reusable. Moreover, no electricity comes in the vicinity of the baby, thereby bringing an additional element of safety (see Box 11.1).

The phase change material (PCM) maintains a stable temperature (with the temperature never exceeding 40°C) that lasts for at least four hours without the need to be reheated. The PCM pouch is placed in a compartment of the sleeping bag that is separate from, but in thermal contact with the baby. The pouch and the sleeping bag work together to maintain a warm microclimate around the baby and provide warmth through dorsal conduction.

While designing the Embrace baby warmer, the end user was consulted throughout the process. Multiple field trips into rural India were made to understand traditional practices, way of living and perceptions of a product such as Embrace. According to Honey Bajaj, the product designer at Embrace, the product was designed keeping the user as the central figure and not the medical community. It seeks to replicate how the baby feels in a womb (see Box 11.2).

The thought was that the product should not feel like an 'alien device' or be considered as some sort of stigma, especially in rural India. It should have a smooth entry so that acceptability is not a problem. The product was designed and styled keeping all this in mind.

The product was put through a clinical trial in an urban hospital in Bengaluru, Karnataka on 20 LBW babies. The trial did not show any adverse effects of the use of the Embrace baby warmer and, thus, was safe to use on babies. With these results, the study has been expanded to a multi-centre study covering 160 stable, LBW babies.

Annexure 2 explains how the embrace baby warmer works.

Image 11.1
Embrace Infant Warmer with Heater and Wax Pouch

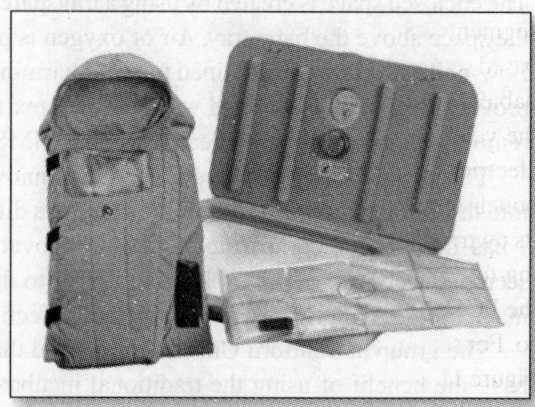

Source: http://www.embraceinnovations.com/, accessed 5 August 2013.

Box 11.1: Types of Embrace Infant Warmers

The Transport Product: The current form of the baby warmer is being also used as a transport device. Here, if the LBW baby is required to be transported intra-hospital or inter-hospital for any laboratory checks or referrals, the baby warmer might be used to keep the baby warm. It is an expensive proposition to use the traditional incubators for transportation within and across hospitals and the Embrace baby warmer is a suitable alternative which is easy to use and cost-effective.

The Rural Product (without use of electricity): Currently, the Embrace baby warmer requires 30 minutes of electricity supply to keep the baby pouch warm for up to four hours at least. Another version of the same warmer is being designed where no electricity usage is required to heat the warm pack. This will typically be used for the rural setting where electricity supply is a problem. This is currently under trial and testing.

Source: Information gathered by PHFI team during site visit at Embrace, May 2011.

Box 11.2: The User's Perspective

'In case of other warmers, they have to only be kept in the hospitals. If it is Embrace then it can be kept at home as well. The parents can be educated and told how to use it at home. Another thing is that other warmers can only be used when there is electricity. With this (Embrace), if there is electricity once, it can be charged and it can be used to maintain temperature for four hours. In these ways it is different from the other warmers ... If we couldn't treat a premature baby at our facility, we need to refer it to another centre for further treatment, to take the baby from here to another place, it would take about an hour and a half. Keeping a baby wrapped only in cloth for that much time does not give us the confidence to maintain the temperature. But after seeing Embrace, we can use it for the babies without any fear and the baby will reach the hospital with the same temperature. Earlier we'd use a 'Bronchator' or other apparatus to maintain temperature and it used to be tough. If we wrap the baby in Embrace, the temperature stays constant and this is very positive.'

Source: Interview with a nurse at Vivekananda Memorial Hospital, May 2011.

Scale-up

Embrace's current outreach strategy is four pronged (see Figure 11.1).

As of now, Embrace is being able to reach segments 1 and 2. In order to reach community-based settings and parents with LBW or preterm babies, it is essential for the team to develop the version of the product which does not use electricity. It may be possible to heat the PCM pouch with boiling water, but that might have its own set of health hazards. The team is working towards devising a simple way of heating the PCM pouch and not using electricity to do so. For scaling-up a product, the cycle shown in Figure 11.2 is followed. In the case of Embrace, the cycle is yet not complete. The technology needs to be piloted, revisions made to the product and then only can it be scaled-up.

Figure 11.1
Embrace's Scale-up Strategy

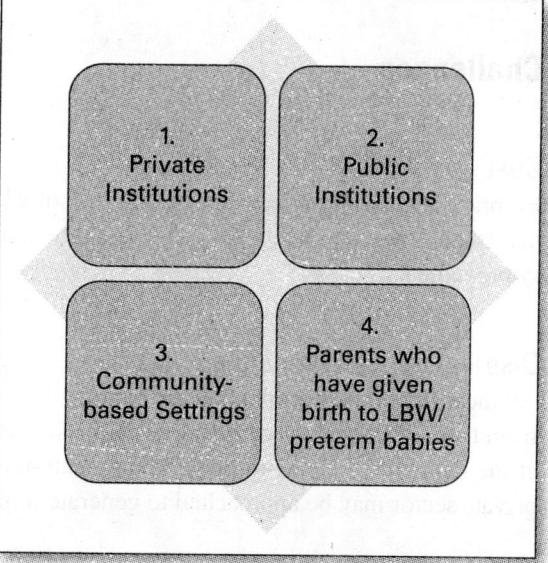

Source: PHFI (2011).

Figure 11.2

Framework for Introduction to Scale-up Technological Innovations

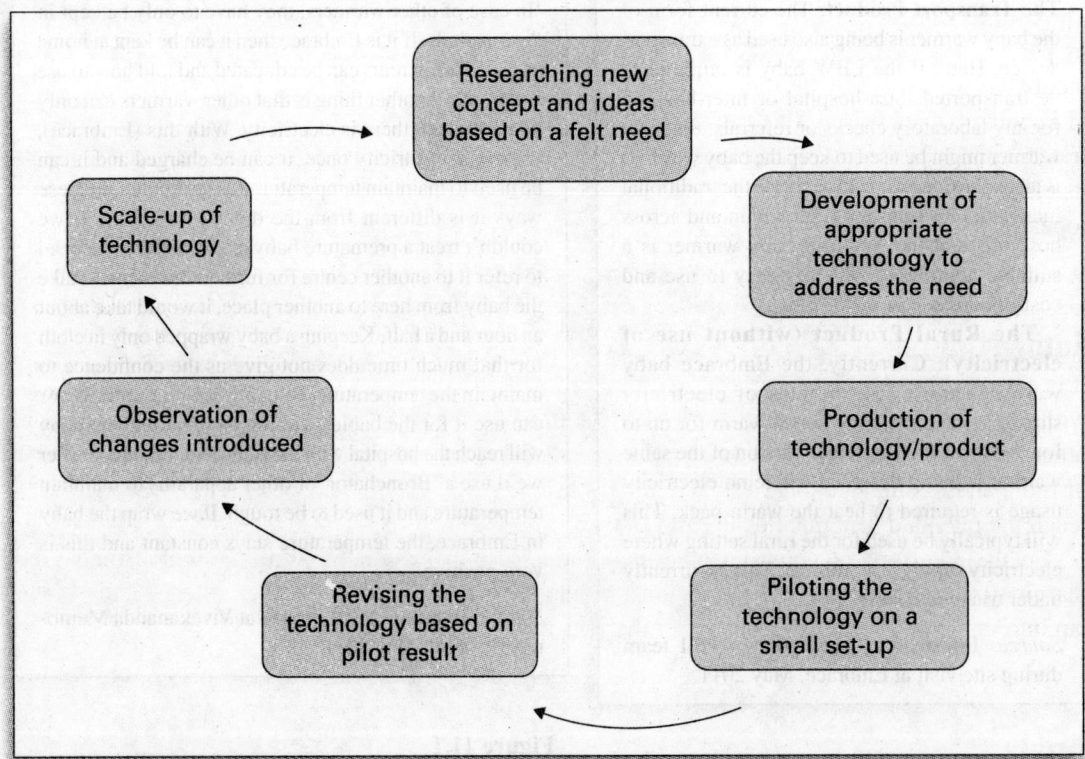

Source: Herzlinger (2006).

Challenges

Cost

Embrace is currently priced at a modest sum of ₹11,000 and can be used up to 250 times. Thus, cost per usage is approximately ₹44. This could be reduced further with increase in volumes and design improvements.

Distribution and Marketing

All the different parts of the unit are put together at an assembling unit in Bengaluru and distributed from there. There is a need for more aggressive marketing and advertising. The strategy employed at the moment is of one-to-one communication and advocating with policymakers. However, the private sector may be approached to generate immediate sales and revenue.

Established methods of care for LBW and pre-term babies and safety concerns of Embrace

The concept of Embrace is new and out-of-the-box. It is a cost-effective method and can be used alike by parents and medical professionals. The established methods such as KMC and use of traditional incubators are trusted by most medical professionals and many are unsure of using the new methods of keeping babies warm. This causes delays in getting the product accepted by the larger medical fraternity. It is primarily for this reason that the various clinical trials are being undertaken to prove its efficacy. Embrace is also ISO 13485 certified and will file for a CE mark to be certified for European standards.

Future Course

It is essential for the Embrace group to now actively distribute their product. Partnerships such as with General Electric (GE) and NOVARTIS will ensure that the product is widely distributed to other cities in India and to different-sized hospitals for wider use. Partnerships with the Government of India and through National Rural Health Mission (NRHM) will be beneficial for this product to reach the intended beneficiaries in rural India.

Focussing efforts on countries other than India, such as Peru and Philippines will also help the marginalized populations in these regions. India is a large country and a huge emerging market to tap into, however, for wider reach other markets may be explored.

Analysis

Embrace is looking to go to scale nationally. The scale-up has been slow so far. Some of the challenges faced in scaling-up by Embrace are that the product still has not been tested in real-life settings as a part of a clinical trial. Experts feel that there is an urgent need for clinical trials on the use and effectiveness of the product prior to marketing and use in real life. The present evidence base in clinical application is inadequate to recommend Embrace in real-life settings in facilities/homes.

The distribution chain of Embrace needs to be strengthened whereby more health facilities can use the product. Partnerships with large companies such as GE and NOVARTIS will be beneficial in the distribution of Embrace infant warmers.

The rural product meant to be used without electricity has not yet been rolled out which is the main need for rural communities and where this innovation will be most beneficial. Embrace will be truly revolutionary when the product is rolled out in communities where it can be used without the use of electricity.

Annexure 1

Table 11A.1
Innovations in Incubators

Project Name	Price	Description	Mechanism
NeoNurture	—	This model was built to address 'access' issues for doctors and caretakers who perform emergency and routine clinical care on at-risk newborns. The prototype includes a detachable bassinette, which can be held in a parent's lap for direct interaction.	Removed from the base, the bassinette can serve as a rocker on any flat surface. The top incorporates button closures and a bacteria-resistant Tyvek® fabric that simulates a blanket covering for the infant and could reduce instances of over-bundling, which is a common problem in Nepal. The bassinette features a clever arrangement of ports and doors, providing doctors, nurses and parents with several access options while minimizing the exposure of the infant to the outside environment. An interior baffle system maintains isolation of the infant's head in all but the most open configuration. Mattress tilt (necessary for relieving acid reflux in newborns) is achieved by shifting the bassinette between carved notches on the curved base. The interface and computer are a modular unit and internal parts, such as heaters and fans, are off-the-shelf components to simplify maintenance. Since power outages are a common occurrence, a backup battery maintains power for the unit until hospital generators turn on.
The Guts	$10	This is a simple replacement for the most vital parts of an infant incubator: a heating element and temperature sensors for the temperature control system and a fan and air filter for air quality and infection control. The system can be used as a substitute for broken heating and filtration elements in existing incubators, which are often donated to hospitals in developing countries without spare parts. The low-cost design would also allow local craftspeople to build their own incubator boxes from locally available materials.	The device consists of a hairdryer heating coil and fan, which is inserted into a rugged Nalgene water bottle, along with an array of thermocouples connected to a controller circuit. The air inlet filter is cut from a standard, disposable, silver-impregnated surgical mask.

(Table 11A.1 Continued)

(Table 11A.1 Continued)

Project Name	Price	Description	Mechanism
mkat	$200	The design is intended to be mounted on a table, saving the materials cost of a base. The hand-access portals feature overlapping neoprene membranes which provide easy access to the child without exposing it to outside elements. The design also features wall panels of translucent plastic that can easily be removed for whole-body access to the child while providing excellent visibility when closed. The entire incubator lid is shaped like a cake box and is easily detachable from the base for emergency access. The housing is designed to be assembled from laser-cut flat stock, meaning that the incubator can be packaged flat for shipping.	
The Life-raft Incubator	$625	This device is a fully functioning incubator prototype that assists in thermo-regulation for a newborn child. This model is designed for easy assembly and repair as it has a detachable heated waterbed, modular electronics (including the alarm signal) which can be swapped out if they break and a cylindrical canopy that can be formed from a single sheet of plastic.	The portals are sealed by a latch that can be opened by elbows and the split canopy is designed to allow medics to access the upper or lower half of the baby, without exposing the whole baby to the open air. The bunting heating trap keeps the baby warm, while a safety strap secures him/her in place. On its base, the incubator has handles for easy transportability and an unambiguous digital display showing vital statistics such as temperature and humidity. To assist with thermo-regulation of the infant, the canopy consists of a double wall of plastic and there is a heated waterbed that acts as thermal mass and provides heat backup in case of a power outage.
Temperature Control System	—	The system consists of stationary thermistors, which are mounted to the exterior and interior of the incubator with a third mounted on a probe that is taped to the infant's abdomen. The existing system will easily incorporate two more thermistors and heat transfer models and experimental results will be used to create a heating algorithm that takes into account all three measured temperatures.	The sensors are interpreted using an Arduino board, which serves as the platform for all of the sensors and controls that make up the basic operation of the incubator. The Arduino board is an inexpensive physical computing platform with its own programming environment. The existing system prototype is able to measure the resistance of one thermistor and convert this value to degrees Celsius. If this value is too low, a light-emitting diode (LED) representing the heater is lit. If the value lies out of a safe range, either too high or too low, an alarm sounds.

Source: http://designthatmatters.org/news/dtm-blog/project/incubator/, accessed on 5 August 2013.

Annexure 2

Figure 11A.1
How to Use the Embrace Baby Warmer

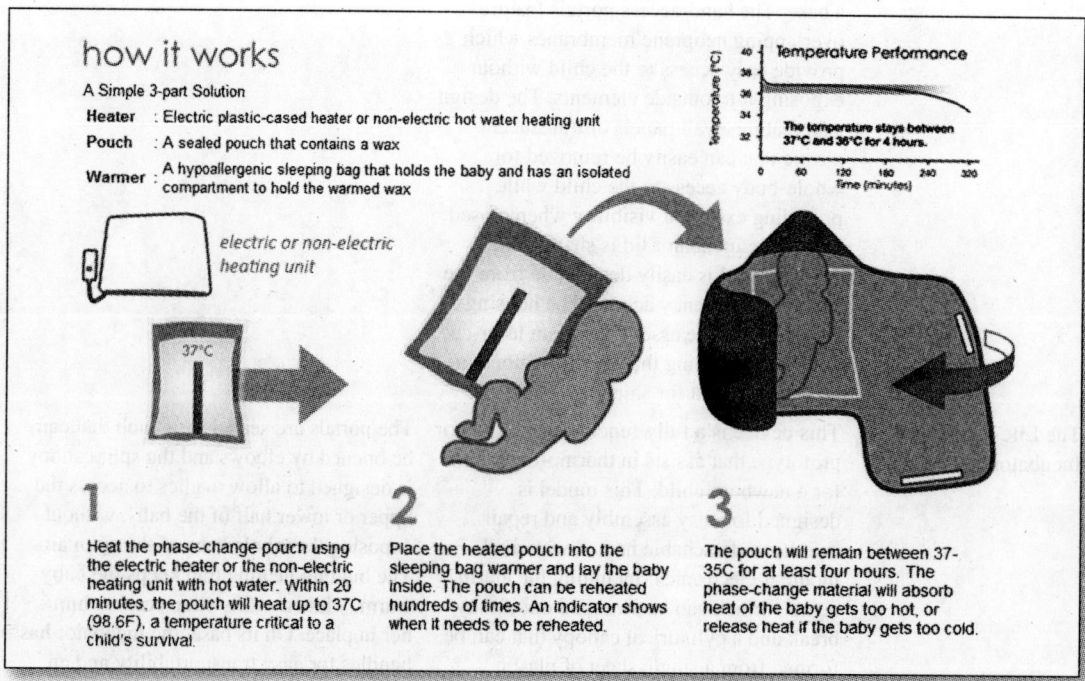

Source: www.embraceglobal.org, accessed on 5 August 2013.

References

All India Institute of Medical Sciences (AIIMS). 2006. 'Incubators'. WHO Collaboration Centre for Training and Research on Newborn Care, Department of Pediatrics, AIIMS. Available at: http://www.newbornwhocc.org/nicu.htm, accessed 5 August 2013.

Brun, C., Stokvad P. and Alsbjorn B.F. 1997. 'Burn Wounds after Resuscitation of a Newborn Girl'. *Ugeskrift for Laeger*, 159(44): 6531–2.

Buczkowski-Bickmann, M.K. 1992. 'Thermoregulation in the Neonate and the Consequences of Hypothermia'. *CRNA: The Clinical Forum for Nurse Anesthetists*, 3: 77–82.

Costeloe, K., Hennessy, E., Gibson, A.T., Marlow, N. and Wilkinson, A.R. 2000. 'The EPICure Study: Outcomes to Discharge from Hospital for Infants Born at the Threshold of Viability'. *Pediatrics*, 106: 659–71.

Christensson, K., Bhat, G.J., Amadi, B.C., Eriksson, B. and Hojer, B. 1998. 'Randomised Study of Skin-to-skin versus Incubator Care for Rewarming Low-risk Hypothermic Neonates'. *Lancet*, 352: 1115.

Gray, P.H., Paterson, S., Finch, G. and Hayes, M. 2004. 'Cot-nursing Using a Heated, Water-Filled Mattress and Incubator Care: A Randomized Clinical Trial'. *Acta Paediatrica*, 93(3): 350–5.

Gunn, T.R. and Gluckman, P.D. 1995. 'Perinatal Thermogenesis'. *Early Human Development*, 42: 169–83.

Johanson, R.B., Spencer, S.A., Rolfe, P., Jones, P. and Malla, D.S. 1992. 'Effect of Post-delivery Care on Neonatal Body Temperature'. *ActaPaediatrica*, 81: 859–63.

Newton, T. and Watkinson, M. 2003. 'Preventing Hypothermia at Birth in Preterm Babies: At a Cost of Overheating Some?' *Archives of Disease in Childhood Foetal and Neonatal Edition*, 88(3): F256.

O'Donnell, J. 1990. 'The Development of a Climate For Caring: A Historical Review of Premature Care in the United States from 1900 to 1979'. *Neonatal Network*, 8(6): 7–17.

Scopes, J.W. and Tizard, J.P. 1963. 'The Effect of Intravenous Noradrenaline on the Oxygen Consumption of New-Born Mammals'. *Journal of Physiology*, 165: 305–26.

Sherman, et al. 2006. 'Optimising the Neonatal Thermal Environment'. *Neonatal Network*, 24(4): 251–59.

Silverman, W., Fertig, J., Berger, A. 1958. 'The Influence of the Thermal Environment upon the Survival of Newly Born Premature Infants'. *Pediatrics*, 22: 876–86.

Smales, O.R.C. and Kime, R. 1978. 'Thermoregulation in Babies Immediately after Birth'. *Archives of Disease in Childhood*, 53: 58–61.

Tafari, N. and Olsson, E. 1973. 'Neonatal Cold Injury in the Tropics'. *Ethiopian Medical Journal*, 11: 57–65.

Post-partum Haemorrhage (PPH)

12. Use of Non-pneumatic Anti-shock Garment (NASG): The Raksha Project

12

Use of Non-pneumatic Anti-shock Garment (NASG): The Raksha Project

Madhavi Misra

Introduction and Background

The biomedical causes of maternal mortality are well recognized (see Figure 12.1). Three quarters of maternal mortalities result from the direct obstetric complications of haemorrhage, infection, obstructed labour, hypertensive disorders of pregnancy and septic abortion. The rest are due to other 'direct' obstetric causes such as pulmonary embolism or ectopic pregnancy or 'indirect' causes that are aggravated by pregnancy, such as malaria, hepatitis, diabetes mellitus and heart diseases. Worldwide, the most common cause of maternal mortality is haemorrhage, but the proportion due to each cause varies between regions.

It is estimated that approximately 40% of women and girls may suffer an acute problem during pregnancy and 9 to 15% may experience a problem needing higher level care. Appropriate and timely intervention from a trained professional could prevent the majority of maternal deaths.

Figure 12.1
Global Estimates of the Causes of Maternal Deaths 1997–2007

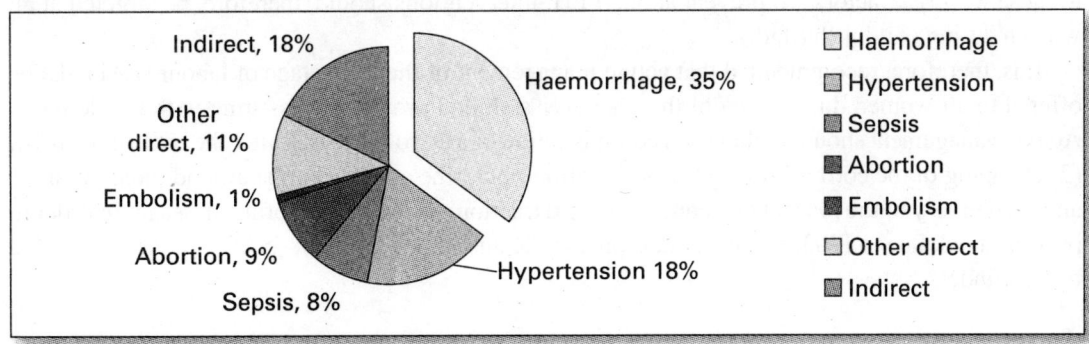

Source: World Health Organization and UNICEF (2010).

Table 12.1
Time to Death for Most Common Obstetric Emergencies

Cause of Death	Time to Death
Post-partum haemorrhage	Two hours
Ante-partum haemorrhage	12 hours
Ruptured Uterus	One day
Eclampsia (severe hypertensive disorder of pregnancy)	Two days
Obstructed Labour	Three days
Infection	Six days

Source: Duffy (2007).

Table 12.1 illustrates that maternal mortalities do not occur instantaneously. If a system is in place to recognize problems promptly and to transport a woman to a health care facility where she can receive appropriate and timely treatment, then the majority of maternal mortalities could be avoided.

As can be seen from Table 12.1, the major cause of maternal mortality (direct) is post-partum haemorrhage, it is also the quickest to cause death (two hours) if left unattended.

Post-partum Haemorrhage

Bleeding after childbirth (post-partum haemorrhage) is an important cause of maternal mortality, accounting for nearly a quarter of all maternal deaths worldwide. Common causes for post-partum haemorrhage (PPH) include failure of the uterus to contract adequately after birth leading to atonic PPH, tears of the genital tract leading to traumatic PPH and bleeding due to retention of placental tissue. Atonic PPH is the most common cause of PPH and the leading cause of maternal death.[1]

According to the World Health Organization (WHO), risk factors for PPH include grand multiparity and multiple gestations. Attempts have been made to identify women at risk of atonic PPH based on historical or clinical factors and steps are planned to prevent it in this allegedly high-risk group of women. Unfortunately, atonic PPH can occur even in women without identifiable, clinical or historical risk factors. Numerically, more women without risk factors have atonic PPH compared to those with risk factors. To prevent atonic PPH, interventions should, therefore, be targeted at all women during childbirth (ibid.).

It is, therefore, recommended that active management of the third stage of labour (AMTSL) be offered to all women during childbirth, whenever a skilled provider is assisting with the delivery. Active management should include: (1) administration of a uterotonic soon after the birth of the baby, (2) clamping of the cord following the observation of uterine contraction (at around three minutes) and (3) delivery of the placenta by controlled cord traction, followed by uterine massage. In order to prevent shock due to PPH, the use of non-pneumatic anti-shock garment (NASG) is recommended by Pathfinder.

---

[1]WHO Recommendations. Available at http://www.who.int/maternal_child_adolescent/topics/maternal/en/index.html, accessed in August 2012.

The use of NASG to prevent shock is the immediate first-aid treatment device for reversing hypovolumic shock in pregnant women suffering from shock due to PPH during transportation and also in the facilities along with other management protocol for the shock.[2]

Raksha Project

The main focus of the project is to improve essential and emergency obstetric care (EmOC) services by addressing the issues of the community and the health system together, systematically, and with close collaboration taking place among all stakeholders. This ensures that communities and health care providers work together to overcome the complex challenges found in the past, with the long-term goal of ensuring that pregnant women receive appropriate and timely care. The community mobilization efforts include establishing partnerships among key community leaders, families, caregivers, front-line health workers and key stakeholders instrumental in expanding the reach of maternal health services, bringing them as close to home as possible.

In light of the fact that post-partum haemorrhage was not being given due importance, Pathfinder International implemented the Raksha Project in 2007 in India to address this. This project was supported by the John D. and Catherine T. MacArthur Foundation using the clinical and community action model to address post-partum haemorrhage. The use of NASG is an important part of this project.

Pathfinder International was influenced by the fact that the great majority of maternal deaths would be preventable if women had access to skilled providers in well-equipped facilities. Unfortunately, poverty, isolation, lack of knowledge and access to a skilled provider or a well-equipped facility continue to pose serious barriers in many countries. While good-quality care must be made available, challenges lie in transforming long-held traditions and entrenched misconceptions that hinder the adoption of healthy behaviours.

Pathfinder International made use of the data on very high maternal deaths due to PPH in order to develop its *Raksha* (meaning protection) Project, to provide Continuum of Care to women to reduce morbidity and mortality associated with PPH. The project focusses on prevention and care from the community level—where women are most likely to give birth at home or in poorly equipped health centres—to higher level facilities where they can receive care for complications. The Raksha Project's community mobilization strategy created an enabling environment by orienting community and household-level decision-makers, as well as by disseminating key health messages through the active involvement of approximately 4,000 front-line health workers and five local non-governmental organizations (NGOs). The Continuum of Care approach to manage PPH in the Raksha model includes the following:

- The active management of the third stage of labour and administration of an appropriate drug (uterotonic).
- Use of a Kelly's Pad (which measures blood loss and can signal when a woman is in danger).
- The NASG which is placed on a woman already in shock to control PPH until she reaches EmOC.
- Improved communication and transportation systems to move women to emergency care on time.

[2]Pathfinder International Project Documents, 2011.

The Raksha Project is currently being implemented in Rajasthan, Bihar, Maharashtra and Tamil Nadu. The project has achieved success in improving maternal health in these four states through building partnerships, supporting and strengthening health systems and promoting skilled attendance during birth at all levels.

Significant Achievements of Raksha Project

- Project evidence shows increased use of AMTSL, timely/proper management of PPH with uterotonic treatment and blood transfusion and use of the NASG for shock cases in intervention facilities.
- Facilities are using guidelines and protocols for improved management of obstetric complications and an improved referral system.
- Six thousand one hundred and fifty three public and private service providers have been trained in the four states. Training of 948 auxiliary nurse midwives (ANMs)/general nursing midwives (GNMs) at the subcentre level emerged as a cost-effective and successful example of task sharing with potential for scale-up to prevent PPH.
- Fifty eight percent of the intervention villages organized a system for transporting emergency referrals.
- Streamlining of procurement systems through use of the Health Management Information System (HMIS) and inventory check lists for ensuring that uterotonics and other essential supplies are in place.
- Supportive ongoing supervision undertaken jointly by project staff and government officials to promote ownership of improving the quality of service at facilities.
- Till date, three memorandums of understanding (MoUs) have been signed (Tamil Nadu, Rajasthan and Bihar) for project scale-up and to provide evidence of Pathfinder's ability and leadership to integrate innovation in the public health system.
- Invested in improving provision of essential equipments such as PPH shock kit, Kelly's Pad, NASG, etc., and strengthening the network for communication and connectivity for emergency and referral transport from home to hospital, by creating a birth preparedness and complication readiness (BPCR) plan at every household in 1,144 villages.

Genesis and Description of Non-pneumatic Anti-shock Garments

The Raksha Project's approach to use NASG to prevent shock goes back a long way. Associate Professor Suellen Miller from the University of California, San Francisco (USCF) proposed a novel first-aid device called the non-pneumatic anti-shock garment originally designed by NASA in the 1970s, to curb blood loss en route to the hospital.[3] UCSF researchers at the Women's Global

---

[3]Pathfinder International Project Documents, 2011.

Image 12.1
Non-pneumatic Anti-shock Garment

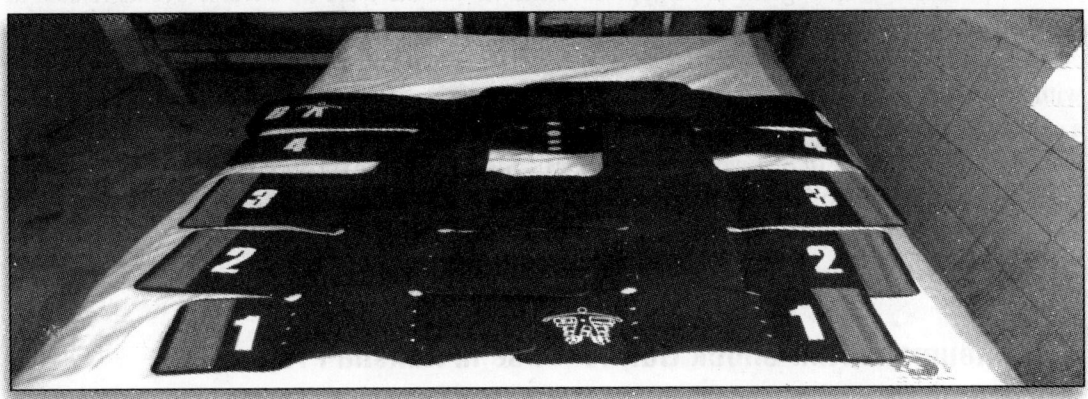

Source: Pathfinder International, 2011.

Health Imperative have been working on an innovative programme of low-cost interventions to treat obstetric haemorrhage in developing countries. The project took a giant leap forward when the MacArthur Foundation pledged $10.75 million to Pathfinder International for the UCSF programme in Nigeria and India.

NASG is made of stretchy, lightweight neoprene. Resembling the bottom half of a wet suit, the garment applies pressure to the lower limbs, pelvis and abdomen via its five velcro closures (see Image 12.1). The NASG is fairly simple and easy to use by any medical or non-medical person with one-hour training in applying NASG. As a part of the Raksha Project, each garment costs only about ₹15,000 or $320 and can be reused up to 50 times. The NASG is safer than traditional anti-shock garments. Because the NASG uses lower pressure, it does not cause compartment syndrome or ischemia (ibid.).

The NASG can be used to manage any condition where there is severe bleeding below the diaphragm. It can be used with all forms of obstetric haemorrhage (in excess of 750 ml) (as long as the foetus is not viable in utero, i.e., the foetus is not alive).

The NASG has a dual mode of action:

1. **Resuscitation of Central Circulating Volume**: Provides mild pressure, pushing blood from the lower extremities into central circulation, making sure there is sufficient blood reaching vital organs, including the brain. This results in translocation of 1.5–2.0 litres of blood from the lower body to the head and chest.
2. **Reduces Haemorrhage in Lower Body**: The foam ball over the abdomen applies pressure to the blood vessels of the uterus, decreasing blood flow. During shock, blood normally pools in the lower half of the body; by applying up to 30–40 mmHg of circumferential pressure, the NASG helps shunt blood back to the organs that need it most: the brain, heart and lungs.

Please refer Annexure 1 for application and removal of NASG.

Non-pneumatic Anti-shock Garment: Evidence from Other Countries

Various pilot studies in Nigeria and Egypt have shown that there are no adverse events related to NASG use. One such pilot study, published in the British Journal of Obstetrics and Gynaecology, compared 158 women given standard treatment (oxytocin + syntometrine)[4] for obstetric haemorrhage with 208 women who received standard treatment plus the anti-shock garment. Results demonstrated a statistically significant 50% decrease in blood loss among those treated with the NASG.

A post NASG study of 854 women in four tertiary centres of Egypt and two facilities in Nigeria conducted from 2004 to 2008 has shown that there is a reduction in measured blood loss by 50% and adverse outcomes decreased from 12.1% to 4.1%.[5]

Non-pneumatic Anti-shock Garment Use in Raksha Project and its Impact

Pathfinder has introduced NASG in a phased manner since 2008 in four states of India—Tamil Nadu, Maharashtra, Rajasthan and Bihar as part of the Raksha Project. As per the project records, it has been significantly instrumental in saving lives.

Pathfinder is working in 53 facilities to ensure the use of project technologies to prevent and manage PPH and also completed clinical training of service providers in March 2010. Subsequently, from April 2010, the project team began tracking quarterly data for clinical indicators.

The Raksha Project has had overall success in the last couple of years. All the technical interventions are being increasingly used (as depicted by the trends analysis since 2010 in Figure 12.2) and there has been a reduction in case fatality rates at the intervention facilities. The incidence of hypovolemic shock has declined over time because of increased usage of NASG and the increasing usage of AMTSL combined with the decrease in the number of PPH and shock cases, which has led to a reduction in maternal deaths attributable to PPH, indicating a promising trend.

As shown in Figure 12.2, data collected in intervention areas from April 2010 to March 2012 indicates that maternal deaths attributable to PPH have reduced by 5%. NASG use per shock case has gone up by 31% and shock cases due to PPH have reduced from 17% to 14%. This indicates that NASG use has seen an upward trend at facility level in the two years after implementation of the Raksha Project.

A significant proportion of Pathfinder-trained providers has accepted the project protocols and technological innovations and has started practicing them routinely. They have access to appropriate information and technologies such as Kelly's Pad and NASG that help prevent PPH, that help in the timely identification of PPH and that also help in the appropriate management of the cases. As a result, there will be changes in the incidence of PPH at the facilities. Initially, PPH incidence was high due to better identification but eventually there was significant decline (7.1 to 5%) because of the better practice of AMTSL (70%) by providers.

---

[4]Available at http://apps.who.int/rhl/pregnancy_childbirth/childbirth/postpartum_haemorrhage/sfcom/en/index.html, accessed 3 August 2013.

[5]Pathfinder International Project Documents, 2011.

Figure 12.2

Annual Trends of NASG Usage and Maternal Mortality (in %)

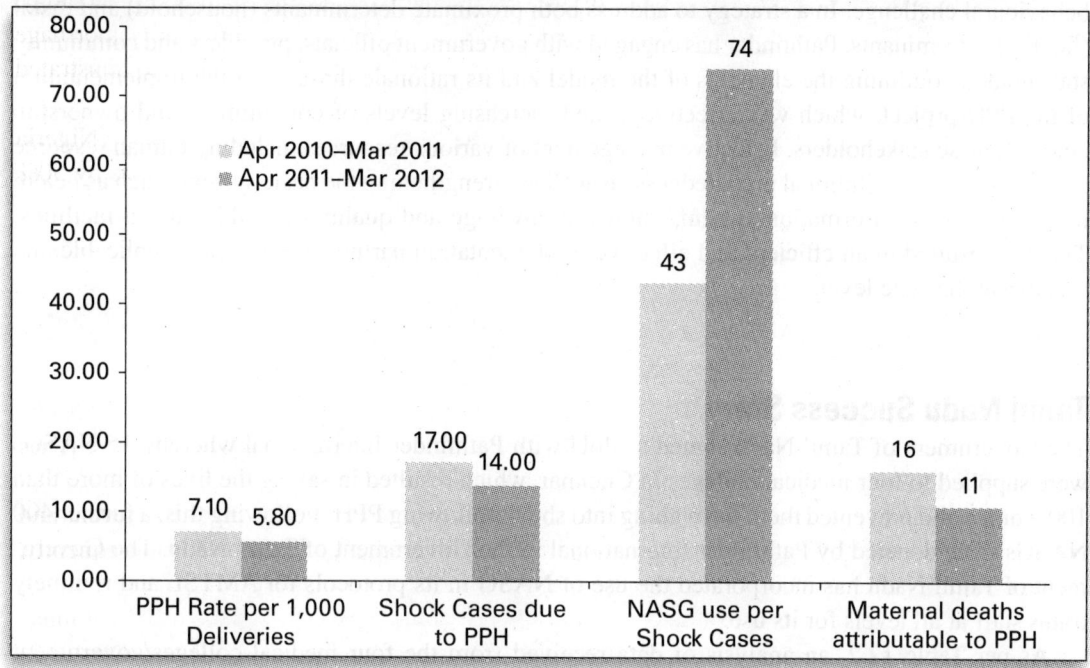

Source: Pathfinder International (2012).

The incidence of shock declined over time during the same duration because of appropriate treatment given to the women who develop PPH. Ninety seven percent of pregnant women are receiving uterotonics and 68% are transfused with blood during the shock.

It is encouraging to see an increased use of NASG for women with shock, which has over time, led to reduced fatality from shock. It is evident that the reduction in maternal death has been due to the multiplicative effect of the reduction in the (a) incidence of PPH, (b) incidence of shock and (c) fatality from PPH due to better management and treatment and the use of NASG. In the intervention facilities, NASG use helps treat shock, resuscitate, stabilize and prevent further bleeding in women with any form of obstetric haemorrhage and helps clinicians to stabilize patients in shock before they get definitive treatment or are transferred to higher levels of health care facilities.

This is a major shift in mindset—a change that has not been easy to bring about. In comparison to the first year of intervention, increased usage of NASG in shock cases can be attributed to:

- Identification of potential champions at the facility level.
- Regular sensitization of postgraduate students/resident doctors of medical colleges who are among the most important stakeholders to improve management for the complication of PPH.
- Increased clarity amongst service providers about actions needed to prevent PPH/shock related morbidity and mortality.
- Sharing of best practices and success stories amongst the facilities, districts and states.

The Raksha model has attracted the attention of health officials and providers in many states because it acknowledges the reality that PPH must be dealt with as both a clinical and a social/behavioural challenge. In a strategy to address both proximate determinants (household) and distal (facility) determinants, Pathfinder has engaged with government officials, providers and community stakeholders, outlining the elements of the model and its rationale throughout the implementation of the PPH project, which was effective in and increasing levels of commitment and ownership amongst these stakeholders. Effective management of various resources including human resource deployment and institutional preparedness, as well as strengthening the basic systems such as health management and information system, improved coverage and quality of health care in facilities. This has resulted in an efficient and effective implementation partnership, which is replicable and scalable at the state level.

Tamil Nadu Success Story

The Government of Tamil Nadu signed a MoU with Pathfinder International whereby 15 NASGs were supplied to four medical colleges in Chennai, which resulted in saving the lives of more than 100 women and prevented them from going into shock following PPH. Following this, a further 400 NASGs were donated by Pathfinder International to the Government of Tamil Nadu. The Government of Tamil Nadu has incorporated the use of NASG in its protocols for AMTSL and routinely trains staff at all levels for its use.

As per Table 12.2, an analysis of data received from the four medical colleges/government hospitals in Chennai over a period of seven months (June to December 2009) revealed a significant reduction of PPH cases and deaths related to PPH. The four institutions were the Tamil Nadu Institute of Obstetrics and Gynaecology, Kilpauk Medical College, RSRM Hospital and the Kasturba Gandhi Hospital, Chennai.

Now the Government of Tamil Nadu is in the process of scaling-up the intervention throughout the state. Following a request from the government, Pathfinder International donated another 800 NASGs and currently all the Emergency Management and Research Institute (EMRI) ambulances in the state, all the comprehensive care facilities and 117 primary health centres (PHCs) are provided

Table 12.2

Data on Deliveries in Four Government Hospitals in Chennai and Use of NASG on PPH Cases

Period	Deliveries	PPH Cases	% of PPH Cases	Total Maternal Deaths	Maternal Deaths from PPH	NASG Applied	% of Maternal Deaths from PPH
2009	28,530	410	1.44%	43	9	2	21%
2010	24,964	274	1.10%	31	6	12	19%
2011	27,702	226	0.82%	27	5	25	18%
2012 (till August)	16,282	136	0.93%	17	3	15	17%

Source: Government of Tamil Nadu, August 2012.

Table 12.3
Consolidated Report from Select Districts in Tamil Nadu from November 2011 to April 2012

Period	PHCs	Deliveries	PPH Cases	Shock from PPH	Total Maternal Deaths	Maternal Deaths from PPH	% of PPH Deaths
PHCs	535	49,721	393	42	95	29	29%
PHCs with NASG	117	9,316	87	15	12	2	18%

Source: Government of Tamil Nadu, August 2012.

with the NASGs. All front-line personnel have been trained in Tamil Nadu on the usage of NASG—its application, removal, disinfection and storage.

As per Table 12.3, consolidated reports received from these districts show a significant reduction in deaths from PPH in the intervention facilities when compared to non-intervention facilities.

The widespread usage of NASGs was made possible through the active support of the Director Public Health and the Health Secretary. The placing of NASG in an ambulance is a unique feature as it is during referral for PPH that the use of NASG is most needed. The statewide use of NASG will ensure reduction in maternal deaths due to shock and has the potential to demonstrate, for the first time in the world, the impact of scale-up of this technology in saving mothers' lives.[6]

The scaling-up of NASG by Tamil Nadu can be attributed to the state having a well-developed public health system with a dedicated public health cadre and adaptive processes. Their willingness to change some of their processes to incorporate the Continuum of Care approach and their willingness to invest in that approach, also contributed to the scale-up. Their public health officials as well as their service providers were willing to accept the capacity building provided and, therefore, the use of NASG to manage PPH became a part of the protocols to be followed by all medical facilities. Rajasthan and Bihar are also very committed to reducing maternal mortality. However, in these states, in terms of the systems, there remain some serious challenges. Pathfinder International's experience was that in Rajasthan and Bihar the service provider's attitudes, abilities and capabilities to accept this Continuum of Care and to practice it consistently were somewhat different from those of the providers in Tamil Nadu. So operationally, Pathfinder was committed to spending a fair amount of time in training and capacity building, not just the providers but also the supervisory staff and the bureaucracy, as well as advocating with the government to make an investment in this intervention.

Discussion and Conclusion

Closely linked with quality of care efforts, the Raksha Project reinforces key health system components such as building human capacity through competency-based training, implementation of standardized and evidence-based practices such as AMTSL and introduction of novel and innovative technologies such as NASG, which most directly affect the quality and sustainability of technical interventions.

[6]Pathfinder International Project Documents, 2011.

Evidence has shown that the increasing usage of AMTSL to decrease PPH and use of NASG to decrease cases of shock are helping lower maternal deaths attributable to PPH.

While it has been effectively demonstrated that NASG has tremendous scope for saving lives, it is quite expensive. It can, however, be used upto 30–50 times and then the cost is about $7.2 per unit. Prior to an all-India scale-up, it is important to ascertain the cost-effectiveness and efficacy of the NASG compared to the alternate forms of preventing PPH. One intervention that has been promoted as effective in preventing atonic PPH is the AMTSL. This intervention was described in the Cochrane Review as a package comprising the following interlocking interventions: administration of a prophylactic uterotonic after delivery of the baby and usually also early cord clamping and cutting and controlled cord traction of the umbilical cord.

According to the International Confederation of Midwives (ICM) and the International Federation of Gynaecology and Obstetrics (FIGO), the usual components of active management include administration of uterotonic agents, controlled cord traction and uterine massage after delivery of the placenta, as appropriate; while in WHO's Integrated Management of Pregnancy and Childbirth Guidelines, the steps in active management of third stage of labour involve giving oxytocin immediately, delivery of the placenta by controlled cord traction and uterine massage.[7]

Misoprostol and oxytocin seem to be the most preferred drugs. Injectable oxytocin has been recommended for routine use in the AMTSL; however, administration of an injection requires skills and sterile equipment for safe administration (Mathai et al. 2007). Oxytocin may be inactivated if exposed to high ambient temperatures. Misoprostol, a prostaglandin analogue with uterotonic effects, is reportedly more stable than oxytocin and has been administered by oral, sublingual and rectal routes in several studies. Suggestions have been made to provide misoprostol tablets, where oxytocin is not available, to non-skilled providers and to women themselves for the prevention of PPH; however, there are concerns that misuse of misoprostol can lead to significant maternal morbidity and even death (Mathai et al. 2007).

Scale-up of NASG as a Frugal Innovation

This combination of challenges and opportunities in emerging markets is producing a cocktail of creativity, which is now referred to as 'frugal innovation'. Because so many consumers are still poor, companies have to go for volume, focus on practical utility and affordable price. The term is used in India and other developing economies to describe innovation that minimizes costs by creating frugal solutions to deliver improved or previously non-existent public services. Frugal innovation has given more people access to a wider range of services. Frugal innovation as a terminology may be used to describe NASG.

The garment is a new technology which has been introduced in emerging markets such as India. The scale-up of such a frugal innovation is dependent on factors such as costs and availability of the product. Currently, the garment is too expensive and hard to procure for many countries with limited resources. To reduce costs, Pathfinder International experts are focussing on the costs of production,

[7]WHO Recommendations. Available at http://www.who.int/maternal_child_adolescent/topics/maternal/en/index.html, accessed in August 2012.

from raw materials through manufacturing, transport and delivery. They are also evaluating regulatory factors that might speed up or slowdown widespread use of the garment. This includes developing an efficient and cost-effective shipping plan to get the garment from manufacturers to the places where it is needed most. Especially for states such as Tamil Nadu which are wanting to scale-up the use of NASG at state level by providing the garments to all the facilities, importing the garment might prove expensive. There seems to be a positive move towards reducing the cost of manufacturing NASG which will be of immense benefit as they will be widely used across underdeveloped and developing countries. NASG is being manufactured currently in India at a cost of $65 which is much less than the cost of the NASG procured by Pathfinder. This is a positive move towards reducing costs. A Chinese manufacturer in Hong Kong is producing it at $57 per NASG.

The NASG has been positioned in a way whereby it fits the Continuum of Care approach. NASG is not an invasive intervention, it is fairly easy to use and anyone with a one-time training can be adept at administering the garment. One is tempted to view the NASG as a panacea for PPH, at the risk of ignoring the other important services that are essential. The garment only sustains a woman in crisis—she still requires the skilled intervention of a trained physician in a facility equipped to deal with an emergency. Blood replacement is essential and a reliable and available blood bank is of the utmost importance.

Annexure 1: Applying the NASG

Figure 12A.1
Applying the Non-pneumatic Anti-shock Garment

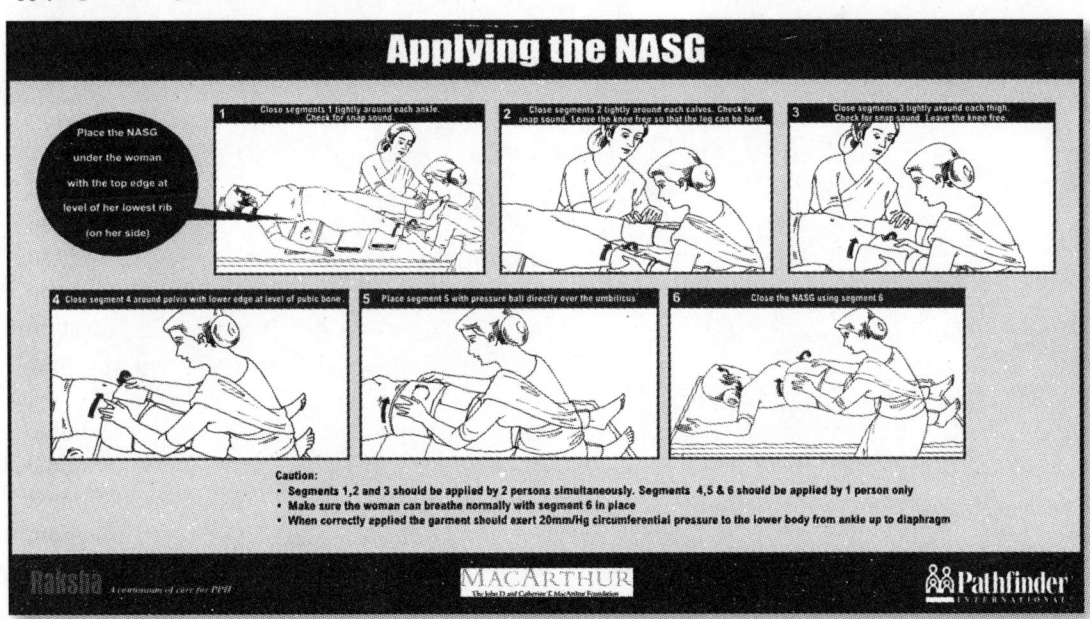

Source: Pathfinder International (2011).

Figure 12A.2
Removing the Non-pneumatic Anti-shock Garment

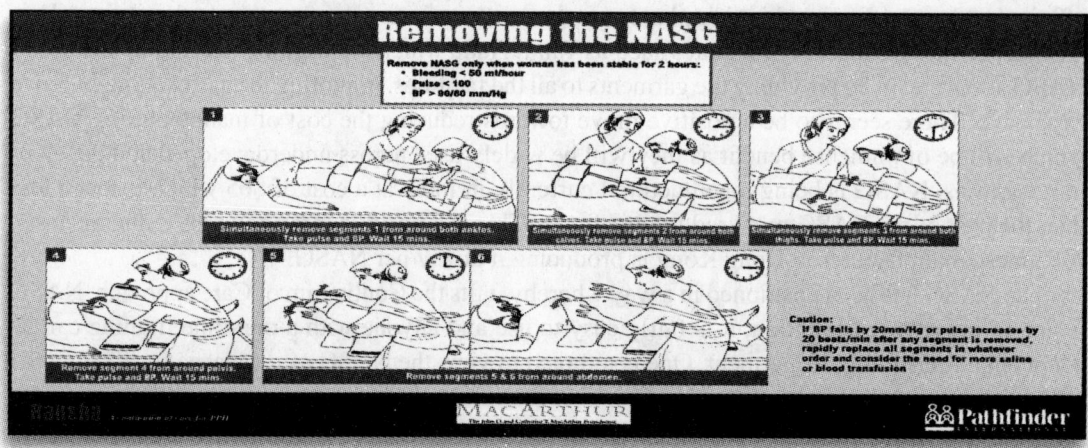

Source: Pathfinder International (2011).

References

Duffy, S. 2007. 'Obstetric Haemorrhage in Gimbie, Ethiopia'. *The Obstetrician & Gynaecologist*, 9: 121–26.

Mathai, M., Gülmezoglu, M. and Hill, S. 2007. 'Saving Women's Lives: Evidence-based Recommendations for the Prevention of Post-partum Haemorrhage'. *Bulletin of World Health Organization*, 85(4): 322–23.

WHO and UNICEF. 2010. 'Countdown to 2015 Decade Report (2000–2010) with Country Profiles: Taking Stock of Maternal, Newborn and Child Survival'. WHO and UNICEF, Geneva.

Section C
Addressing Indirect Causes of Maternal and Newborn Mortality

Sub-themes

Family Planning
Community-based Intersectoral Interventions in Health
Youth Reproductive and Sexual Health

Section C
Addressing Indirect Causes of Maternal and Newborn Mortality

This section presents innovations—clinical, non-clinical and programmatic—that target areas that impact the health and development of a community and the individual indirectly, often through a distal route. Intervention at this level can impact the health and well-being of mothers and their newborns. Innovations such as these, addressing indirect causes of maternal and newborn health, include education and awareness on health issues, community-based interventions, sanitation, family planning and youth health in the larger directory.

Intersectoral interventions in health seek to bring together different areas of public health towards achieving common health goals. Two programmes illustrated in a case study under the sub-theme of intersectoral interventions in health attempt to describe the use of community-based interventions targeting women, men and adolescents, health and sanitation programmes, nutrition and awareness towards creating overall behaviour change that indirectly impact social factors influencing health (level of education, status of women, early marriage, early childbirth and others). The case study on Comprehensive Rural Health Project, Jamkhed (CRHP) and the Community-led Initiatives for Child Survival (CLICS) from Maharashtra are examples of intersectoral interventions in health with an emphasis on the use of the community towards improving maternal and newborn health indicators.

Family planning is crucial towards empowering men and women to delay birth of their first child, space out children and prevent pregnancies—all crucial towards ensuring a healthy pregnancy, healthy delivery and a healthy newborn. The PRACHAR Programme by Pathfinder International seeks to improve family planning by creating awareness on family planning, making family planning socially acceptable and empowering men and women on their reproductive rights, along with improving other intersectoral elements such as education of young girls, menstrual and reproductive health knowledge of young women and men and other issues. This case study is a glimpse into the activities of the PRACHAR Programme in the Gaya District of Bihar.

Interventions in the area of Youth Reproductive Sexual Rights are crucial towards ensuring that young people develop into healthy adults—healthy parents with healthy children. This case study features three kinds of youth-friendly clinics or centres—operated by an NGO, tertiary-care hospital and government—that aim to provide young people with a safe space to learn about reproductive health and to access clinical and non-clinical health services.

Family Planning

13. Promoting Change in Reproductive Behaviour: PRACHAR

13

Promoting Change in Reproductive Behaviour: PRACHAR

Sanghita Bhattacharya and Radhika Arora

Background

Maternal health continues to present a challenge at both the national and global level. It's not just the large numbers of women affected that is worrying, but also the fact that almost 99% of these deaths take place in developing countries and almost all these deaths are preventable (WHO 2010).

Primarily the following approaches can reduce these deaths:

- Making pregnancy and delivery safer.
- Reducing the number of pregnancies through family planning (FP).

FP not only reduces the number of unintended and unwanted pregnancies but also can defer pregnancy in women of higher parity, who face higher risk during pregnancy.

India is one of the first countries in the world to start its FP Programme (in 1952). The programme started with awareness and information activities to clinical services and later on to a time-bound target-oriented programme. After the International Conference on Population and Development (ICPD) in 1994, India's policy on FP Programme moved away from target-oriented programmes and got integrated as part of Reproductive and Child Health (RCH) Programme (see box titled 'An Integrated Approach to Improve Reproductive Health').

> **An Integrated Approach to Improve Reproductive Health**
>
> 'Measures that are required to improve child and maternal health, sexual and reproductive health services, includes access to family planning, pre and postnatal care (PNC), emergency obstetric services and access to information, as well as to resources necessary to act on that information.'
>
> *Source:* The UN Committee on Economic, Social and Cultural Rights.

The National Population Policy, adopted in February 2000, further supported the paradigm shift to client-based services. State governments have also framed state-specific population policies, thereby, broadening the scope for experimenting with interventions. In several states, innovations have focussed on delivery of services through public–private partnership (PPP) mode; involvement of male adolescents in programmes and information education communication (IEC) efforts to enable clients to exercise informed contraceptive choice.

In 2002 Pathfinder International tested the PRACHAR model (the Hindi word *prachar* means: 'to let people know' or 'to disseminate') in the state of Bihar targeting multiple stakeholders and devising innovative IEC/behaviour change communication (BCC) strategy to delay and have a better spacing between children (Wilder et al. 2005). The model provides reproductive health (RH) information to adolescents and young couples, their parents, in-laws and influential community members, creating an enabling social environment conducive to innovative ideas that improve health and quality of life (see Box 13.1).

The model has been tested in three phases and learning from each phase helped in devising strategy for the next phase (see Table 13.1). Currently, the innovation is in its last phase aiming towards scalability and integration within the government programme.

The following section describes key features of each phase of this model.

> **Box 13.1: The PRACHAR Way**
>
> - Change behaviour through communication.
> - Achieve impact and effect sustainable change.
> - Implement in phases.
> - Structure the implementation process.
> - Build capacity to implement.
> - Improve access to RH services.
> - Monitor vigorously.
> - Provide technical support.
>
> *Source:* PRACHAR Programme Document.

Table 13.1

PRACHAR Project's Different Phases

Phases	Intervention Area	Key Features
Phase I (2002–05)	Three districts in Bihar (Patna, Nalanda and Nawada).	Key target groups included adolescents and young couples between the ages of 12 and 24. It worked with local NGOs and trained more than 400 partner staff to work as change agents, carrying out intensive training and public education activities in their communities.
Phase II (2005–09)	Two districts (Gaya and Shekhpura) in addition to the existing three districts of Phase I.	Target groups remained the same. The project tested several communication approaches to identify the most effective sets of tools and approaches for engendering behaviour change in this phase.
Phase III (2009–12)	Ten blocks in Gaya District.	With 'scale-up' and 'sustainability' as a key approach, the project is being implemented through the government, community front-line worker (ASHA) and civil society partnership model.

PRACHAR I

In 2001, Pathfinder International launched the Promoting Change in Reproductive Behaviour in Bihar (PRACHAR) project with the support of the David and Lucile Packard Foundation. The main objectives of the model were:

1. Change the beliefs held by young people between the ages of 12 and 24 regarding RH and FP, challenge traditional behaviour patterns of early childbearing and inadequate spacing between children and promote informed and healthy reproductive behaviour.
2. Change beliefs held by parents of adolescents and influential community adults about RH and FP, provide them with knowledge and education to discourage early marriage of their daughters, curb the pressure that they place on young couples for early childbearing and encourage adequate spacing of subsequent children.
3. Increase the use of contraceptives among young married couples, particularly to delay the first child until the mother is 21 years of age and to space subsequent births by at least three to five years.
4. Enhance the capacity of 30 non-governmental organizations (NGOs) in Bihar to design, implement and monitor quality RH and FP programmes.
5. Enhance the quality of basic maternal and child health care, RH and FP services delivered by community-based traditional birth attendants (*dais*) and informal rural medical practitioners (RMPs).

Intervention Area

- The programme started in 19 intervention areas of three districts in Bihar (Nalanda [7], Nawada [7] and Patna [5]).
- Intervention villages were geographically demarcated for each of the 19 intervention areas and one non-intervention, control area was identified in Nalanda District which comprised a group of villages covering equivalent population in the respective block.
- Community-based interventions were organized around groups of 20 to 30 villages, each with a population of about 30,000. Each intervention area was subdivided into three clusters, each covering a population of 10,000 and then further subdivided into field units, each of 2,500 people. Every two to three villages represented a field unit.

Target Group

The programme not only targeted adolescents and young couples but also other decision-makers, such as in-laws, parents and also service providers such as traditional birth attendants (TBAs) and RMPs.

A wide range of stakeholders were targeted as programme strategy to reach out to varied audience for achieving effective RH and FP behaviour change and addressing harmful traditional customs and beliefs that influence early childbearing.

One of the main aims of the programme was to delay the age of first childbirth and increase spacing between children.

- Newly-weds were encouraged to delay their first child until the wife reached the age of 21 and to space subsequent children by three years. Nearly 2,886 couples learned about reproductive health care, contraception and healthy timing and spacing of pregnancies (HTSP) as a couple. Follow-up home visits to women and group meetings with men made sure that the couples understood how to use the contraceptives.
- Young couples with one child and the groom's parents were educated on the importance of child spacing and the adoption of post-partum contraception within 45 to 90 days after delivery. A total of 34,168 men and women and 5,320 mothers-and-fathers-in-law were covered through home visit and group meetings (54% of all mothers and fathers of newly-wed husbands). With this saturation, adoption of contraception among women with one child within 90 days of childbirth rose from 2% to 25% percent.
- Young adolescent girls (12 to 14 years) received preparation for puberty with information on menstruation and hygiene. Nearly 18,641 girls were trained (97% of girls this age).
- Adolescent girls and boys (15 to 19 years) were trained separately on sexuality, RH, FP and spacing of children, human immunodeficiency virus/acquired immunodeficiency syndrome (HIV/AIDS) and its prevention and the importance of sharing and negotiating decisions within marriage. During Phase I nearly 17,451 girls and 16,136 boys were trained (more than 60% of these groups in the community).
- TBAs (dais) deliver 66% of the 80% of babies delivered at home in Bihar. They are generally illiterate, having learned through apprenticeship. 1,378 dais were trained in safe delivery procedures, post-partum counselling and promoting use of contraception for birth spacing.
- RMPs (village doctors) have no formal training, but they provide services, give injections and prescribe medicines to patients. Pathfinder trained 470 RMPs to support the RH and FP needs of the youth.
- In addition to education and training for primary target groups, whole communities attended street theatre performances using 'folk media' that acted out the RH crises of women, particularly highlighting maternal and child mortality. Dramas sought to show people what was going wrong in their lives and then the steps they might take to remedy the problems.

Output and Outcome

Some outcomes of the programme based on evaluation conducted at the end of Phase I are described in the following paragraphs (see also Table 13.2).

Reach

- Built management and technical capacity in 30 NGOs, trained 1,378 dais and 470 RMPs
- Trained and selected 342 change agents
- Trained 227 cultural team members
- Trained 17,451 girls and 16,136 boys
- Trained 900 NGO staff in RH and FP
- Total of 2,886 couples attended newly-wed meetings (64% of all newly-weds)
- Around 70% target population had undergone some form of education/training in the area

Table 13.2
Phase I Summary

Project Reach	Key Strategies
• Total population covered: 636,803 people • 86,398 adolescents and young couples • About 100,000 parents and other adults in the community • 1,378 dais • 470 RMPs • 900 staff of 30 NGOs, out of which 342 were change agents (one female for every two villages (5,000 population) and one male for every four villages (10,000 population). • 227 cultural team members	• Partnering with local NGOs • Capacity building of local NGOs and staff • Community engagement/assessment • Programmes with targeted populations • Cultural teams and use of folk media for communication • Training community influencers in reproductive health leadership groups • Improving access to quality RH services • Monitoring information and evaluation systems

Key Components
- Phased programme implementation
- Selection and training of NGO partners
- Recruitment and training of male and female change agents
- Project launch/community mapping
- Outreach programmes for targeted populations (for example, *Nav Dampati Swagat Samaroh* (NDSS) for newly-weds, ARSH training for adolescents)
- Training cultural performers—folk media
- Outreach workshops for community influencers
- Efforts to increase access to RH services through auxiliary nurse midwives (ANMs), dais and RMPs
- Performance monitoring and use of data for programme planning and management
- Rigorous evaluation

Source: PRACHAR Programme Document.

Outcome

- Around 92% of primary target audience groups recalled receiving BCC messages.
- Percentage of population (all respondents) who believe that contraception is both necessary and safe increased from 38 to 81. Among adolescents, this figure increased from 45 to 91.
- Percentage of newly-weds who use contraception to delay their first child went up four times from 5% to 20%.
- Percentage of first-time parents who used contraception to space their second child increased from 14% to 33%.
- Percentage of newly-wed adopters who began to use contraception within three months of consummation of marriage increased from 0% to 21%.

PRACHAR II

PRACHAR II was designed based on evidence of Phase I to yield key information needed for subsequent replication and scale-up (Pathfinder International 2009). The objectives of Phase II were to identify: (1) a set of appropriate and essential interventions that are effective, affordable and easily implementable through the existing government health delivery system, (2) an optimal duration (two, three or five years of duration) of intervention required to attain a critical level of behaviour change (contraceptive use) and (3) sustainability of intervention effects over time, in this case two years after discontinuation of a three-year Phase I intervention.

Methods and Reach

- New activities included training and enlisting the assistance of elected members of local self-government groups called *Panchayati Raj*, who are in an excellent position to encourage healthy behaviour and promote access to services.
- More than 485 dais have also been trained in FP to improve access to services, as have other local providers such as 333 RMPs.
- Where chemists and medical stores do not exist, local grocers are urged to stock condoms and oral contraceptive pills. Partners worked with social marketing agencies to supply contraceptives to these outlets (Parivar Mitra) to ensure a steady supply.
- Finally, overcoming cultural inhibitions, Pathfinder developed a curriculum to train RH biology teachers and provide accurate information about human biology, RH and FP.

Highlights of Phase II:

- Forged new NGO partnerships and expanded to new intervention areas.
- Increased NGO capacities to implement sexual and RH programmes.
- Trained a new cadre of 2,324 voluntary contraceptive counsellors (*Parivar Kalyan Salahkars*) to promote FP within their communities.
- Trained and enlisted the assistance of local self-government institutions (*Panchayati Raj* Institutions), who are in an excellent position to encourage healthy behaviours and promote access to services.
- Worked with social marketing agencies to ensure a steady availability of contraceptives.

PRACHAR III

The goal of the current phase of PRACHAR is to delay marriage and first births and to promote birth spacing between first and second births in 10 blocks of Gaya District, Bihar (see Figure 13.1). The objective is to increase contraceptive use for delaying, spacing and limiting births. Phase III, which is being supported by the David and Lucile Packard Foundation and United Nations Population Fund (UNFPA), builds on successes and lessons learned from Phases I and II. The project is being implemented through a government and civil society partnership model to promote ownership by the state government and encourage the replication and institutionalization of the most cost-effective and successful approaches for large-scale implementation.

In Phases I and II, PRACHAR used multiple pathways such as reaching parents of the couple, in-laws, community leaders, influential people, newly married couples and also the unmarried adolescents. In Phase III, the main aim is to work with the government. The focus of the programme

Figure 13.1
Components of PRACHAR

Pattern of Group Meetings

Target Group	# Meetings	Meeting Objectives
Newly-married men	3	Delay first child; use FP consistently; STI prevention
Father-in-law	3	Not to demand early child-bearing; reinforce importance and support delaying first child
Husbands of first time pregnant women; fathers w/1 child	3	Understand need to space births; use post-partum contraception; care during pregnancy; STI prevention
First time pregnant women	5	ANC; two TT injections; exclusive breastfeeding/colostrums importance; post-partum contraception
Mother-in-law	3	Not to demand early child-bearing; reinforce importance and support delaying first child
Mother of 1 infant child (46 days to 28 months old)	4	Importance of spacing; regular use of contraception; avoid abortion

Pattern of Home Visits

Target Group	Number of Home Visits
Newly-married women w/o children	1st visit immediately after learning of marriage, 2nd visit two weeks later, 3rd visit four weeks after 2nd, once monthly thereafter until woman conceives or adopts contraception
First time pregnant woman	At least 3 (immediately after learning of pregnancy, 4 weeks later, during 8th month of gestation)
First time post-partum women	3 (within 10 days of delivery, 20 days later, 4 weeks later)
Married women within 1 child under 28 months old	Once a month until she conceives her second child or first child attains 28 months
Contraceptive users	1st visit two weeks after staring the method, 2nd visit two weeks after 1st, 3rd visit four weeks after 2nd, once monthly thereafter

Source: PRACHAR Programme Document.

was narrowed down so that the best lessons of PRACHAR could be integrated into the government system. In this phase, the programme is working with a large number of front-line workers, primarily Accredited Social Health Activists (ASHAs), but also ANMs and *Anganwadi* Workers (AWW) to communicate on how to convince couples with no child and couples with one child on delaying and spacing births and to use contraceptives. Through performance improvement training of 1,100 ASHAs, the project tries to demonstrate the potential of scaling healthy timing and spacing initiatives for population stabilization. The project also tries to advocate at the state, national, regional and international levels urgent increased attention to programmes that address youth RH and fertility.

Key features of this phase are:

- Develop and test an effective hybrid government-civil society partnership model for delivery of youth RH and fertility interventions at scale in one district of Bihar.
- Change the beliefs of young couples (of zero and one parity) regarding RH and FP and increase the contraceptive use among them to delay the first child until the mother is 21 and space subsequent births by at least three years.
- Advocate with policymakers, donors, governments and NGOs for addressing issues of youth fertility.
- Tested in 10 blocks of Gaya District.

Target Groups

- Unmarried adolescents
- Married women (with focus on zero and one parity)
- Married men (with focus on zero and one parity)
- Enablers (PRI, village influencers and parents-in-law)
- Front-line workers

> For women: Government appointed Pathfinder-trained ASHAs
> For men: Pathfinder-trained male communicators (MCs)

Project Design

The overall goal of the PRACHAR Phase III is to have significant impact on youth fertility by delaying and spacing births in Gaya District through adopting the following steps:

Community Sensitization and Interventions with Young Married Men through Trained Male Communicators

Under PRACHAR, MCs are deployed to organize small group meetings with husbands of women being counselled by ASHAs to permit candid discussion about FP and to address any lingering misgivings and concerns they might have. These meetings are conducted at convenient times and in centrally located spaces. With the zero and one parity men, MCs discuss the outcomes of early marriage, untimely childbearing and various methods of contraceptives. With two and two+ parity men, MCs stress upon consistent use of condoms and provide information on permanent methods for limiting family size. Fathers of adolescents are sensitized about healthy age of marriage and the importance of allowing their children to attend the PRACHAR adolescent trainings. In these small groups, men are invited to ask candid questions, practice skills such as condom use and voice their opinions on gender issues. So far (up to December 2011), 160 MCs have reached 21,881 men of zero parity, 21,967 men of one parity and 57,584 men of two and more than two parity at least once through group meetings.

Interventions with Young Married Women through Project Trained ASHAs

In 10 blocks, a total of 1,295 ASHAs have been trained extensively under PRACHAR Phase III. There are 19 ASHAs remaining to be trained in essential blocks as they have not been recruited yet. ASHAs are trained for four days in eight essential blocks and for two days in two stand-alone blocks. The various topics covered during ASHA trainings are roles of ASHA in development and health of mothers and babies; sexual and RH; FP; knowledge and understanding regarding pregnancy; knowledge and understanding of various methods of contraception; information about reproductive tract infection (RTI), sexually transmitted infection (STI) and HIV and AIDS awareness, prevention and treatment; conducting effective home visits for disseminating messages regarding sexual health and contraception methods and how to do listing of the targeted beneficiaries for home visits. Careful monitoring and registration skills are also taught as ASHAs record each visit.

These trained ASHAs work with Pathfinder to develop relationships with women of different parities and go to their homes to discuss a wide range of gender-specific issues related to FP and RH. With women of two and more parity, ASHAs conduct group meetings. As a starting point for dialogue, ASHAs use a set of flipcharts to discuss both FP and RH, but then tailor the information to the clients' personal needs.

Motivating ASHAs to host group meetings with women who have two or more children continues to be a challenge because ASHAs do not see these meetings as their responsibility and prefer to reach clients during routine home visits or informally in the normal course of the day. In addition, although they are trained and fully aware of how to conduct meaningful home visits with zero and one parity women, the ASHAs sometimes do not follow the guidelines in totality. As such, Pathfinder is continuously reinforcing the importance of group meetings as a mechanism for empowering young women to learn and make healthy decisions about FP/sexual and reproductive health (SRH).

So far (up to December 2011), through group meetings, ASHAs have reached 21,557 women of zero parity and 23,547 women of one parity through home visits. In addition, 72,467 women of two and more than two parity have been reached through group meetings by ASHAs. PRACHAR's 360 support systems for reaching, motivating and encouraging ASHAs and rigorous supervision of MCs to reach eligible couples have already generated an increase in method acceptance: 15.4% of zero parity and 21.2% of one parity young couples are now using a contraceptive method, as compared to 3.3% and 11.2% in the baseline survey.

Capacity Building, Technical Assistance and Supportive Supervision of ASHAs and Male Communicators

Rigorous validation and verification of data from home visits and group meetings is done by project staff. MCs conduct verification of minimum of 20% of ASHA's home visits while consultant block officers conduct verification of minimum of 20% of ASHA's home visits records and MCs records on a monthly basis. Corrective actions are made based on weekly discussions between PRACHAR and Pathfinder Country Office team to address variance issues as noticed. Also incentives paid to ASHAs and MCs are linked to their monthly deliverables and deductions where necessary.

Rigorous efforts are made to have continuous improvements. From front-line workers to state project staff to country office staff dedicated to PRACHAR, everyone has a clear scope of work and is held accountable for meeting deliverables. Performance is routinely monitored closely by the Pathfinder India Country Office. A results-based work plan for the project has been developed and is utilized for internal monitoring. Pathfinder regularly conducts internal review meetings where activities accomplished are reviewed against the PRACHAR timeline and work plans.

Unmarried Adolescent Training

Under PRACHAR, separate RH trainings are conducted for adolescent boys and girls, aged 15 to 19. This intensive programme (15 hours over the course of three days) provides information and provides opportunities to practice skills that are needed to make responsible sexual and reproductive choices as they transition to adulthood and marriage. Topics such as the process of growing up, menstrual hygiene, unwanted pregnancy, infection and FP, proper nutrition, relationship-building with spouses are covered. Because these adolescents are at the age of marriage common in Bihar, training also emphasizes the dangers of early marriage and childbirth, as well as the importance of a woman postponing the birth of her first child until the age of 21. Discussions and exercises are intended to help adolescents resist family and community pressures to marry and conceive at a young age. A total of 62,883 adolescents have been trained in the essential blocks and 16,771 adolescents in stand-alone blocks. According to the beneficiary listing, there are 1,23,305 adolescents in essential blocks and 37,107 in stand-alone blocks. Hence, so far PRACHAR trainings have covered 51% of adolescents in essential blocks and 45% in stand-alone blocks out of those listed.

Contraceptive Assurance in the Intervention Blocks and Villages

Under the project, Pathfinder's NGO partners organize subcentre-level meetings for ANMs, ASHAs and MCs, across various blocks to collectively discuss issues related to the availability and distribution of contraceptives. ANMs, MOs and ASHAs are reached through these meetings. The PRACHAR team facilitates their discussion to build good coordination among them. Using a questionnaire, contraceptive availability at various health facilities such as subcentres and PHCs and with various health functionaries such as ASHAs and ANMs was determined. It has been found that 60% of ASHAs have condoms and oral contraceptive pills available with them and they are distributing them on demand. The ASHAs receive these contraceptives from the *Anganwadi* Centres or ANMs, who get these contraceptives from PHCs.

The focus of the PRACHAR Programme was to bring behaviour change in the community, men and women towards the use of contraceptives—for delay in first child and other FP purposes. Contraceptives are provided by the government through health facilities and community-level workers.

Taking the Project to Scale

Pathfinder is working with the Government of Bihar in this phase by constituting a project steering committee at state-level involving Bihar State Health Society and at district-level with district health society, district magistrate and civil surgeon. The main goal is not only to keep them updated about the programme but also to advocate for inclusion of MCs in the health system as well as for incentivizing ASHAs to provide messages on RH and FP.

One of the key aspects of this phase is to scale the programme by integrating into existing government scheme. In this respect, PRACHAR is providing training to ASHA on communicating about delaying marriage, delaying the first birth and spacing and till date 1,295 front-line workers (ASHAs) have been imparted training. At present, incorporation of training materials as part of overall ASHA training is under process. But the challenge lies in monitoring and evaluating the training programme. So to address this issue PRACHAR is working closely with community-based organizations and NGOs and capacitating them so they can work closely with the front-line worker, when the PRACHAR Project ends.

The PRACHAR Model and Its Impact on Reproductive Health Based on Result for Phase I and II

PRACHAR's mission is threefold:

- Increase girls' age at marriage.
- Delay the first birth after marriage until the age of 21.
- Ensure spacing of at least three years between the first and second births.

PRACHAR interventions have been highly effective in increasing contraceptive use both before and after a first birth among young couples in Bihar. They have also increased the age at marriage and first birth. The principal vehicle of PRACHAR intervention is increased awareness, knowledge and understanding of RH issues related to timing and spacing of pregnancies. PRACHAR's audience is unmarried adolescents, young couples, their guardians (parents and in-laws) and influential community members. Information is given to them through targeted channels but no direct services are provided.

PRACHAR has completed two phases of implementation. Phase I, from 2002 to 2005, tested the full model (with all the elements of the intervention already described) in 19 blocks in Patna, Nalanda and Nawada Districts of Bihar. Phase II, from 2005 to 2008, tested four different approaches, with varying elements of the interventions in nine Phase I blocks and additional four blocks, in Gaya and Shekhpura Districts to find elements that produce best outcomes with minimal inputs. Phase III is currently scaling-up the evidence-based approaches of PRACHAR model in the government health system, with local NGO involvement, in an additional 10 blocks in Gaya District of Bihar.

The impact of PRACHAR interventions has been assessed at both Phase I (2002 to 2005) and Phase II (2005 to 2008) through baseline and follow-up surveys. Surveys of young couples (whose wives' ages are below 25) were conducted in intervention blocks and comparison blocks all in three districts of Bihar (Rahman and Elkan 2010).

Impact

- In the intervention blocks, contraceptive use increased significantly from 4% to 21% between the baseline and follow-up period (PRACHAR Phase I) while, in the comparison blocks, it only increased from 3% to 5%.
- Disaggregated by the number of children, contraceptive use for women with no children increased from less than 4% to 16% and that among women with one child increased from 6% to 25%. These increases, as well as increases in demand for contraception and indicators of knowledge and understanding of RH, were significantly greater in the intervention blocks than the comparison blocks (Daniel et al. 2008).
- PRACHAR's impact on delayed marriage and childbearing, based on a study of 300 girls and 300 boys, selected from the list of trainees, was conducted to examine the impact of the PRACHAR in 2008. The age of respondents was between 19 and 24 during the study. A control sample of 600 age-comparable females and males was selected for the study from the PRACHAR comparison blocks. Results show that RH behaviour among adolescent girls and boys who received training was significantly better than the comparison group. Age at marriage for trained girls was 2.6 years higher than for those girls who did not receive training (22.0 years versus 19.4 years). For trained boys it was 2.8 years than comparison group (24.1 years versus 21.3 years). Age at first birth among trained girls was 1.5 years higher than those who did not receive training (23.1 years versus 21.6 years). Respondents who received training had significantly higher use of contraception before the first birth. The delay in first birth was, thus, achieved through delayed marriage and higher use of contraception by the trained respondents.
- PRACHAR interventions improve contraceptive service utilization for all socio-economic groups, but the least advantaged benefit the most. While analyzing usage of contraceptive based on level of schooling, in the intervention areas, the increase in contraceptive use was around 2.5 times for the groups with one to 9 years of schooling and 10 or more years of schooling. In sharp contrast, the increase was over six times for those who had no schooling. The results show that information provision is extremely powerful in increasing contraceptive use across socio-economic groups but the least advantaged benefit more from the information as the relative increase of contraceptive use is much higher among them than among others.

Pathfinder sought to promote major attitude and behaviour changes in youth—as well as their parents and influential community members—related to delaying the first child and spacing subsequent children. The hypothesis underlying programme implementation was that if at least 80% of the members of each primary target group were reached with appropriate and understandable messages, it would maximize the chances of changing the beliefs and behaviour of at least 20% of the members of these groups. The conversion of this critical mass would ensure that the new beliefs and behaviours would be sustained and continue to grow in the community.

References

Daniel, E.E., Masilamani, R. and Rahman, M. 2008. 'The Effect of Community-based Reproductive Health Communication Interventions among Young Couples in Bihar, India'. *International Family Planning Perspectives*, 34(4): 189–97.

Pathfinder International. 2009. 'PRACHAR II Results', Paper presented at the David and Lucile Packard Summit, Gaya, Bihar, India, March 2–4.

Rahman, M. and Elkan, E.D. 2010. 'A Reproductive Health Communication Model That Helps Improve Young Women's Reproductive Life and Reduce Population Growth: The Case of PRACHAR from Bihar'. India: Pathfinder International.

WHO. 2010. '10 Facts on Maternal Health'. Available at www.who.int/features/factfiles/maternal_health/maternal_health_facts/en/index.html, accessed on 7 November 2010.

Wilder, J., Masilamani, R. and Daniel, E.E. 2005. 'Promoting Change in the Reproductive Behaviour of Youth: Pathfinder International's PRACHAR Project, Bihar, India'. Watertown, MA, USA: Pathfinder International.

World Health Organization. 2010. Available at www.who.int/topics/maternal_health/en/, accessed on 7 November 2010.

Community-based Intersectoral Interventions in Health

14

The Silver Lining: Community-led Initiatives for Child Survival (CLICS)

Radhika Arora

Introduction

The Community-led Initiatives for Child Survival Programme (CLICS) is a five-year-$2-million project co-funded by the United States Agency for International Development (USAID) and the Aga Khan Foundation USA (AKF USA) under the 2003 Child Survival Health Grants Program (CSHGP). The goal of the project is to bring sustainable improvement in the health status and well-being of children below three years and women in the reproductive age group (15–44 years), in a beneficiary population of 88,128 residing in 67 villages across Wardha District, Maharashtra, India.

CLICS seeks to facilitate 'community-ownership' of a package of health services by refining and applying a 'social franchise model' that is demand-driven, inherently sustainable and suitable for expansion. As construed by CLICS, a social franchise model is one where a contractual obligation between two parties is entered into for the purpose of producing a 'social product' of a particular kind and quality. The model, as such, is an efficient means for the 'franchiser', in this case the Department of Community Medicine (DCM) at the Mahatma Gandhi Institute of Medical Sciences (MGIMS) to interact with and build the capacity of potential 'franchises' (village communities) to produce an integrated package of affordable and high-quality child survival and health services. Interventions under CLICS remain focussed on maternal and child health.

Background

Three major factors contribute to poor health in Wardha.

Poverty

About 44.4% of the people in this primarily rural district fall below the poverty line (BPL). Most households consume less than adequate calories, lack access to safe drinking water and live in houses without solid construction.

Gender Inequality

As in other parts of India, Wardha shows skewed literacy rates between men and women (86.3% males and 67.5% females), reflecting unequal access to schooling.

Insufficient Health Care for Women, Newborns and Infants

The amount of money spent on health care for women is about half of that spent on men. This unequal access to care results in a higher mortality rate for women aged 15–19.

In October 2003, the AKF began a programme called the Community-led Initiatives for Child Survival (CLICS), a five-year initiative, specifically focussed on improving the health of women of reproductive age and young children. The AKF, in collaboration with the DCM at the MGIMS, is creating a sustainable health care system at the village level in the district of Wardha. Keeping in mind the social and economic factors that contributed towards poor health of the people in the area, long-term community involvement was essential for the success and sustainability of the programme. Both partners work to build the capacity of local communities to develop, manage, fundraise and ultimately achieve ownership of village-based child survival and health services. The programme's overall goal is to create a community-owned sustainable health system at the local level that continually improves the health status and well-being of children under the age of three and women of reproductive age (15–44 years).

Objectives

- To provide affordable, high-quality health care through effective partnerships at the village level.
- To build the capacity of coalitions of local partners to sustain child survival activities and health gains.
- To refine and test a social franchising model for the delivery of child survival interventions.
- To document, disseminate and share key programme lessons and results to facilitate adaptation, replication and policy advocacy.

Programme Activities

The CLICS Programme is an initiative to bring about improvements in the health and mortality indicators of children below the age of three and women in the reproductive age group through a community-based, intersectoral approach to health. The programme was initially supported by USAID and AKF USA.

Sustainability of the programme and the involvement of the community were essential to its design, to ensure more effective impact and long-term benefits. Elements of the CLICS Programme such as the community-based groups and Kiran Clinic continue today, guided by the Dr Sushila Nayar, School of Public Health.

Community-based Groups

Self-help Groups

The CLICS Programme has formed an average of three to four self-help groups (SHGs) per village. A total of 263 such groups were in place on 30 September 2006. The members themselves have learnt to manage the groups, which, with the help of trainings and over a period of time, have developed as member-owned and member-managed institutions. The programme provides assistance to add a health action agenda to the primary financial function (finance +) of the SHGs so that the women are able to determine health priorities and to play a proactive role in health care delivery in their villages.

Thirty seven income-generation activities have been started by the SHG members. The income generation activities include sale of vegetables, hiring out equipment required for marriages and other public functions, catering, embroidery, tailoring, dairy farming, grocery shop, sale of stationery, farming, herbal insecticide preparation and motor winding. The capital for these ventures has been acquired through loans from the groups or from banks.

Kisan Vikas Manch

The *Kisan Vikas Manch*s (KVMs), which are farmers' groups, have been formed to involve men in health activities. A total of 72 KVMs have been formed. The programme provides learning opportunities for the members to improve their agricultural yield and thus improve their economic status. A health action agenda has also been added to the primary purpose of the *manchs*, to empower them to actively participate in the health programme. Two special training programmes for 'master trainers' were organized during the reporting period which were attended by identified persons at village level.

Kishori Panchayats

As of 30 September 2006, the programme achieved the formation of 64 *Kishori* Panchayats (KVs), which are adolescent girls' groups, in the programme area. These have become platforms for adolescent girls to share their ideas, views and problems and indirectly for the development of their personalities. The adolescent girls are provided training in income generation activities and on health. Apart from gaining knowledge for their future lives, a number of group members have taken up the responsibility of imparting health education to pregnant women and postnatal mothers.

Various training programmes on nutrition, pregnancy and newborn care, health and sanitation, menstrual hygiene, safe motherhood and first aid were organized for the groups. Under the CLICS Programme, keeping in view adolescent behaviour, various programmes are being taken up among the members of the KVs for enhancing awareness on reproductive health (RH).

Village Coordination Committees

In addition to 32 village coordination committees (VCC) formed earlier, 31 new ones have been formed, bringing the total number to 63. All committees have their *Gram Swasthya Kosh* (Village

Health Fund) which is deposited in a bank. On an average, there are 21 members in each committee. Each of these committees has done a village health needs assessment and subsequently developed a village health plan. Later on, the VCC were transformed to village health and sanitation committees under National Rural Health Mission (NRHM).

Village Health Fund

To implement child survival activities at the village level, the VCC has collected a *Gram Swasthya Kosh* through community contributions, according to a set fixed amount per family member. A prerequisite of setting-up the fund is that at least 75% of households in the community contribute to this fund.

Selection of CLICS *Doot*

Another important achievement was identification of village health workers, known as CLICS *doots*, in all the project villages with a VCC. During the current reporting period, a total of 45 new CLICS *doots* have been identified. Presently there are 88 CLICS *doots* working in all the programme villages and training for them has been completed. Later on with advent of NRHM, the majority of CLICS *doots* have been selected as Accredited Social Health Activists (ASHAs).

Community-based Organizations

Community-based organization members obtained their information on important health issues through being involved in community-level programmes, *melawas* (meeting sessions), cooking competitions and celebration of events such as International Women's Day. During their monthly meeting the community organizers discussed and educated the community-based organizations members on important health issues.

Panchayati Raj Institutions

One-day training programmes for the panchayat members mainly focussed on the role of *Panchayati Raj* Institutions (PRIs), on CLICS Programme's issues and interventions and on government health policy and relevant national health programmes.

Capacity Building

Integrated Management of Neonatal and Childhood Illnesses Training for the Health Providers

One important development during this period was a training workshop on Integrated Management of Neonatal and Childhood Illnesses (IMNCI) for the master trainers of the programme. Initially a

10-day training workshop was conducted at MGIMS, Sewagram. Subsequently, two IMNCI training programmes were organized for the training of government health providers.

Clinical Interventions

Community Health Clinics

The project has four community health clinics under the programme called *Kiran* Clinics. These have been set-up with the help of the community and the VCC. The clinics provide essential health care services to members of the community at affordable rates. Essential medicines are also dispensed at lower rates. Maternal and newborn health is prioritized with the clinic conducting antenatal care (ANC) check-ups (with referral services, if needed). Awareness campaigns with members of the community, especially women's groups, have helped many women overcome social barriers in accessing health care services.

Other Initiatives under CLICS*

Bal Suraksha Diwas

CLICS has promoted *Bal Suraksha Diwas* (BSD), Child Survival Day, on a monthly basis in the programme villages. The BSD is an expanded activity of the immunization day organized in villages through the primary health centres (PHC) with village health and sanitation committee as nodal agency. The CLICS *doots,* members of the SHGs and adolescent girls are being encouraged to participate actively in the BSD, during which growth monitoring and promotion is being done every month for more than 80% of children in the age group of 0–3 years.

Campaigns

During the current reporting period, 138 *Suraksha Aaichi Aani Balachi Mohim* (Mother and Child Safety Mission) and 58 *Mulgi Wachawa Mohim* (Save the Girl Child Mission) were conducted covering all the programme villages. The activities basically included community-based events and programmes in which the causes of the mother and child were promoted. The programme staff took special efforts to involve local leaders, opinion makers, public and private health care providers and members from the media. *Melawas* for mothers-in-law and males were organized at each subcentre. People were educated about problems of maternal and child health, immunization, adverse sex ratio, the prenatal diagnostic techniques (PNDT) Act, human immunodeficiency virus/acquired

---

* Based on interviews with members of the CLICS team and members of community-based groups in Wardha, Maharashtra. ©PHFI, 2011.

immunodeficiency syndrome (HIV/AIDS), reproductive tract infections/sexually transmitted infections (RTI/STI) and family planning.

Management Information System

CLICS has developed a management information system (MIS) based on information equity, which will ensure that awareness and knowledge of an issue, health problem or programme is shared among different individuals within a group and among different groups in a community. The practice also ensures that the community has access to corresponding information sources. In general, communities in India have little or no access to reliable health information or sources. CLICS ensures information equity by involving community institutions in the design, collection and use of data from the MIS. This enables community institutions to monitor and understand changes in health status, crucial for sustainability of programme gains.

Communications

CLICS also worked on behaviour change through communications, which has been crucial for achieving its objectives of creating awareness of the preventive and promotive health practices to promote safe motherhood and child health behaviours and utilization of the services. Using a behaviour change communication (BCC) strategy was critical for effective community mobilization to improve access, availability and equity of health services under the project.

Key Achievements

- Completion of household and baseline surveys.
- Development of the detailed implementation plan.
- The creation of SHGs, KVMs and KVs helped the organization build partnership at the village/community level.
- Sixty-three VCCs covering all villages have been formed; social franchise agreements have been signed with 23 VCCs; 88 *doot*s selected by VCCs are in place; community health clinics are functional in eight villages; training needs assessments have been carried out for staff, VCCs and public health providers; training of trainers has been done on IMNCI; community mobilization and appraisal exercises; health facility needs assessment has been done and quality assurance tools development and testing have been completed.

Impact

During the second half of the programme (2006–2008), CLICS has been able to concentrate more on improving health indicators. For example, previously the majority of women gave birth at home. Now nine out of 10 births in the project area take place in health facilities. The infant mortality rate (IMR) decreased significantly—for the years between July 2006 and June 2007 and July 2007 and

June 2008, there was a reduction in IMR from 49.3/1,000 live births to 37.8/1,000 (a drop of 23%). The neonatal mortality rate (NMR), showed a 21% decline from 38.5/1,000 live births from mid-2006 to mid-2007 to 30.4 from mid-2007 to mid-2008. Malnutrition in the under-three population also reduced: in January 2007, severe malnutrition was observed in 17.8% of the targeted age group, by February 2008 this reduced to 9.8%.

Discussion and Conclusion

CLICS deploys a multipronged strategy, working in several areas and with several people to bring about an improvement in the health indicators. It must be noted that CLICS does not work exclusively on maternal or child health even though that is its main target, but as with any other intersectoral intervention, it keeps in focus all the dimensions of health. CLICS has rightly identified poor child and maternal health to be rooted in poverty and gender equality. Accordingly, groups such as *Kishori* Panchayats help empower women about their rights and raise awareness, which in turn helps them make healthier and more informed choices in life regarding their own and their baby's health. Similarly, *Kisan Vikas Manch*s help farmers raise their income by helping them increase yields and an increase in income is the path to better nutrition and better health.

Community-based initiatives such as CLICS have an added advantage of fostering a sense of ownership of the intervention by the community and allow them a forum to bring their concerns to the fore. Yet the challenge of a community-based programme, especially a 'demand-driven' one, lies in the fact that the needs of the poorest of the poor must consistently be kept in view or they will get obscured. Communities are never homogeneous and community-based forums can end up being dominated by those most powerful within the community and this can lead to a distortion of priorities where only the interests of the powerful get represented. The concept of inclusive development becomes especially important in this scenario and if CLICS can provide not only a wide range of services but also reach a wide range of vulnerable people, it can go a long way in making a macro impact.

While the CLICS Programme funded by USAID and the AKF ended in 2008, successful elements of the programme such as the community-based groups continue even today. The communities have taken on ownership of these groups, the responsibility for sustaining them and also for initiating new ones in the intervention areas. The programme continues to be supported by the MGMIS.

Suggested Readings

Annual Report, Community-led Initiatives for Child Survival Program (CLICS). 2004. The United States Agency for International Development, the Aga Khan Foundation, USA and Department of Community Medicine, Mahatma Gandhi Institute of Medical Sciences, Sewagram. Available at http://pdf.usaid.gov/pdf_docs/PDACA727.pdf, accessed on 6 August 2013.

Endline Study for Community-led Initiatives for Child Survival (CLICS). ORG Centre for Social Research. Available at http://pdf.usaid.gov/pdf_docs/PNADN791.pdf.

15

Community for Care: Comprehensive Rural Health Project (CRHP)

Radhika Arora

Introduction

Over 40 years ago, a young couple from Maharashtra, Dr Raj Arole and Dr Mabelle Arole, returned to India after completing their higher education in medicine and public health from the United States. Their vision was to use a community-based primary health care approach to improve the health and lives of people living in some of the poorest parts of the country. In 1970, the Aroles established the Comprehensive Rural Health Project (CRHP) in Jamkhed, Maharashtra (see Map 15.1).

Their mission was to ensure that health, a universal human right, is not denied to the people and that in the long term they are able to achieve access to health care and freedom from poverty, hunger and violence. The women are the focus and the goal of the initiative was (and is) to meet

Map 15.1
Map of Maharashtra

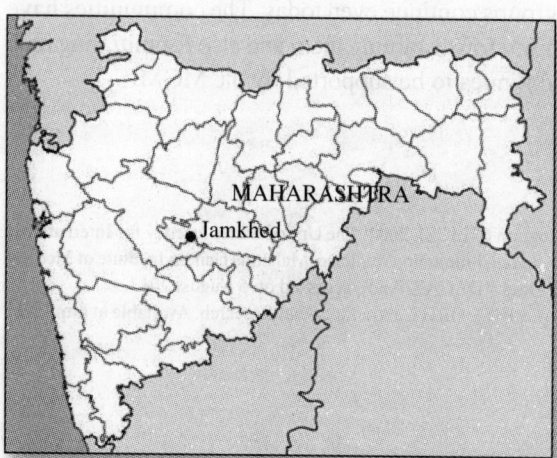

Source: Wikimedia Commons (2011).

Interview Bytes: Ravi Arole

'About 80% of problems that cause death in rural areas can be prevented. You have to have the involvement of the community. The community has to be educated and most illnesses are because of three things: the first is safe drinking water; the second is nutrition and third is environment. All three of these can easily be taken into the hands of the community, therefore, giving health knowledge as well as knowledge of social structures, greatly influences and impacts your mortality rates.'

Source: Ravi Arole, Director, CRHP
Interview conducted in Jamkhed, Maharashtra, November 2011.

their special immediate and long-term needs through expansion of local knowledge and resources, by partnering with village communities.

Background

The CRHP was established by the Aroles before the Alma Ata Conference of 1978 on primary health care. The three main objectives of the project are[1]:

1. Universal health care for all.
2. Poverty alleviation for the poor and marginalized.
3. Freedom from caste, religious and gender inequality.

At the time the CRHP was established, the Aroles aimed at achieving the following targets in the first five years (Arole and Arole 1994):

1. Reducing infant mortality by 50%.
2. Reducing maternal mortality and morbidity.
3. Bringing down the crude birth rate by 10 points.
4. Working on chronic diseases such as leprosy and tuberculosis (TB).
5. Providing basic curative care.

Jamkhed and its neighbouring areas are in a rain shadow area, thus known to be drought-prone and poor. The region also had high rates of malnutrition and maternal deaths, along with high rates of infectious and chronic diseases (at the time of CRHP's establishment in the 1970s). The infant mortality rate (IMR) was 176 per 1,000 live births and levels of antenatal care (ANC) and safe delivery practices in the area were negligible (FutureGenerations 2011). Access to health care services, their availability and information on them were low. Keeping these factors in mind, the Aroles decided to establish a health programme in this region, despite initial suggestions of collaborating with a medical college or research establishment.

In the few years between the establishment of CRHP and the Alma Ata Conference, the Aroles' work was said to have become one of the inspirations for the International Conference on Primary Health Care and its Declaration of Alma Ata.[2] Over the last four decades that CRHP has worked in and around Jamkhed, the community has seen major transformations in health indicators in the area and a change in attitudes and awareness on health issues.

Physical Coverage of the Comprehensive Rural Health Project

The CRHP began its work in eight villages covering a population of 10,000 people; by 2011, approximately 500,000 people in 300 villages were covered by CRHP's work. The organization operates in 45 villages at any given point of time; handholding and supporting the community until the community

[1] www.jamkhed.org, accessed on 6 August 2013.
[2] http://www.apha.org/NR/rdonlyres/D7630DFD-3129-44E9-A240-67EEE738C64E/0/Carl_Taylor_Raj_Arole_2010.pdf, accessed on 6 August 2013.

develops the ability and confidence to provide primary health care services to its people without the constant handholding by CRHP. However, village health workers and community-based organizations formed during the intervention period continue to be supported by CRHP, even after the intervention village is left to operate independently.

Beyond the CRHP campus and intervention villages, the organization has worked in other parts of the Maharashtra and India. This has involved work with the tribal population in districts of Maharashtra; they are also presently working with the Government of Andhra Pradesh towards replicating elements of the Jamkhed Model in that state. Focus on training, capacity building (including for the government and the NGO sector) and continuing education is high at the CRHP.

Figure 15.1

Key Elements of Successful IAH

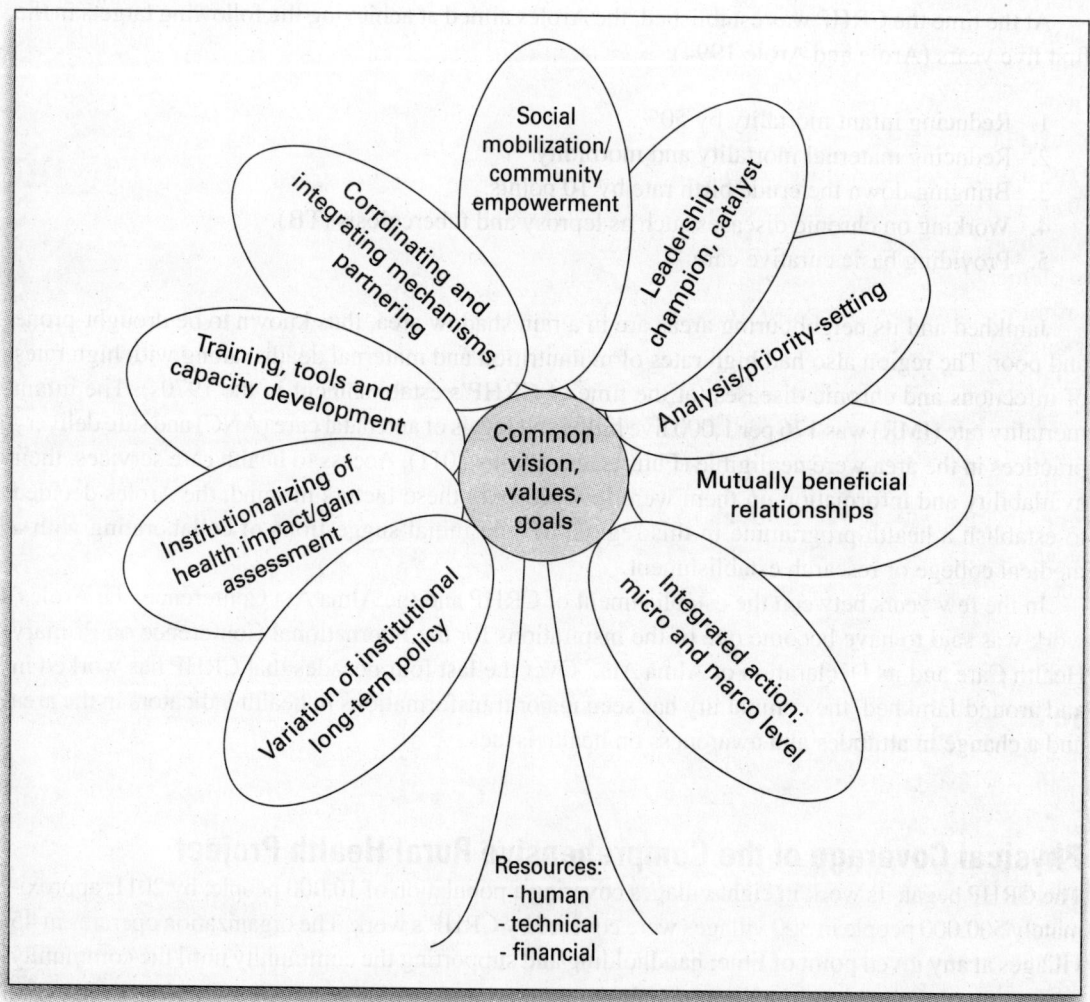

Source: WHO (1997).

Intersectoral Action for Health

The realization of the importance of an intersectoral approach towards improved health care for all perhaps originated around the time of the Alma Ata Conference in 1978. In 1986, a technical paper by the World Health Organization defined intersectoral as a recognized relationship between part or parts of the health sector with part or parts of another sector which has been formed to take action on an issue to achieve health outcomes (or intermediate health outcomes) in a way that is more effective, efficient or sustainable than could be achieved by the health sector acting alone (WHO 1997). The audio-visual case study accompanying this document highlights the elements of 'social mobilization/community empowerment' required for successful intersectoral action for health (IAH), adopted by CRHP as one of the tools to improve health care of the community (see Figure 15.2). This case study will highlight the community-based components as well as the development of human resources, nutrition, education, behavioural system and capacity development aspects of the CRHP intervention.

Figure 15.2
Conceptual Framework of IAH Represented as a Flower, Dr Rita Thapa Diagram on the Experience of WHO-SEARO in IAH

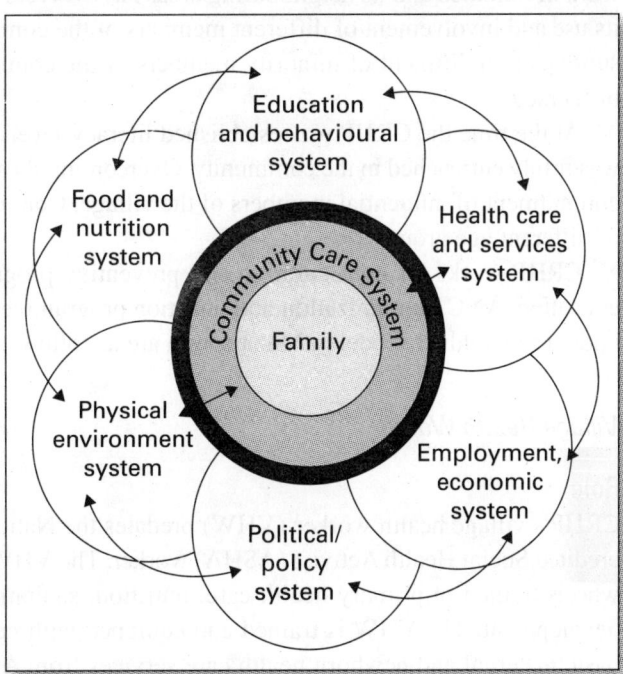

Source: WHO (1997).

Figure 15.3
The Jamkhed Model

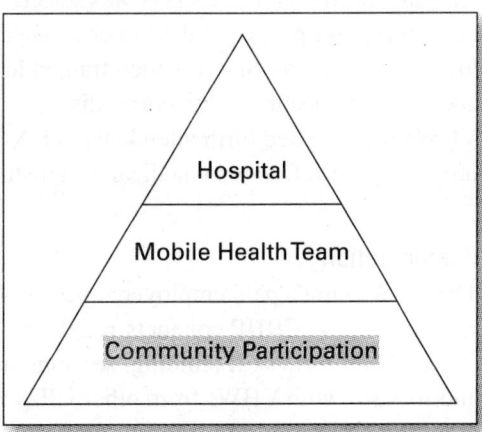

Source: Author's own.

The Jamkhed Model

The CRHP's three-tier approach to health care was formally recognized by the World Health Organization (WHO) and the United Nations Children's' Fund (UNICEF) in 1974 (see Figure 15.3). The Jamkhed Model as it came to be known was soon adapted for implementation in other parts of the world by the WHO and UNICEF.

The Jamkhed Model works at three levels which are described in the following paragraphs.

Community Participation

Community involvement is integral to the Jamkhed Model. It forms the base upon which CRHP's work in Jamkhed and its neighbouring areas has evolved. The strength of the Jamkhed Model lies in its use and involvement of different members of the community, especially in the involvement and subsequent upliftment of minority members of the community, women and those with low levels of literacy.

At the time the CRHP was established literacy levels in the area were low and the caste system was firmly entrenched in the community. Overcoming these challenges required the cooperation and commitment of influential members of the village. Community involvement included both genders of different age groups.

CRHP works on both curative and preventive programmes, with focus especially on health education, ANC, immunization and nutrition programmes. The major community-based initiatives under the Jamkhed Model in Maharashtra are as follows:

Village Health Worker

Role

CRHP's village health worker (VHW) predates the National Rural Health Mission's (NRHM) Accredited Social Health Activist (ASHA) worker. The VHW is a female, a member of the community, who is trained in primary health care, nutrition, sanitation and some other aspects of health and development. The VHW is trained and equipped with necessary tools and information to provide basic maternal and newborn health care services from ANC to delivery, postnatal care (PNC) and family planning (FP). She monitors the growth of children in the community, tracks their growth, ensures immunization and addresses nutritional needs.

Selection

At the time of the creation of the VHW, the caste system in the community was especially rigid. Keeping this in mind, the VHW was selected from the lowest caste of the community (as at the time of its inception people of the upper classes would not have been willing to work for people from lower social strata). She was then trained in aspects of primary health care in the areas of maternal and newborn health, water borne diseases, sanitation and communicable diseases among others. VHWs were trained birth attendants (TBAs) and were also trained to identify signs of danger in a pregnancy for referrals to medical establishments.

Remuneration

The VHW is not a paid employee; once established in the community she is paid in cash or kind by her clients. The CRHP conducts regular training sessions for the VHW at their Jamkhed training centre. Apart from skill building, sessions such as these give the workers an opportunity to interact and socialize with VHWs from other villages. This is also the time when she can restock her supply of basic medication, delivery kits, etc., which are provided by the CRHP for use.

Mahila Vikas Mandal (Women's Group)

Role

One of the most important organizations to have evolved is the *Mahila Vikas Mandal* (MVM) or women's development group, which have been founded in all project villages. In each village, women from different castes and religious groups come together to share health knowledge and improve their socio-economic status.

The women are given training and assistance in operating various economic programmes to improve the condition of their families and communities. Women's groups discuss issues of nutrition, health and hygiene, safe drinking water, kitchen gardens, afforestation, microcredit and income generation. The VHW builds links with the village MVM for information sharing.

Impact

At present 107 self-help groups (SHGs) with 1,187 members are operational in the intervention areas. Resource pooling by the SHGs have given the women of the community the opportunity to build savings as well as get loans for businesses and other needs. The average savings in the bank of a women's group is almost ₹1.3 million (CRHP 2010–11).

Information sharing, reaching entire families through the women has improved the health of the people of the community, as well as improved the use of FP.

The MVMs succeeded in breaking down the socio-economic barriers by bringing together women from all castes to form one group in the village. The groups have now become a place where women can turn to for financial support; it has given them a platform to voice their needs, demand their rights and hold discussions on health and social issues. It has facilitated improvements in their economic and social status in the village.

Farmers' Club

Role

Male involvement in improving the overall health and development of a community is crucial. Male members of the community were reached through farmers' clubs which brought together village men from different socioeconomic backgrounds. The farmers' clubs addressed social issues such as alcoholism, caste, improving the environment and sanitation. Health issues such as nutrition, maternal health and FP are also addressed through group meetings and training sessions.

Impact

The farmers' club created a space for the men of the village to discuss issues related to farming, animal care, government programmes and even organize cooperatives to level the land, construct check dams, etc. At the same time, the club succeeded in imparting crucial health information and sensitized the male members of society towards the need for improving the health needs of the women and children of their community.

Adolescent Girls and Boys Programmes

Role

Young people of the community are reached through the adolescent girls and boys programmes. The Adolescent Girls Programme (AGP) was started almost 10 years ago. Weekly or biweekly meetings are organized for the AGP by the VHWs or the MVM. The AGP has helped organize adolescent girls groups in 54 villages with an average of 25 girls per village participating. The AGP now works on a peer model with five girls from each village being trained to become peer educators. The objective is to cover all girls above the age of 12 in 20 villages in three years. Weekend training sessions are held at the CRHP centre where girls are also trained in computers, craft and self-defence.

The aim of these meetings and groups is the empowerment of young girls through information and knowledge. The rationale is that better informed women are also able to make healthier and more responsible choices regarding their body, pregnancy and the like. This has tremendous impact on maternal and newborn health outcomes.

The Adolescent Boys Group (ABG) is less than a year old (as of November 2011). Training and sensitization of young adolescent boys (14–16 years) towards women's health was important for Mabelle Arole, as they would be the future generations of men. The group has a 16-week training period on awareness regarding abusive behaviours, attitudes and beliefs towards women and developing social skills. Future plans for the programme include developing livelihood opportunities and practical skills, with the help of SHGs.

Activities

Both programmes use training sessions, peer group leaders and group meetings to discuss and educate young people on sexual and reproductive health, mental health, rights, maternal and child health as well as FP.

Not only are these meetings a good place to socialize, but also include health education (nutrition, sex education, FP and menstruation, hygiene, sanitation and environment, common diseases and their remedies), social and cultural issues (social and legal rights), self-defence, presentations on various issues covered and creative activities (singing, dancing, creative writing etc.).

The boys' group is relatively new, but changes in behaviour of participants before and after being part of the ABG were observed by the organizers.

Impact

With the AGP, CRHP managed to reach out and create awareness among the women of the community at a young age. This resulted in better informed adolescents, who, when they got married, were better informed on taking care of their own needs, of the needs of their families and caring for their newborn children.

The ABG is less than a year old, but interaction with the young members indicated that reaching out to boys at this age was making a difference in sensitizing them on sexual and reproductive health issues, crucial at the time of puberty. It also provided a platform for the young boys to clarify doubts, ask questions and become sensitized to the needs of women/girls.

Sustainability

Acknowledging the social structures which implied that young girls had less access to money than the boys—CRHP structured the adolescent groups in a way in which, much like the SHGs, there would be pooling of finances. However, in the adolescent groups the amount contributed would go towards a savings account. Boys are required to contribute ₹50 a month, whereas the amount is flexible for adolescent girls.

Mobile Health Team

The second tier is the CRHP's Mobile Health Team (MHT), which acts as a liaison between each project village and the CRHP. The MHT provides periodic support for all health and development activities when needed and conducts extensive project monitoring. The MHT also serves as a link in CRHP's health referral network.

The MHT comprises a nurse, social worker, medical doctor and driver. The team visits the villages periodically—covering each village at least once a month. The women's groups in the village help the MHT in organizing health check-ups.

The MHT supervises new VHWs and assists and trains the others as needed. It also ensures that pregnant women are visited, providing pre and postnatal care, including check-ups for the newborn and provides assistance on FP. The team helps in identifying cases (including maternal) for referral to the hospital if needed.

Hospital and Training Centre

The third tier is the hospital and training centre located in CRHP's Jamkhed compound. It is here that local, national and international training in community-based health and development takes place and the trainees, including VHWs, are housed. The non-profit hospital provides many medical and surgical referral care services for the populations of the project villages and also receives patients from other areas outside Jamkhed Block. The aim is provision of low cost secondary care where minimum cost ensures quality of care.

The Julia Hospital is a 50-bedded facility serving a population of 500,000 from nearby villages. The hospital provides general surgeries and critical care; it was recently upgraded with new equipment and facilities. Services provided include emergency maternal and newborn care, normal deliveries, FP services, snake bites, general surgeries, burns, eye camps, cataract surgeries, etc.

Care is provided free of charge to poor people at the hospital and at a low cost to those who can afford to pay.

Other Intersectoral Initiatives by CRHP That Impact Health

Appropriate Technologies

Based on the utilization of locally available resources, effective traditional remedies and methods are encouraged and expanded upon. One example is the Jaipur foot, an artificial lower limb. CRHP also advocates the use of and research into, low cost and efficient methods of energy production to address chronic water and energy shortages, thereby increasing productivity, improving the local economy and reducing poverty. Some examples include installation of solar panels and wind turbines in the CRHP compound. CRHP is also in the process of developing a water filter, which is a variant of the more traditional slow sand filter, at $25 per unit. This has great potential to improve health.

Child Development Programme

A preschool programme known as Joyful Learning is run for disadvantaged and poor children with an aim to increase their self-esteem, improve their health and provide them with social and health education (the child-to-child programme especially focusses on this). To prevent the disruption of studies of the children during the seasonal migration of parents for work outside the village, a hostel has been built. It ensures uninterrupted studies, proper hygiene and balanced nutrition.

Environment and Sanitation

The CRHP recognized the improvement of agricultural techniques and practices as a necessary step towards the promotion of better nutrition and health. To this end, CRHP has often partnered with government agencies, universities and other NGOs to obtain financial as well as technical support for water and land-related development projects, as well as to organize relevant seminars for local farmers. The main objective of the Watershed Development Programme is to ensure the proper use of rainwater and to reduce its wastage, along with the associated erosion of topsoil.

Personal and domestic hygiene is promoted by the VHWs who are taught effective ways to reduce the spread of water-borne diseases that occur through faecal-oral contact as well as the use of unsafe drinking water, combined with proper ways to treat, follow-up or refer infections and illnesses if they occur. This information is subsequently disseminated by the VHWs.

Nutrition

Apart from community-based interventions, one of the ways in which CRHP is seeking to improve nutrition in its intervention villages is through improving agricultural knowledge, not just through the farmers' clubs but also through a demonstration farm. Despite the harsh environmental conditions of Jamkhed, the demonstration farm—the Khadkat Farm—is about 50 acres of cultivated land where nutritious crops are grown, both indigenous and otherwise.

The farm also serves to demonstrate how, in a hot and dry area such as Jamkhed, it is possible to cultivate healthy crops with the help of appropriate technological interventions. Empowering ordinary people to cultivate nutritious crops, especially those that could be grown all year round, instead of plants with a longer crop cycle or those that deplete an already inadequate soil is an important element of CRHP's intersectoral approach towards health.

Impact and Achievement

This case study focusses on the impact of an intervention on maternal and newborn health; which relates to the achievement of Millennium Development Goal (MDG) 4 (reduction of child mortality) and MDG 5 (improvement in maternal health).

CRHP has aimed to reduce child mortality through educating mothers about nutrition, improving kitchen and vegetable gardens, monitoring the weight of the children, emphasizing home remedies such as steam inhalation, cold sponging and oral rehydration salts (ORS) and encouraging understanding about sanitation and communicable diseases.

The IMR dropped from 176 per 1,000 live births in 1971 to 24 per 1,000 live births in 2004 (CRHP).[3] Immunization in villages with CRHP intervention went up.

Improvements in maternal health, such as ANC coverage went up from 0.5% in 1976 to 99% in 2004 (ibid.). CRHP's data indicates that 90% of the pregnancies are registered within the first semester, 80% of the pregnancies are managed successfully through VHWs, there is acceptance of the need of ANC and safe deliveries, high-risk pregnancies are identified in time and referred to secondary-care facilities, there is provision of community emergency transport, there are less than 5 to 10% caesarean sections (C sections) and there has been only one maternal death in the last five years in the project villages. Even sexual health has been impacted and the human immunodeficiency virus (HIV) prevalence is less than 1% in the general population and 0.07% in pregnant women.[4]

As indicated by the figures, the number of women using FP has increased from less than 1% in 1976 to 68% in 2004; there has been a resultant decrease in the number of births (see Figure 15.4). The increase in FP methods does not just impact women's health by reducing unwanted pregnancies but also protects them from sexually transmitted diseases and gives them greater control over their bodies.

Figure 15.4
Percent of Married Women Using Family Planning

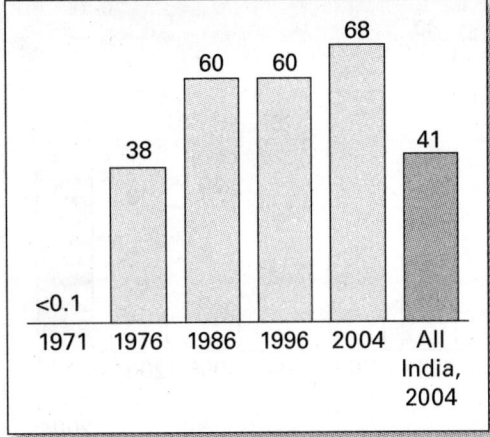

Source: http://www.prb.org/Articles/2007/ LessonsLearnedCommunity-BasedProject.aspx, accessed on 6 August 2013.

Looking Ahead

CRHP has taken up scaling-up as one of its goals and has chosen to do so by the sharing of knowledge and experience that the organization has gained over the years.

Training is one of the most important tools of scaling-up that CRHP uses to inform and pass on lessons from the decades of experience it has in community health.[5] CRHP has focussed on the role of trainer and facilitator to enable other community-based organizations and government agencies to implement such projects in areas where the need is apparent. The organization conducts residential and non-residential (on-site) training of grassroots workers, government and CRHP staff at various

---

[3] Data sent over email by CRHP to PHFI.
[4] Data sent over email by CRHP to PHFI.
[5] Interview with Ravi Arole held in November (2011) at Jamkhed, Maharashtra.

Figure 15.5
Births per 1,000 People

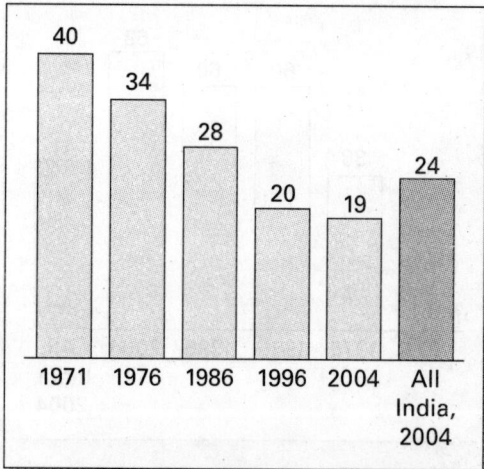

Source: http://www.prb.org/Publications/
Articles/2007/LessonsLearnedCommunity-
BasedProject.aspx, accessed on 6 August 2013.

levels of the health system. Over the past 30 years, CRHP has trained over 100,000 community health and development (grassroots) workers. The training centre receives approximately 2,000 trainees per year from NGOs and government agencies from nearly every state in India and about 100 other countries.

The work by CRHP has extended beyond the geographical borders of Maharashtra. For example, CRHP is working with the Society for the Elimination of Rural Poverty (SERP) in Andhra Pradesh. The state government is sending project coordinators, health professionals and grassroots workers from every district for the 10–14-day training at the CRHP training centre in Jamkhed. CRHP acknowledges the role of governments and NGOs in scaling-up programmes such as its own to country-wide dimensions. The Jamkhed Model has also been replicated in some Latin American and African countries. Organizations seeking to replicate the model from these countries sent their representatives to spend a couple of years to train at the CRHP centre and take back the learnings to their countries.

The idea behind scaling-up through training, as argued by the CRHP, is that this approach is more cost-effective and has more significant and sustainable impact on the community than attempts to recreate the project in remote areas. There is little evidence to test the validity of this statement (whether one is better than the other); however, the creation of human capital (through training) does have a significant impact on health outcomes.

Conclusion

The CRHP adopts a multi-sectoral approach to address various interrelated health problems. As can be seen from the results, it does manage to create an impact through direct interventions such as nutrition, planned and assisted pregnancies and encouraging home remedies and through indirect ways such as improving sanitation and adopting green technologies, which impact health in a broader sense.

If one critically examines CRHP it can be noted that while improvement is visible, it has happened over 30 years. This is a long duration and it can be assumed that during this time several other factors, unrelated to the project, such as improvements in roads and transport, advances in technology, influx of media even in remote villages and on a large scale and increase in the autonomy of women after three decades might have also impacted maternal and newborn health. It is difficult to evaluate the counter factual (what would have happened in the absence of the intervention) and, thus, measure the exact impact of CRHP. It is also difficult in multi-sectoral interventions to evaluate the pathways through which different methods (direct and indirect) impact maternal and newborn health or to quantify the exact degree of impact.

Perhaps more rigorous evaluation of the project with control groups and study of the impact of various factors in isolation will assist the programme managers in designing the most cost-effective and sustainable method for impacting maternal and newborn health.

References

Arole, R. and Arole, M. 1994. *Jamkhed—A Comprehensive Rural Health Project*. Macmillan Publishers.

Future Generations. 2011. A Tribute to Raj Arole of the Comprehensive Rural Health Project in Jamkhed, India. Available at: http:// www.future.org/news/20110609/tribute-raj-arole-comprehensive-rural-health-project-jamkhed-india, accessed on 7 August 2013.

World Health Organization (WHO). 1997. 'Intersectoral Action for Health: A Cornerstone for Health for All in the Twenty-First Century'. Report of the International Conference. Halifax, Canada. WHO. Available at: http://whqlibdoc.who.int/hq/1997/ WHO_PPE_PAC_97.6.pdf, accessed on 6 August 2013.

Youth Reproductive and Sexual Health

16. Growing-up Healthy: Anwesha Clinics, Friends Clinic and Safdarjung Hospital Adolescent Health Network (SHAHN)

16

Growing-up Healthy: Anwesha Clinics, Friends Clinic and Safdarjung Hospital Adolescent Health Network (SHAHN)

Radhika Arora

What Is Adolescent Health and How Is It Linked with Maternal and Newborn Health?

Adolescence is defined as the period in the human life cycle that lies between puberty and adulthood. Usually between the ages of 10 to 19 years, this transitory period is marked by physical, emotional, psychological, sexual and mental maturation. The duration of the perceived 'adolescent period' (UN-FPA 2003)—which in turn affects the impact of adolescent behaviour on health—is often influenced by socio-cultural factors.

Young people, as different from adolescents are those between the ages of 10 to 24 years of age. For the purpose of this case study, we will focus on services which focus on populations belonging to this age bracket.

Why Focus on Youth Health

The adolescent–youth period is marked by significant mental and physical changes; in addition, social and cultural responses to the individual also change during the adolescent period, creating a complex socio-cultural context for a young person to navigate the changes that s/he is undergoing. Inspite of this, young people tend to present less morbidity and mortality than children and older people.

Young people are more vulnerable to sexual violence, exploitation, drug abuse, etc. In some aspects of health, such as mental and sexual health, adolescents suffer disproportionately. Youth is also the period when lifelong health-related behaviours, such as smoking, eating habits, sexual behaviours and help-seeking behaviours develop (Bayley 2003). Social response to puberty and adolescence is often influenced by external factors such as education, awareness and access to information and services. Sociological factors can also define and influence the way an adolescent copes with the changes and the way puberty is addressed (UNFPA 2003), which in turn could influence and determine a young person's health status, needs and health seeking behaviour.

Socio-cultural practices that encourage early marriage and childbirth and low levels of education, awareness and empowerment, make women of this age group especially vulnerable to early marriage, early and unsafe pregnancies, nutrition issues and risk of sexual disease and abuse.

The need for adolescent health services in India is particularly urgent. India has more adolescents than any other country in the world (243 million), making up almost one-fifth of the country's population. Various national policies affecting youth health

> **Box 16.1: National Policies Affecting Youth Health in India**
>
> - 1974: National Policy for Children
> - 1976: Child Marriage Restraint Act
> - 1985: National Youth Policy
> - 1986: National Policy on Education
> - 1997: Reproductive Child Health I
> - 2000; National Population Policy
> - 2001: National Policy for Empowerment of Women
> - 2002: National AIDS Prevention and Control Policy
> - 2002: National Health Policy
> - 2003: National Youth Policy
> - 2005: Reproductive Child Health II
> - 2008: Right to Education
>
> *Source:* Result of various searches and documents.

in India have been implemented over the year (see Box 16.1). Almost 47% of India's adolescents are women. Forty four percent of adolescent are married before the age of 18. Adolescent mothers are at a higher risk of miscarriage, maternal mortality and stillbirths (Government of India 2006) as compared to women who have children at a slighter older age; 36% of women in India were pregnant or delivered their first child by the age of 19 years of age (NFHS-3 2005–06). Approximately 50% of adolescent girls in India are underweight and approximately 30% anaemic, which affect maternal and newborn health.

Given this context, the need to provide integrated and appropriate youth services has perhaps never been more important.

How Can Youth Health Services—through Youth-friendly Health Centres—Impact Maternal and Newborn Health?

There are a variety of innovative youth health programmes in India. These range from behaviour change communications (BCC) strategies to education and livelihood programmes (see Box 16.2). Programmes targeting young people may also be a component of larger initiatives such as youth health programmes that are components of larger community-based or maternal health interventions. This case study will focus on 'adolescent clinics' or 'youth-friendly health centres'. The two terms are used interchangeably throughout this case study.

Between 2010 and 2011, as part of the ongoing PHFI-MacArthur Foundation project on documenting interventions in maternal, newborn and adolescent health, a directory of innovations implemented and ongoing in India was compiled. Of the 218 innovations in the directory, 34 interventions specifically focussed on youth reproductive and sexual health (YRSH). From these, the idea of providing health services and information targeting young people through 'adolescent clinics' or 'youth-friendly health centres' was selected for documentation as a film and print case study.

'Adolescent clinics' or 'youth-friendly health centres' are physical spaces created especially for the provision of youth-friendly health information and services. These spaces may be stand-alone dedicated clinic-style spaces or may be developed as part of an existing health facility, either as a separate room or separate time slot dedicated for the provision of youth health services within a larger health, educational or community space.

There are some key distinguishing features of a youth-friendly health centre. These are to provide health services tailored to the needs of this demographic, as well as to encourage and improve access to youth health services, especially to deliver services effectively within local socio-cultural contexts.

Adolescent or youth-friendly health centres provide a variety of clinical and non-clinical health services. These may include, but are not restricted to:

Box 16.2: Types of Adolescent Health Programmes in India

- Adolescent clinics
- BCC strategies
- Community-based, peer-group model
- Education and livelihood programmes
- Emotions and stress counselling
- Family planning
- Family planning—availability of information on and methods of contraception
- Growth and development monitoring
- Gynaecological services
- Health: Clinical interventions
- Immunization
- Medical termination of pregnancy: counselling and referrals
- Menstrual health
- Mental health services
- Nutrition: For boys, girls and young women
- Preventive counselling against injuries, substance abuse and high-risk sexual behaviour
- Promotion of healthy lifestyle
- Reproductive sexual health programmes (including RTI/STI): information and counselling
- Soft-skill development: Personality and personal presentation development, language skills, personal grooming, etc.
- Vocational skills
- Weight management
- Youth affairs and sports

Source: Dr Roza Olyai, Chairperson, Adolescent Health Committee, FOGSI.

Clinical and Non-clinical Health Interventions (information and services)

- Reproductive and sexual health
- Family planning: Information and services
- Reproductive and sexually transmitted diseases
- Medical termination of pregnancy
- Counselling—physical and mental health issues
- Menstruation
- Mental health
- Nutrition

Other Interventions

- Life-skills development
- Education—academic and vocational
- Social support

- Domestic violence
- BCCs
- Targeting social issues: Delay in age of marriage, delay in first pregnancy, birth spacing, women's health, etc.

Some of these interventions may be common to other related areas of public health services. However, adolescent/youth health services are set apart not just by the menu of services they offer, but also in the way in which the services are delivered (see Figure 16.1).

Essential Characteristics of Youth-friendly Health Services (through a centre/clinic setting)

- **Ensuring privacy**: To improve access to services that might be culturally sensitive or taboo.
- **Confidentiality**: Towards creating a space where young people are able to discuss their issues in a safe space.
- **Unbiased services**: Towards ensuring that services delivered are free of social, cultural, racial, religious or economic prejudices and do not reflect negative socio-cultural perspectives, if any.

With a socio-cultural context that encourages early marriage and childbirth, as well as makes discussing issues of reproductive sexual health tricky, there is a need to make reliable, appropriate adolescent health services accessible and available for India's large youth population. Focus on improving youth health—especially reproductive and sexual health among young people, empowering young women through education, as well as creating awareness on social-cultural practices—can help delay the age of marriage and first pregnancy in young couples, improve use of contraception and encourage birth spacing and also reduce incidence of reproductive tract infection/sexually transmitted infections (RTI/STI)—contributing towards improved maternal, neonatal and perinatal health indicators.[1]

Adolescent Friendly Health Centres

For the purpose of highlighting the case of providing youth-friendly health services through adolescent health centres or clinics, three different kinds of adolescent clinics were visited in Delhi and West Bengal. These have been used to demonstrate different aspects of initiatives towards establishing youth-friendly health centres in India. The three clinics featured as a case study in this document are:

1. **Safdarjung Hospital Adolescent Health Care Network (SHAHN):** One of the first adolescent clinics to be set-up by the government with support from the World Health

---

[1] Swach Report titled 'Use of a public health approach to adolescent friendly health services in a rural community in Haryana'. Available at ftp://203.90.70.117/searoftp/WROIND/whoindia/linkfiles/Adolescent_Health_and_Development_(AHD)_swach_report.pdf, accessed 6 August 2013.

Figure 16.1
Strategy Paper on Family Welfare

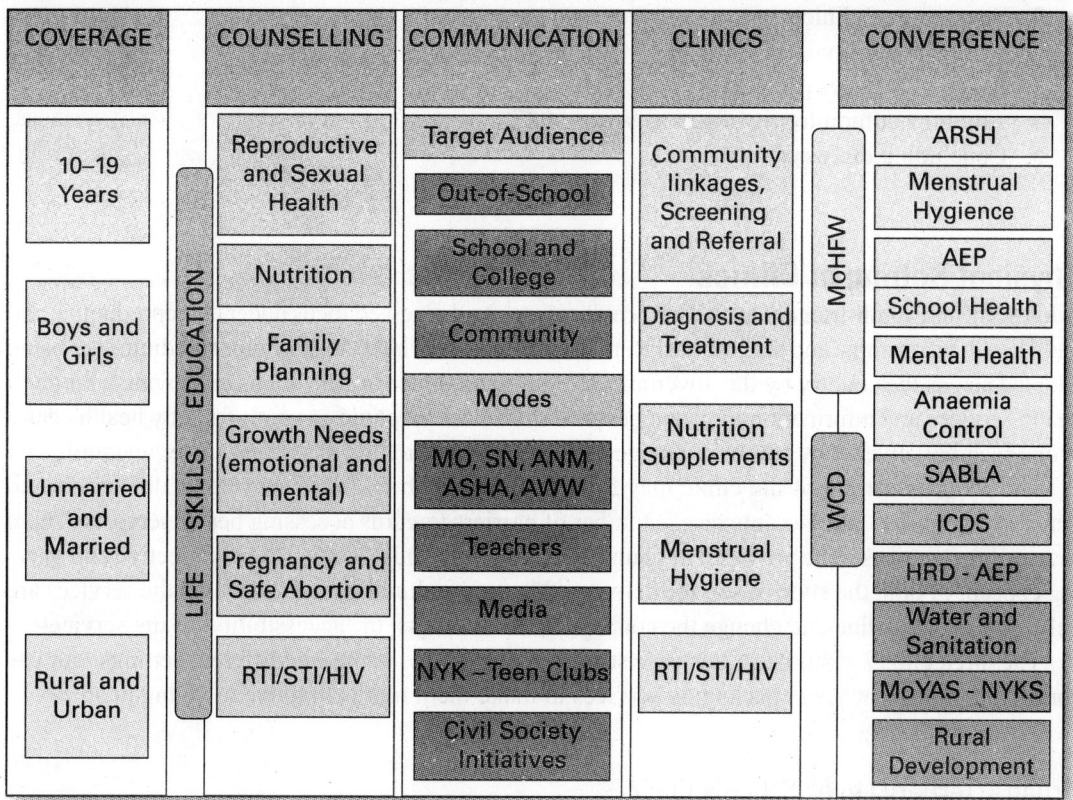

Source: Gupta and Nair (2010).[2]

Organization (WHO), SHAHN provides health care services for adolescents within the tertiary-level Safdarjung Hospital.

2. **Friends:** An initiative by the NGO MAMTA with support from the Swedish International Development Cooperation Agency (SIDA), the Friends' clinic was set-up in an urban slum in Delhi for young people to access clinical and non-clinical services.

3. **Anwesha:** An initiative by the Government of West Bengal, the Anwesha clinics provide clinical and non-clinical services through clinics set-up at primary health centres (PHCs) and district-level hospitals and also outreach services in schools.

Three clinics were selected for developing this case study to illustrate the use of youth-friendly services through a facility-based setting in different social, geographical and financial contexts. The case study is divided according to the emerging themes of:

[2] Available at http://pglibrary-publichealth.wikispaces.com/file/view/4+Health+%26+Family+Welfare+(II)+swot+gantt.pdf, accessed on 6 August 2013.

1. Physical setting of clinic
   • Geographical coverage
2. Financing of clinics
   • Sustainability
3. Kinds of services provided
4. Any impact/monitoring of services—results
5. Concluding discussion

Physical Setting of Clinics

Adolescent and youth-friendly health services have received renewed focus under the reproductive and child health programme and the National Rural Health Mission (NRHM). Different mediums are being adopted across the country by the government, NGOs and donor organizations to provide a range of health services and information to young people. An adolescent clinic or youth-friendly health centre is one such initiative. They combine a range of clinical and non-clinical services under one roof.

The physical setting of the clinic may differ. While health facilities provide health services to general populations, adolescents face a number of barriers towards accessing health services. There is a need for services to be provided to young people in a 'friendly' setting. The subjective and varying concept of both the style of service delivery, the socio-cultural context in which the services are delivered would define and change the concept of 'friendliness' or 'accessibility' of the services.

The three clinics featured in this case study are physically located in different settings, but use some similar approaches in packaging services to make them more attractive to young people.

Urban + Tertiary Level: SHAHN Clinic

The SHAHN was set-up in the year 2000 by the Safdarjung Hospital (1,500-bedded tertiary-level hospital in New Delhi) along with the WHO and the Ministry of Health and Family Welfare. SHAHN was one of the first initiatives of its kind towards developing specialized adolescent-friendly health services (AFHS) in the country (Government of India 2005). Ten such AFHS were established by the Government of India (GoI). A need for a separate space to provide clinical and non-clinical health-related care for young people was felt by doctors at the department of pediatrics. Traditionally, health care services at the hospital and elsewhere, were geared towards the needs of children or adults, with very limited services customized to the needs of adolescents and young people.

The intervention was selected to illustrate the use of existing resources in creating an adolescent clinic in an urban, tertiary-hospital setting. The physical infrastructure for the clinic and human resources were largely drawn from the existing hospital pool of medical doctors and non-medical staff, with some assistance from supporting organizations.

The decision to set-up the clinic within the hospital was also made in order to retain and maintain links with patients from the department of pediatrics and at the same time attract new younger clients to utilize necessary services and information on health care issues, it was decided to open an adolescent clinic within the existing infrastructure of the tertiary-level Safdarjung Hospital in Delhi with technical assistance from the WHO and support from the Ministry of Health.

Urban + Community Level: Friends' Clinic

The NGO MAMTA had been working in the area of sexual and reproductive health (SRH) since the 1990s. The organization primarily worked in the resettlement colony of Tigri in Delhi. MAMTA established a youth-friendly centre called Friends in Tigri, Delhi in 2006.

Studies indicate various barriers that adolescents faced towards accessing and utilizing public health services. These include lack of privacy, confidentiality, availability of same-sex doctors among other elements preventing adolescents from accessing public health facilities. The study also highlighted the need for the health system to cater to the needs of adolescent reproductive and sexual health.

The Friends' Clinic is located in a community setting. The clinic focusses on three areas: raising awareness on SRH issues, clinical health services—for both SRH issues and general health issues (including diagnostics and referral services) and also outreach services to create awareness and sensitize other members of the community (towards reducing barriers for young people to access health information and services).

Rural + Community + Primary Level: Anwesha Clinics

Anwesha (the Bengali word for quest) is a chain of adolescent clinics run by the Department of Health and Family Welfare, Government of West Bengal. The clinics were started when it was realized that women above the age of 19 years and children below the age of six had some access to health services but there were no health care facilities available that provided specialized care for those between the ages of 10–19 years. This was especially relevant for creating awareness on nutrition, menstruation and menstrual hygiene for young women and addressing the issue of RTI/STIs among young men and women of the community.

Acknowledging the gap in services for young people, the Government of West Bengal started adolescent clinics in 2004 at the community health centre (CHC) level. District-level clinics were set-up in 2006, but by 2007 it was evident that a single district-level adolescent clinic could not cater to the needs of the society. By 2008, adolescent clinics were established at PHCs at the block level.

This form of adolescent health services through a clinic setting provides care at multiple levels and settings, such as outreach in schools and community towards generating demand at adolescent clinics in PHCs to providing a network of referrals to provide more comprehensive health services.

Discussion on Location of the Clinic

The physical location would play a crucial role in the addressing issues of access to health services for young people. Physical access, such as having a clinic in a space where young people might be hesitant to visit, is one of the barriers towards accessing age-appropriate health services. This is essential towards addressing issues of privacy, confidentiality and accessing youth-health services even in social spaces that might not be encouraging towards accessing these services. It would influence the demographic profile of clients that use the clinic; it would impact the kind of services that the clients use the clinic for—especially in the context of what might or might not be acceptable socially.

Just as important as the physical and geographical location of the clinic, is enabling access and acceptability of youth health services by reaching out to guardians or 'gatekeepers'. Given the often sensitive nature of SRH needs, socio-cultural perceptions (for example, privacy while accessing health services, especially for young girls) would be a matter of concern.

Take for example, the Friends' Clinic which is based in a community setting needed to blend in comprehensive outreach and awareness activities in its intervention areas to sensitize gatekeepers of the community on the kind of services provided by the centre, the need for it and remove taboos related to accessing services. The Friends' Clinic also provides general health services to the community enabling it to develop a more inclusive approach towards providing comprehensive adolescent health services for young people.

The Anwesha Clinics are held at a specific time, within a primary health centre in a rural setting. Outreach in the community and in educational establishments is an essential component towards generating demand for youth health services. The Anwesha Clinics are also located at health centres at different levels: at PHCs, district health centres (DHCs) and also at the tertiary level. The availability of youth-friendly health services at different tiers allows the clinics to cover young people living in different physical and social spaces. It also allows for improved tracking of young people who may move and also for referrals.

Financing of Clinics

All three clinics featured in this case study present examples of different ways to finance the establishment and operations of adolescent clinics. The issue of sustainability would be important towards ensuring continuous provision of relevant youth health services in a community.

The SHAHN clinic was set-up using existing resources of the Safdarjung Hospital. Technical advice was provided by the WHO and the initiative was supported by the Ministry of Health and Family Welfare. The SHAHN was one of the first initiatives of its kind in the country. In the 11 years since its establishment it has served as a demonstration of providing youth-friendly services in a cost-effective way within a tertiary-care facility. Even after partnerships with other organizations ended, the location of the clinic meant that it could be sustained within the hospital premises and operations.

The Friends' Clinic was set-up and is operated by the NGO MAMTA with support from SIDA. The clinic also charges a nominal user fee for clients. However, the questions that may be discussed here is how can one ensure sustainability of such clinics without external funding?

The Anwesha Clinics of West Bengal are supported and operated by the government under the NRHM. The Kolkata Medical College is the nodal centre for adolescent-health related activities (NRHM 2010). The clinics are located in existing health care facilities at primary, district and tertiary-level government health care facilities, thereby optimizing and adding to existing resources.

Kind of Services Provided

Services provided by youth-friendly health centres include a range of services that cover the needs of young people. These would include both clinical and non-clinical services, covering general health issues, SRH issues as well as counselling and information provision services (see Table 16.1).

This section presents a table of services provided by the three adolescent clinics featured in this case study, along with a brief discussion section.

Table 16.1

Comparison Table of the Three Adolescent Clinics Featured in This Case Study

	Anwesha	Friends	SHAHN
Target Age Group	Youth: 10–24 years	Youth: 10–24 years	Adolescent: 13–19 years
Marital Status	Married-Unmarried	Married-Unmarried	Unmarried
Gender	Boys and girls	Boys and girls	Boys and girls
Financing	Government (under NRHM)	Donor-funded (NGO)	Government (initial technical support by the WHO)
Location	• Community-based (PHC level) • District level • Tertiary level • Rural and Urban	• Community based • Urban (lower socio-economic)	• Tertiary level • Urban
Outreach: • Target • Geographical Coverage	• Community-based outreach • Peer-to-peer • Gatekeepers: Community leaders, teachers, parents • Dedicated outreach personnel	• Community-based outreach • Peer-to-peer • Gatekeepers: community leaders, teachers, parents • Dedicated outreach personnel • Drop-in centre	• In-school adolescents
Family Planning	• Prevention of pregnancies • Prevention of RTI/STIs • Counselling • Emergency contraception • Advocacy—age of marriage • Advocacy—age of birth of first child	• Prevention of pregnancies • Prevention of RTI/STIs • Counselling • Emergency contraception • Advocacy—age of marriage • Advocacy—age of birth of first child	• Prevention of pregnancies • Prevention of RTI/STIs • Counselling • Emergency contraception • Advocacy—age of marriage • Advocacy—age of birth of first child
MTP	• Counselling	• Counselling	• Counselling • Reference towards safe accessing safe MTP services
Nutrition	• Counselling on nutrition • Food habits • Target youth and parents of young people towards ensuring nutritious diet • Distribution of IFA tablets		• Counselling • IFA

(Table 16.1 Continued)

(Table 16.1 Continued)

	Anwesha	Friends	SHAHN
HIV/AIDS	• Integrated counselling and testing centres (ICTC) by NACO • Information and services • IEC	• Information and services • IEC	• Information and services • IEC
General Health Services	• No: General health services by other providers at health care facility	• Yes: Provide general health services	• No: General health services by other providers at health care facility
SRH	Yes	Yes	Yes
Referrals	Yes	N/A	Yes. Links to other departments within the hospital setting, including, but not restricted to: • Dermatology • Gynaecology • Endocrinology
Capacity Building	N/A	N/A	• Development of adolescent-friendly health services • Facilitation of adolescent programmes across the country • Encouraging medical students to use adolescent health subjects for their thesis work
Menstrual Health	• **Awareness:** On issues of menstrual health and hygiene • **Sanitary Napkins:** Access to sanitary napkins, therefore, reduces UTI/RTIs caused by old and used cloth. Supply cost: ₹8.50 to ₹7.50 per packet • Addressing menstrual health issues	• **Awareness:** On issues of menstrual health and hygiene • Addressing menstrual health issues • **Sanitary Napkins:** Access to sanitary napkins	• **Awareness:** On issues of menstrual health and hygiene • Addressing menstrual health issues
Mental Health	Yes	Yes	Yes
Privacy and Confidentiality	• Training of health care personnel to provide youth-friendly care • No separate timings for boys and girls	• Training of health care personnel to provide youth-friendly care • Separate timings for boys and girls to ensure privacy	• Training of health care personnel to provide youth-friendly care • Privacy concerns acknowledged

(Table 16.1 Continued)

(*Table 16.1 Continued*)

	Anwesha	Friends	SHAHN
	• Separate room from general health services for counselling • No concept of privacy in waiting area	• Separate waiting area	• No separate timings for boys and girls • Separate room from general health services for counselling • No concept of privacy in waiting area
Pregnancy Care for Young Mothers	• ANC counselling • Immunization • Counselling on breastfeeding	N/A	N/A
Information Education Communication (IEC)	Information leaflets: Parents, teachers, young people, issue-based	Information leaflets available	Information leaflets: Parents, teachers, young people, issue-based
Other			• Tetanus toxoid (TT) vaccine

Source: Information on clinics based on secondary literature, organization reports and field interviews.

Discussion

The services provided by all three clinics are almost similar in nature and type. The kind of services and the way in which these services are provided would depend on various factors including, but not restricted to goals of the clinic, target audience or context, physical location of the clinics, client profile and evidence-based need.

While the three clinics provide similar services, emphasis on each differs according to local contexts. For example, the Anwesha Clinics focus more on UTI/RTI/STIs which is a common health complaint among young girls and boys at the PHC-level at the Barasat District which we visited. For the Friends' Clinic providing general health services along with focussed SRH and menstrual issues helped it gain acceptability in the community area. The SHAHN clinic focusses on addressing clinical and non-clinical complaints specific to adolescents, using an intensive network of referrals available to the clinic because of their location at a tertiary health facility, to provide specialized care to clients when needed.

Any Impact/Monitoring of Services—Results

This case study seeks to look at the need for and the provision of youth-friendly health services through the lens of its impact on maternal and newborn health. Impact as discussed in this case would largely be based on utilization of services at the clinics.

In this regard, provision of youth-friendly services can impact maternal and newborn health through a distal route (see Table 16.2).

Table 16.2
How Can Youth Friendly Services Impact Maternal and Newborn Health

Counselling, Information Dissemination	• Delay the age of marriage • Delay the age of first pregnancy • Improve information on and adoption of family planning methods for young, married adolescents • Improve awareness on SRH • Improve and create awareness on mental health issues • Awareness on nutrition—girls and boys • Community BCC • Counselling and awareness on maternal and child care for young people with newborn babies
Clinical Services	• Provision of primary health care services • Provision of health care services related to menstruation and SRH • Management, treatment and information on sexually transmitted diseases, reproductive health, HIV/AIDS • Health care referrals
Non-clinical Services	• Nutrition • Menstrual health • Referrals for further health services if needed

Source: Based on information presented in this case and secondary literature on adolescent-friendly health services.

Not much information on utilization and coverage of the Anwesha Clinics was found at the time of documentation for the purposes of this case study. Based on interviews with field staff and clients of services at the Chhotogulia PHC in the Barasat District of West Bengal as well as observations at a local middle school it was found that the clinic was well-known in the area. Utilization of the clinics, especially for girls, was largely for RTIs, common to the area and also for menstrual health services and counselling. Outreach activities in the school influenced and facilitated better communication between young people and outreach personnel, as well as better understanding between the two genders in the school setting. Group discussions with students from Grade 8 indicated their awareness of the need to delay marriage until the specified 18 years of age for girls and 21 years of age for boys was high. Issues of sanitation and menstrual health were also comfortably discussed.

In terms of access to clinics, there are 342 Anwesha Clinics at the block level in the state, 16 adolescent health clinics at the district level and three at tertiary-level medical colleges. These are served by one counsellor, one general nurse midwife (GNM) and one medical officer.

The Friends' Clinic has been running in the community since 2006; it has, over the last five years, provided services to 688 clients (over 1,791 visits in 2006–08; Das et al. 2009)—giving access to both medical and non-medical services and counselling to the young people between the ages of 15 and 19 years from the community. Most clients came with general health complaints and gradually began using the health services to discuss sensitive issues. SRH complaints were expressed by 17.2% male and 36.9% female clients at the time of first medical history recording. Menstrual health was presented as one of the primary concerns of female clients—72% of female clients indicated concerns regarding menstrual health.

The need for promoting safer sex was highlighted; there was an increased awareness on the proper use of condoms. Information on this increased by 82% among males and 92.9% among females over multiple visits.

Clients were assessed for their knowledge about condoms and its correct use—the results improved over the number of visits of each client, bringing about behaviour change in terms of increased knowledge on safer sexual practices and prevention of HIV and other STIs. Men and women, 12.4% and 11.2% respectively, reported symptoms of STIs. Approximately 76% of clients felt that discussions on SRH were necessary.

Most clients, almost 95% did not face any difficulty in visiting the clinics and accessing services. Visiting hours were convenient and time spent by health care providers was sufficient, as expressed by 96.8 % male and 83.4 % female clients. Majority felt they had sufficient privacy and almost 91% indicated satisfaction with the nature and quality of services provided.

Information on the impact of services according to each service for the SHAHN clinics was scant at the time of documentation. Based on information accessed on utilization it was found that the clinic receives almost four to five new clients every week, though the number of clients visiting the clinic reduces during the months of March–April due to school and university examinations.

A network of referrals, from the department of pediatrics to the SHAHN Clinic and from the SHAHN Clinic to other departments within the hospital network such as gynaecology, endocrinology, dermatology, etc., was established. Outreach activities in nearby schools were conducted to create a demand for services. This was an essential component of SHAHN's activities. It was used to conduct awareness activities on adolescent health in schools and colleges and also generate demand for services among young people. Clients also find out about the SHAHN Clinic through word of mouth and referrals from within the hospital.

The initial response to the clinic was lukewarm with one or two new clients being registered every session; the numbers gradually increased and the clinic sessions had to be increased to two to three times a week.

Concluding Discussions

The SHAHN was one of the first initiatives of its kind in the country. In the eleven years since its establishment. it has served as a demonstration of providing youth-friendly services in a cost-effective way within a tertiary care facility.

Lessons from SHAHN's operations along with other similar initiatives, over the last decade have been used towards supporting the development of other similar adolescent clinics as well as other forms of adolescent-friendly health care services in India. Lessons from SHAHN reinforced the need for context appropriate, well-designed and effectively implemented youth health services. It highlighted the intersectoral nature of the health care needs of this population.

It is through pilot interventions such as this that issues of features of adolescent-friendly services have emerged from easy-to-miss issues of accessibility to training to health care providers and kinds of services provided.

One of the most important lessons for youth health issues to have emerged from this initiative was to integrate community outreach and sensitization of stakeholders to increase demand for youth-friendly services.

As with the SHAHN Clinic, the Friends' Clinic realized the importance of community outreach and sensitization towards reducing barriers that young people faced during accessing youth health services. While the Friends' Clinic is well-established within the community, challenges emerged in terms of scaling-up of services and suitability. Apart from the issues faced while scaling-up, operating an adolescent clinic such as this can be faced with certain challenges as well. Developing the capacity of people working at the centre towards providing adolescent-friendly services was essential towards building a friendly and safe environment. For the clients, this was the first time that many of them had the opportunity to use a facility such as this and also get the opportunity for one-on-one interactions with medical practitioners.

Political will and government support gives the Anwesha Clinic the opportunity to extend its services to remote and larger populations, largely in underserved rural areas. Here as well, outreach and community mobilization proved to be crucial in gaining acceptability and reducing barriers towards accessing adolescent-friendly health services.

Adolescent-friendly health services can have a distal impact on MCH. India's demographic and present maternal and child mortality figures indicate an urgent need for health care provision customized for this demographic. Sustainability and reaching out to larger populations are concerns of adolescent clinics. As indicated by all three clinics featured in this case outreach and community awareness is crucial in removing barriers, improving access and improving awareness on both the need for, as well as, kind of youth health services available.

Snapshot of a Clinic

Anwesha Clinic

Chhotojagulia Block Primary Health Centre, Barasat District, North 24 Parganas, West Bengal

Less than an hour's drive from Kolkata, a short drive from the Barasat District Hospital is the Chhotojagulia Block Primary Health Centre. Here, amidst the greenery and ponds of the villages is a well-equipped PHC.

It's 11am, and in a cheerfully painted bright green building just outside the main PHC building block, crowd starts gathering. There are a number of young people in the queue which is now extending outside the doors of the building. And there are visibly more young girls than boys—its Anwesha Day. Held three times a week on Monday, Wednesday and Friday the Anwesha Clinic provides health information and services to the young people of this community.

Inside the building, there is a large airy room where a medical doctor sits; there is also a smaller room, lined with colourful posters on adolescent-health related issues—this is where the adolescent health worker/counsellor sits. Young people are encouraged to come to the centre to meet the counsellor for both medical and non-medical related health issues. Whether its acne or menstrual problems—the Anwesha Clinic is available for the young people. Often, the counsellor conducts

Image 16.1
Name of Clinic and Timings Displayed Prominently in Chotogulia Block, Primary Health Centre, West Bengal

Image 16.2
Counsellor Conducting a Session on Menstrual Health at the Anwesha Clinic

Image 16.3
Reproductive Sexual Health Awareness Session Conducted at the High School Level, West Bengal

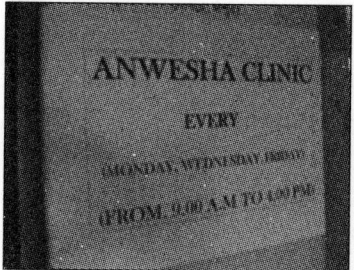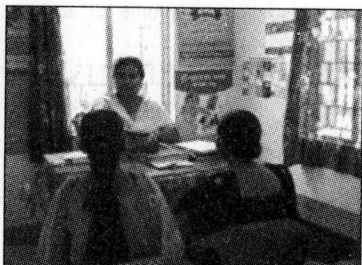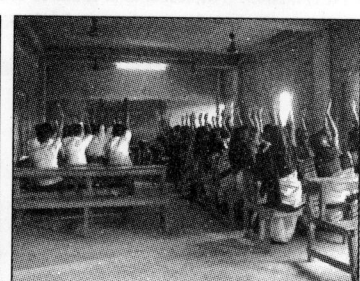

Source: Radhika Arora, PHFI (2011).

awareness sessions—young people of the community are informed ahead of time to attend these sessions. Today's topic is on menstrual health, and the counsellor stands at the head of the table to address the 15 to 20 young girls sitting inside the room. Outside, the girls referred to the medical doctor meet with him for the recommended medical check-up (see Images 16.1, 16.2, and 16.3).

In terms of health-issues presented at the clinic, one of the most common complaints of young people here, we are told, is that of reproductive tract infections (RTIs) caused by young people's tendency to bathe in the many stagnant ponds of water in the area. Other complaints include urinary tract infections (UTIs), menstruation and related health issues, puberty-related questions and general health issues.

Along with clinical services, the Anwesha Clinic has a counsellor who provides outreach services. S/he visits schools within an assigned area to conduct counselling sessions with school students as well as create awareness on the Anwesha Clinics and the services provided by it. Outreach activities play a crucial role, especially in rural areas, towards bringing young people to the Anwesha Clinics, as well as towards providing sexual and reproductive health (SRH) education in schools.

References

Bayley, Olivia. 2003. Improvement of Sexual and Reproductive Health Requires Focusing on Adolescents'. *Lancet*, 362(9386): 830–31, 6 September. DOI: c10.1016/S0140-6736(03)14281-XCite or Link Using DOI http://www.thelancet.com/journals/lancet/article/PIIS0140-6736(03)14281-X/fulltext, accessed 6 August 2013.

Das, S., Lakhara, K., Agrawal, D. and Mehra, S. 2009. 'A Culture of Trust and Confidence "Friends" Youth Friendly Health Center'. New Delhi: MAMTA Health Institute for Mother and Child. Available at http://www.yrshr.org/adolescent/PDF/YHFS%20Full%20Report.pdf, accessed 8 August 2013.

Government of India. 2005. Safdarjung Hospital Adolescent Healthcare Network: Establishing Adolescent Friendly Health Services at Safdarjung Hospital, New Delhi. End of Term Report. Ministry of Health and Family Welfare, Government of India. Available at http://www.whoindia.org/LinkFiles/Adolescent_Health_and_Development_(AHD)_SHAHN_End_Term_Report_2005.pdf, accessed 6 August 2013.

Government of India. 2006. 'Implementation Guide on RCH II ARSH Strategy'. Available at http://india.unfpa.org/drive/ImplementationGuideFinal-RCH2ARSH.pdf, accessed 6 August 2013.

NFHS-3. 2005–06. 'Marriage and Fertility'. Available at www.nfhsindia.org/NFHS.../PPT/NFHS-3%20Key%20Findings.ppt, accessed 27 March 2012.

National Rural Health Mission (NRHM). 2010. 'Reaching the Unreached: A Presentation under the National Rural Health Mission, West Bengal'. Presented at Bhopal, Madhya Pradesh. Available at http://nrhm.gov.in/mediamenu/presentations/nrhm-workshop-conference/bhopal-workshop.html, accessed 6 August 2013.

UNFPA. 2003. 'Adolescents in India: A Profile'. UN Inter Agency Working Group on Population and Development. Available at http://web.unfpa.org/focus/india/facetoface/docs/adolescentsprofile.pdf, accessed 6 August 2013.

Section D
Accountability of Programmes

Section D
Accountability of Programmes

Sub-themes

Monitoring and Evaluation
Social Accountability Initiatives

Section D
Accountability of Programmes

Enhancing accountability is often used as a tool in health systems for improving health system performance. The notion of better accountability might seem straightforward, but it contains a high degree of complexity. Accountability maybe defined using three categories: financial, performance and political/democratic accountability (Brinkerhoff 2003). Using an accountability lens can: (1) help to generate a system-wide perspective on health sector reform and (2) identify connections among individual improvement interventions. These results can support synergistic outcomes, enhance system performance and contribute to sustainability.

To improve maternal and child health in India many health programmes have been designed and implemented by both government and non-government institutions. While considering scale-up of programmes which demonstrate encouraging results, it is crucial to note whether these programmes have been successful. This could be done through systematic analysis of the programme. Information brings accountability and helps to improve performance. In the Ekjut, MAPDIER and MDR case studies, the importance of collection of information and how it helps to improve performance is the underlying theme. The Ekjut case study, discusses the importance of design before the intervention begins. The case studies on MAPDIER and MDR discuss the processes involved to undertake verbal autopsy and use of information to improve the existing systems and community practices.

In India, government is the primary health care provider for most people, although there is a strong presence of private sector as well. Both public and the private sector need to acknowledge being held accountable by society (WHO).[1] Social accountability is a method through which one creates a more accountable system to perform based on existing resources. The White Ribbon Alliance for Safe Motherhood (WRA) is a global movement which builds alliances, strengthens capacity, influences policies, harnesses resources and inspires action to protect the lives of women and newborns around the world. In India, the WRA unites individuals, organizations and communities who are committed to increasing public awareness on how to prevent maternal deaths and promote safe motherhood. This case study documents the various techniques advocated by the WRAI to elucidate the role that the tools of social accountability can play in creating a rights-based mass movement directed towards safe motherhood for all.

---

[1]Defining and measuring social accountability of medical records, WHO, Geneva. Available at http://apps.who.int/iris/bitstream/10665/59441/1/WHO_HRH_95.7.pdf, accessed on 5 August 2013.

References

Brinkerhoff, D. 2003. 'Accountability and Health Systems: Overview, Framework and Strategies'. Bethesda, MD: The Partners for Health Reformplus Project, Abt Associates Inc. Available at http://www.who.int/management/partnerships/accountability/AccountabilityHealthSystemsOverview.pdf.

WHO. 'Defining and Measuring Social Accountability of Medical Records'. Available at http://apps.who.int/iris/bitstream/10665/59441/1/WHO_HRH_95.7.pdf.

Monitoring and Evaluation

17

Collection of Evidence through Randomized Control Trial Setting: Ekjut Trial

Sutapa B. Neogi and Sourav Neogi

Background

More than 20% of the population of Jharkhand and Orissa belong to the Scheduled Tribes (STs) and 12 percent to the Scheduled Castes (SCs). Indigenous communities have higher mortality rates and poorer access to health services as compared to the non-indigenous population. Both maternal and neonatal mortality rates are high in these two states and urgent efforts are needed to reduce them. As per the Sample Registration System (SRS) 2009 estimates, Jharkhand's neonatal mortality rate (NMR) is 28 and the maternal mortality ratio (MMR) is 261. Orissa's NMR is 43 and MMR is 258. The all-India figures are NMR 35, and MMR 212.

The prevalence of maternal depression is an increasing public health concern in low-income countries because of its wide ranging implications for the health of the mother and infant. Delivery of appropriate interventions to prevent or treat maternal depression through health workers is a major challenge, especially in countries with under-resourced health systems, despite evidence of the effectiveness of these interventions.

Neonatal mortality is also a major concern in developing countries. Participatory interventions are considered to be effective and have lasting impact (see box titled 'Then and Now: Excerpts from a Traditional Birth Attendant'). Large improvements were noted in birth outcomes in a poor rural population in Makwanpur, Nepal after a low cost, potentially sustainable and scalable participatory intervention was conducted with women's groups. A note on the intervention is attached in Annexure 1.

In India, many such interventions have been carried out with women's groups, but there is little documented evidence regarding effectiveness. However, an intervention conducted by Ekjut in Jharkhand and Orissa provides documented evidence.

Then and Now: Excerpts from a Traditional Birth Attendant

'In the earlier days, deliveries used to take place in dark and unclean rooms without ventilation. Deliveries were done on mats or old clothes whichever was available at that moment. Earlier we used to assist the mother without washing our hands and used to keep the newborn a little away from the mother to avoid the newborn from taking in amniotic fluid and we cut the cord only when the placenta came out completely. We used to use roof tiles (Khapra) along with the old blade or knife to cut the cord. After separating the placenta we used to give honey and pig fat orally to the newborn and apply pig fat on the whole body of the newborn and bathe the newborn with stale rice water (*basimard*). We did not wrap the newborn with clothes but just let the baby lie over any cloth that was available.'

Since Ekjut started organizing meetings with the community things started changing. According to the same dai behaviours and practices started changing. She said,

'The practices are changing due to the meetings. Now, we cut our nails, remove the bangles, finger rings and wash hands with soap before helping in deliveries. Simultaneously, we advise to boil the thread and blade before use. Instead of bathing the newborn, we apply mustard oil and wrap the newborn with clean and dry cloth and do not apply pig's fat on the newborn's body.'

Source: During a discussion regarding home deliveries with a village dai (traditional birth attendant) in a remote tribal village of West Singhbhum District of Jharkhand.

Ekjut, meaning 'coming together for a cause', is a non-governmental organization founded by Dr Prasanta Tripathy and Dr Nirmala Nair. It was founded to tackle the high levels of child deaths in the states of Jharkhand and Orissa. Ekjut, in partnership with the Institute of Child Health at University College, London and with funding from the Health Foundation, a UK-based charity, initiated a cluster randomized controlled trial to assess the impact of community mobilization through participatory women's group on birth outcomes in poor rural communities.

Where Is Ekjut Operational?

According to Dr Prashant Tripathy, a founding member of Ekjut,

The partnering communities of Ekjut belong to the indigenous communities (Adivasis), who live in the underserved areas of Jharkhand and Orissa. The terrains are difficult and health facilities are quite far away from where they live. Most deliveries happen at home. These communities belong to Hoe, Santhal, Juwang, Paraon and various other ethnic groups. We also work with SC communities and people belonging to the other backward castes and the poor people living alongside them. About 73% of women who participated in Ekjut trial had not gone to school and many were asset-less and belonged to below poverty line. (As told to PHFI research team, Chakradharpur, Jharkhand, June 2011)

Jharkhand (Ekjut presently works in six districts) and Orissa (Ekjut works in three districts) are two of the poorest states in eastern India (see Map 17.1). The average life expectancy among women in both states is about 60 years and around 63% are illiterate.

The Ekjut Model

Ekjut's intervention model is divided into four phases. These are: (1) Identifying and prioritizing the problems, (2) finding appropriate solutions and strategies together, (3) implementing the prioritized strategies and (4) evaluating the impact of the intervention. These four phases are interlinked. Inputs and findings from each phase help to plan and build the next one. A flow chart (see Figure 17.1) demonstrates how each phase works and how these phases are interlinked.

Map 17.1
Jharkhand and Orissa State Political Map Highlighting the Districts Where Ekjut Is Working

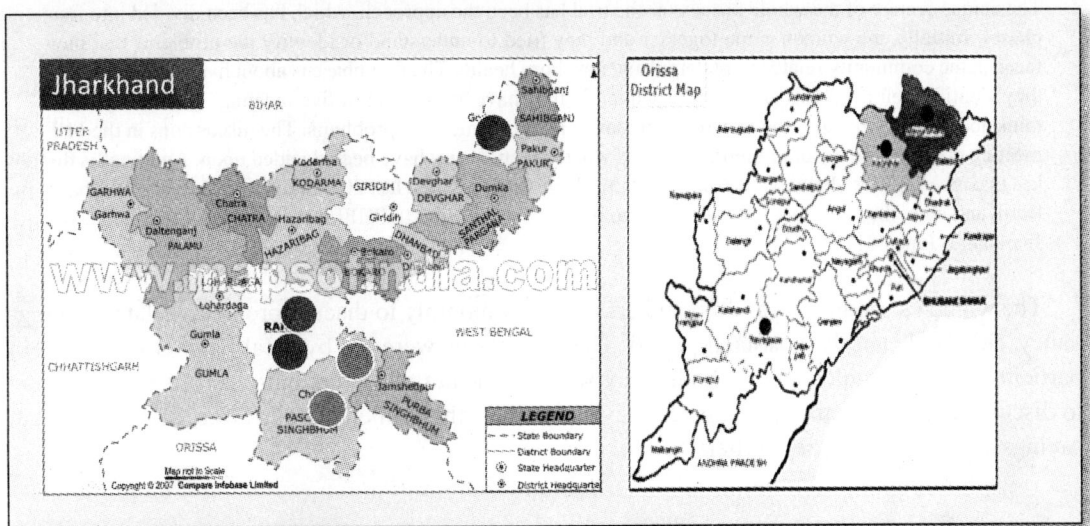

Source: Maps of India.

Figure 17.1
The Ekjut Model Cycle

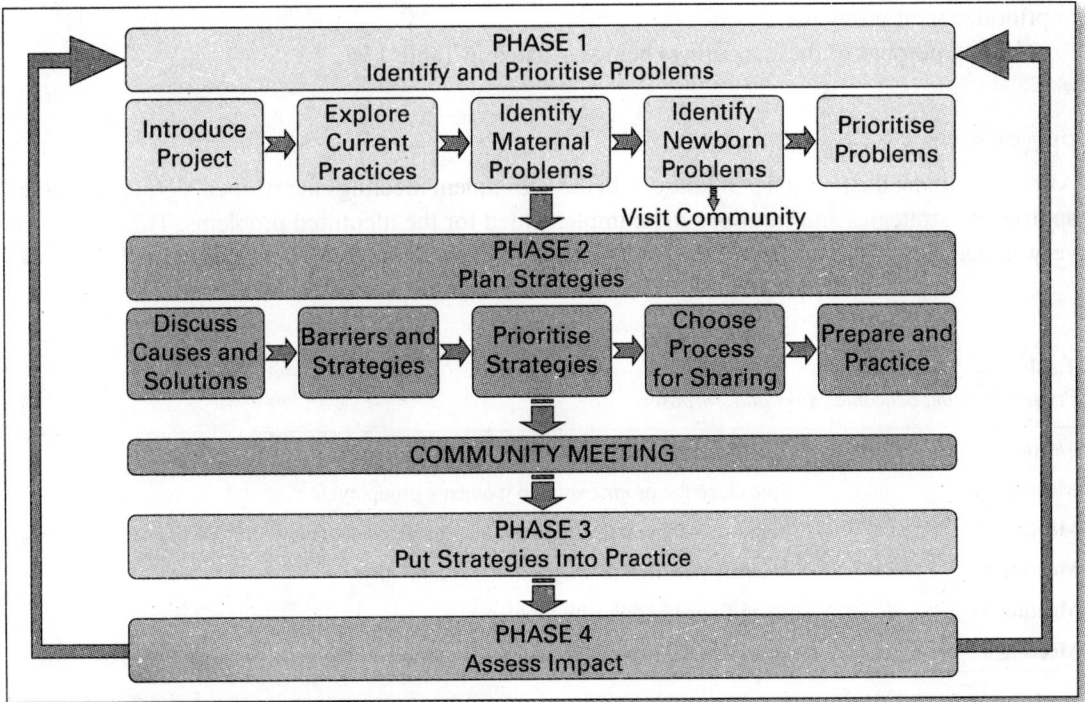

Source: Rath et al. (2010) and Tripathy et al. (2010).

According to Dr Nirmala, founding member of Ekjut,

The unique feature of the whole process or the trial has been the approach, which has been divided into four phases. Initially, the women came together and they tried to understand or identify the problems that they faced in the community related to maternal and new born health. The first phase is about five meetings where they identify their problems and then subsequently they have another set of five meetings where they try to think about what strategies they need to implement to overcome their problems. The discussions in the 11th meeting onwards are about implementation of whatever strategies have been decided upon. And finally, the last two meetings are about evaluation. What they have done over the last 20 months, what lessons they have learnt and what they have actually been able to implement. (As told to PHFI research team, Chakradharpur, Jharkhand, June 2011)

The women's groups of 15–20 members each met monthly to discuss problems related to pregnancy, childbirth and the postnatal period. These meetings were led by local facilitators trained in participatory communication methods; they were not health educators but received basic training to discuss health problems during pregnancy and childbirth. Women's groups were also involved in savings and credit activities earlier.

PHASE 1: Discussions around Identifying and Prioritizing Problems

A series of interactions happened at the monthly meetings; the facilitators from Ekjut took the women's group through a 'five-meeting participatory learning and action cycle' process. Facilitators, who were all women, encouraged the community women to discuss maternal and newborn problems using visual aids such as picture cards and at the end of the five meetings they were able to prioritize their problems.

The aim/purpose of these meetings being as stated in Table 17.1.

PHASE 2: Plan Strategies

After prioritizing the problems in Phase 1, in the subsequent meetings the women's group discussed appropriate strategies and solutions to be implemented for the identified problems. This phase was very important as it encouraged the community to think about possible solutions for their own

Table 17.1

Phase 1 Meeting Schedule: Aims and Purposes

Meeting	Aim/Purpose
Meeting 1	Introduce the project and the women's group cycle.
Meeting 2	Explore local practices and beliefs linked to pregnancy, childbirth and motherhood.
Meeting 3	Identify maternal problems in the community.
Meeting 4	Identify newborn health problems.
Meeting 5	Prioritize the maternal and newborn problems the group wants to focus on.

Source: Rath et al. (2010).

Table 17.2

Phase 2 Meeting Schedule: Aims and Purposes

Meeting	Aim/Purpose
Meeting 6	Discuss causes and solutions to local maternal and newborn health problems through storytelling.
Meeting 7	Identify strategies arising out of the solutions and understand opportunities and barriers before prioritizing them using the bridge game.
Meeting 8	Discuss the process of sharing information on problems and strategies with the community.
Meeting 9	Prepare a community meeting.
	COMMUNITY MEETING

Source: Rath et al. (2010).

problems. In this phase, storytelling, games such as the bridge game, role plays were performed so that the women gained a critical understanding of the specific issues.

A total of five meetings were held with these women's groups in the Phase 2, the aim/purpose of these being as stated in Table 17.2.

At the culmination of the nine meetings, a community meeting was held to inform the larger community about how the women had arrived at a solution over the last nine months and decided on the possible strategies and to seek necessary support from the wider community.

PHASE 3: Implement Strategies

In this phase identified strategies were implemented using participatory learning and action cycle of meetings with the women's groups. Materials for individual meetings such as participatory games and strategies were included. Here the group members undertook responsibilities either individually or as a group to ensure that the prioritized strategies were implemented and they also tracked the progress of the work. Information about clean delivery practices and care-seeking behaviour was shared through stories and games, rather than presented as key messages. They also discussed issues such as inadequate care, unhealthy household environment, household food insecurity, etc.

A total of 10 meetings were held with women's groups in the implementation phase, the aim/purpose of these being as stated in Table 17.3.

PHASE 4: Assess Impact

Two meetings were organized with the women's groups during this phase. In these meetings, the group members discussed their achievements (see Table 17.4).

The women's group members towards the end of the cycle evaluated their performance regarding the meetings they liked the best and what they found useful, what impact the intervention had on the members themselves and also on the non-members/non-attenders/men and the larger community. They also explored what changes in key practices they had seen over the two years of the intervention and the support they had received from the family/community.

The use of a structured and phase-wise content in the meeting cycle and the emphasis on collective problem solving contributed to learning and confidence building. This appears to have been a key

Table 17.3

Phase 3 Meeting Schedule: Aims and Purposes

Meeting	Aim/Purpose
PHASE 3 : IMPLEMENT STRATEGIES	
Meeting 10	Discuss the implementation of strategies and undertaking responsibilities for implementation.
Meeting 11	Review the progress of strategy implementation.
Meeting 12	Discuss how maternal problems can be prevented.
Meeting 13	Discuss how newborn problems can be prevented.
Meeting 14	Discuss the home-care solutions for selected problems.
Meeting 15	Discuss facility-based care for selected problems.
Meeting 16	Identify which problems are emergencies, prepare the group for emergencies and discuss ways of addressing delays in care-seeking.
Meeting 17	Identify emergency and non-emergency problems, appropriate responses and referrals.
Meeting 18	Learn about the activities of other groups and prepare for a cluster-level community meeting.
	CLUSTER-LEVEL COMMUNITY MEETING

Source: Rath et al. (2010).

Table 17.4

Phase 4 Meeting Schedule: Aims and Purposes

PHASE 4: ASSESS IMPACT	
Meeting 19	Review the cluster community meeting, discuss the activities and achievements of the group and evaluate each phase of the cycle.
Meeting 20	Discuss possible behavioural changes linked to the intervention that occurred in the wider community.

Source: Rath et al. (2010).

determinant of the intervention's efficacy and acceptability. Local acceptability of the intervention, a participatory approach and community involvement are the key factors of the model. Acceptability was enhanced due to the deployment of local facilitators, use of appropriate discussion materials while keeping visual literacy in mind and flexibility in the timing and content of meetings. Three additional features of the intervention, built on the participatory principles inherent to the women's group intervention, were unique to the trial—involvement of the wider community, including local community health workers and the active targeting of marginalized groups and pregnant women. Involvement of the wider community meant that the existing groups which were closed because they dealt with microcredit activities, became open to all community members with the addition of the participatory cycle. Second, group members shared their problems and strategies with the wider community during village and cluster-level meetings. Third, community members including men offered support in the implementation of the groups' strategies.

In order to implement this model a strong workforce was put in place by Ekjut (see Box 17.1). Figure 17.2 is a snapshot of this.

Box 17.1: The Surveillance System Set up for the Ekjut Trial

Facilitators were selected after holding discussions with opinion leaders, elders, headmen and women. Preference was given to local, literate married women, preferably a daughter-in-law, from selected villages.

They were trained in two phases: the first lasting for five days and the second lasting for two days after an interval of six months. Production and iterative adaptation of locally appropriate picture cards, stories and games increased acceptability and catalyzed learning and planning within groups.

Three to four identifiers were selected for each cluster (one for 250 households); they were selected from the same pool (trained birth attendants [TBAs], family members of TBAs, men). Education was not a precondition for their selection. Identifiers received a one-day formal training on recruitment. They identified births in their cluster and reported to monitors two to three times a month.

From this same pool again, some women were selected as monitors. For selection as monitor one criterion was having around 10 years of schooling and another criterion was having a bicycle for mobility. Monitors arranged appointments with the mother/family member to gather information within 42–45 days, for live births. In cases of a still birth/neonatal death/maternal death there was flexibility in the appointment schedule.

Monitors received four days of training on recruitment. Their performance was reviewed on a weekly basis. They also received one refresher training and postnatal depression training, besides on-the-job training.

Source: Information shared by the Ekjut team.

Figure 17.2
Schematic Diagram to Depict Surveillance System Followed during the Ekjut Trial

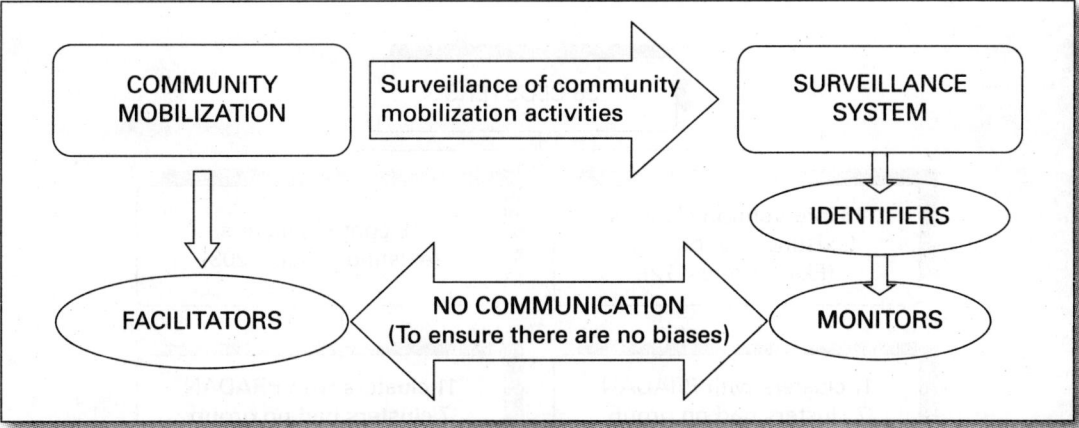

Source: Prepared by the research team based on the information obtained during the interview with the Ekjut team.

The Surveillance System

Randomized controlled trials are considered the most rigorous method to evaluate the impact of complex interventions. Attention must be given to the contextual and process factors that affect the efficacy of such interventions in order to determine how results might be replicated in non-trial settings

Note: Surveys should always be done by the people not involved in the intervention, no communication between facilitators and monitors to avoid biases during information gathering.

(Oakley et al. 2006). Community mobilization interventions raise specific evaluation challenges because their development, implementation and success involve a range of actors, activities and processes, often over prolonged periods of time (Butterfoss 2006).

In the community mobilization intervention of the Ekjut Model, three contiguous districts of Jharkhand and Orissa—Saraikela Kharswan, West Singhbhum and Keonjhar—were selected. The proportion of Adivasis (tribals) within the study clusters was 58% to 70%. Twelve rural clusters per district were identified, with a mean population of 6,338 per cluster (see Figure 17.3). The estimated population in these 36 clusters was 228,186 (2001 Indian Census projections).

All the 36 cluster villages benefitted from the health service strengthening interventions.[1] However, the women's group intervention took place in only half of the clusters (see Box 17.2). A system was put in place in which every mother who delivered was identified and they were interviewed by the monitors after 42 days of their delivery. A detailed questionnaire was filled in by the monitors and input into a database for analysis at a later date (see Box 17.3). In all 36 clusters, all the births and

Figure 17.3

The Surveillance System Model—RCT

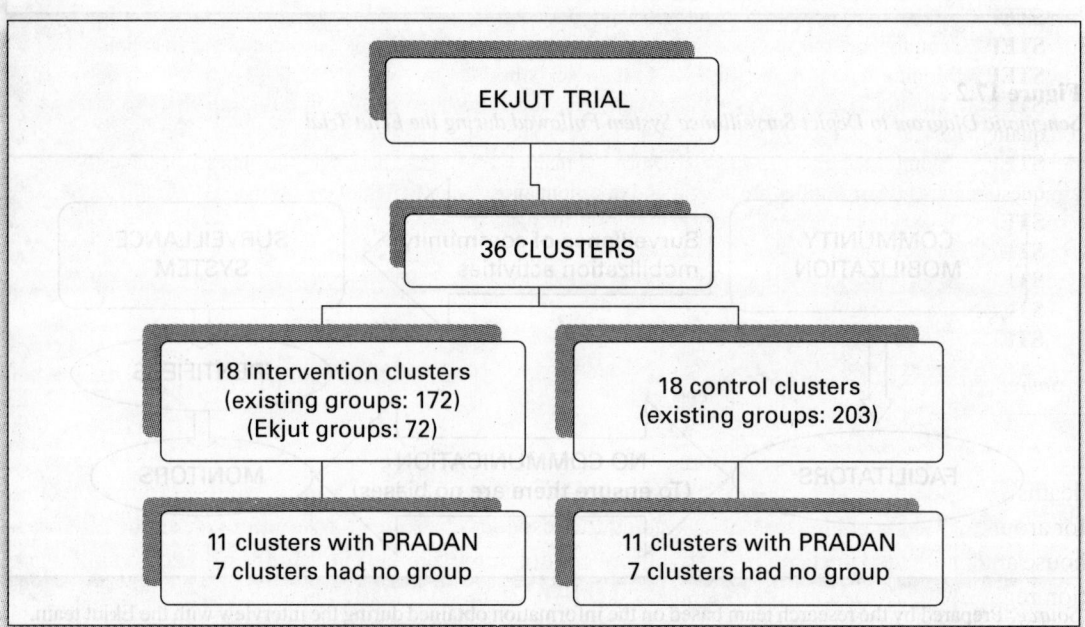

Source: As shared by the Ekjut team with PHFI.

[1] Ekjut formed health committees in all intervention and control clusters so that community members would have the opportunity to express their opinions about the design and management of local health services. About 10 village representatives within every cluster met once every two months and used a structured action cycle to discuss maternal and newborn health entitlement issues. As a result, committee members became more knowledgeable about the government health system and assisted with the formation of village health committees as part of the National Rural Health Mission programme. In addition to the creation of cluster-level health committees, Ekjut provided workshops for appreciative inquiry with front-line government health staff from seven clusters per district in Jharkhand. Participants assessed the programme qualitatively at the end of every training session.

Box 17.2: Cluster Selection

Under the Ekjut trial the selection of clusters had its own significance. It was very important to select the cluster in a scientific manner with defined criteria. The following criteria were used to select a cluster:

Eight–10 villages per cluster
Cluster population = 5,000–7,000
High proportion of tribal (greater than 50%)
Preferably with existing SHG groups
Buffer zones in-between all clusters
Physically and functionally remote from health services

Source: Tripathy et al. (2010).

Box 17.3: Monitoring and Surveillance Process

A 10-step process was followed under the surveillance system. Following is a description of each step.

STEP 1: All births identified by identifiers and reported to the monitor.
STEP 2: Monitor confirms the event, pays a token remuneration to the identifier and arranges an appointment.
STEP 3: Monitor reports to the supervisor on a weekly basis.
STEP 4: Monitor interviews the family members; supervisors are present in 10% interviews to perform quality check.
STEP 5: Monitor submits the completed questionnaire on a weekly basis and the supervisor rechecks the questionnaires (clarifications are sought and questionnaires resent to field if necessary).
STEP 6: Supervisors fill the district-level register formats.
STEP 7: Questionnaire submitted for data entry.
STEP 8: Data entry done by the three data-entry operators.
STEP 9: Data cleaning and analysis.
STEP 10: Dissemination of results.

Source: As shared by the Ekjut team with PHFI.

---

deaths were identified by the key informants—identifiers. These key informants were responsible for around 250 households and they assisted the respective monitors. A monitor visited the mother's house and confirmed the birth or death before conducting the interview. Monitors collected information regarding the birth/stillbirth/neonatal death (0–28 days)/maternal death/woman's death.

Ekjut also formed health committees in all intervention and control clusters so that community members would have the opportunity to express their opinions about the design and management of local health services.

Impact/Findings

Assessment of the impact noted a 32% reduction in NMR during the three-year trial, after adjusting for clustering, stratification and baseline differences (see Table 17.5). MMR was also lower in the intervention than in the control clusters.

Table 17.5

Impact on Mortality Figures

	Baseline		Year 1†		Year 2†		Year 3†	
	Intervention	Control	Intervention	Control	Intervention	Control	Intervention	Control
Births	2,457	2,235	3,171	3,052	3,404	3,135	3,195	3,073
Stillbirths	109	73	98	92	118	100	85	88
Maternal deaths	16	7	20	30	22	18	7	12
Stillbirth rate per 1,000 births	44.4	32.7	30.9	30.1	34.7	31.9	26.6	28.6
NMR per 1,000 live births	61.8	53.6	55.6	53.4	37.1	59.6	36.3	64.3
Perinatal mortality rate per 1,000 births	85.1	68.4	67.4	65.2	57.0	75.0	47.5	73.5
MMR per 100,000 live births	681.7	323.8	650.8	1013.5	669.5	593.0	225.1	402.0

Source: Tripathy et al. (2010).

Note: Data are unadjusted. †Including migrated mothers and infants.

Qualitative evidence from the study of the trial's process showed that community mobilization through women's groups might have contributed to avoidance of maternal deaths, though the study was not powered to detect differences in maternal mortality. No significant differences were noted in health-care seeking behaviour between control and intervention clusters. However, home-care practices showed substantial improvements. Improved hygiene and care practices were the most likely mechanism of mortality reduction (see Table 17.6). The most striking reduction in mortality rate was noted in early neonatal deaths.

Although there was no significant effect on maternal depression, reduction in moderate depression was 57% in the third year (see Table 17.7). It has been hypothesized that the large reduction in moderate depression seen in the third year could have occurred through improvements in social support and problem-solving skills of the groups. Adequate social support reduces the risk of depression during pregnancy and is an important social determinant of mental health. Group meetings also strengthened problem-solving skills, a component of psychotherapeutic interventions that has been shown to affect depression in other settings.

The acceptability was evident from the high population coverage. In the Ekjut trial, the coverage of women's groups was one group per 468 population, highest among other comparable trials (1:756 in Makwanpur, 1:1414 in Bangladesh).

Challenges and Learnings

The team initially experienced difficulties in building a rapport with marginalized tribal communities and dealing with expectations of financial gains. Facilitators had to contend with dominant group members and cancellations during festivals and cultivation periods. They had to deal with the presence of men during sensitive discussions. They also had to ensure participation during internal conflicts within villages. Group members were sometimes constrained by in-laws and TBAs in the implementation of strategies, as some felt that the contents went against traditional beliefs and practices.

Table 17.6

Changes in Care

	Intervention Clusters	Control Clusters
Births‡	9,468	8,867
Any antenatal care (ANC)	74%	75%
≥3 antenatal care visits	32%	41%
Institutional deliveries	14%	20%
Birth attended by formal provider (doctor or nurse)	16%	23%
Home deliveries	8,084	7,034
Birth attended by TBAs	33%	38%
Birth attendant washed hands with soap	41%	23%
Safe-delivery kit used	32%	18%
Plastic sheet used	26%	8%
Cord tied with boiled thread	32%	11%
Cord cut with new or boiled blade	83%	79%
Live births (home deliveries)	7,890	6,873
Cord undressed or dressed with antiseptic	84%	89%
Infant wrapped within 30 minutes	36%	43%
Infant not bathed in first-24 hours	27%	22%
Infants alive at one month	8,807	8,119
Any of three infant illnesses (cough, fever, diarrhoea)	20%	29%
Care-seeking behaviour in event of infant illness	54%	44%
Exclusive breastfeeding for first six weeks	80%	69%

Source: Tripathy et al. (2010).
Note: Data are number (%), unless otherwise indicated. ‡Excludes births to migrated mothers and twins; 1,739 for intervention clusters and 2,388 for control clusters.

Table 17.7

Mental Health

	Year 2		Year 3	
	Intervention	*Control*	*Intervention*	*Control*
Mothers (n)	3,332	3,016	3,120	2,963
No or mild depression (10–15)	88%	87%	95%	90%
Moderate Depression (16–30)	11%	13%	5%	10%
Severe Depression (31–50)	<1%	<1%	<1%	<1%

Source: Tripathy et al. (2010).

Improvement in care seeking was slower; marginalized groups, tribal communities and more so the poorest among them, had difficulty in accessing services. The remoteness of the villages, poor access to transport and bad road conditions compounded these communities' social isolation.

Scaling-up

After the successful demonstration the model has been tried in other parts of the country, recently in Madhya Pradesh. Ekjut started the operation of the model in these places.

Credibility of the Model

This model is based on sound evidence. The trial was registered as an International Standard Randomized Controlled Trial. The results have been published in *Lancet* and *BMC International Health and Human Rights*. The trial has been recognized as Trial of the Year by the Society for Clinical Trials. This award is given annually to the clinical trial that best embodies the following aspects:

- It improves the lot of mankind.
- It provides the basis for a substantial, beneficial change in health care.
- It reflects expertise in subject matter, excellence in methodology and concern for study participants.
- It overcomes obstacles in implementation.
- The presentation of its design, execution and results is a model of clarity and intellectual soundness.

The model has been successfully implemented in rural tribal settings in underdeveloped districts. The impact is tangible and clearly associated with the intervention.

Relevance

The model is relevant in the national context. Reducing the high NMR is a priority and government is actively looking for solutions. It is hypothesized that the Ekjut intervention was successful because the interventions were operationalized with local adaptations and the intervention had adequate population coverage. Scaling-up this community mobilization intervention will require detailed understanding of the way in which changing contexts, delivery mechanisms and implementation styles will affect key characteristics of the intervention.

Scalability

The model is effective in reducing NMR. The intervention requires a training and support structure to manage facilitators in charge of 12–14 groups per month, with every group responsible for a population of about 500 and for recruiting up to half of newly pregnant women. Scaling-up this community-based intervention will require a detailed understanding of the way in which changing contexts, delivery mechanisms and implementation styles will affect key characteristics of the intervention. The researchers estimated that the additional cost of introducing support to these groups per newborn life saved was around $910. While government of Jharkhand has begun scaling-up of this model through the ASHAs (Accredited Social Health Activists) called Sahiyas in Jharkhand, in Odisha this approach is now being scaled-up in Western Odisha by the state government through trained facilitators.

Annexure 1

Effect of a Participatory Intervention with Women's Groups on Birth Outcomes in Nepal: Cluster-randomized Controlled Trial

Neonatal deaths in developing countries account for the largest contribution to global mortality in children younger than five years. Ninety percent of deliveries in the poorest quintile of households happen at home. It has been postulated that a community-based participatory intervention could significantly reduce the neonatal mortality rate (Manandhar et al. 2004).

The intervention pair-matched 42 geopolitical clusters in Makwanpur District, Nepal, selected 12 pairs randomly and randomly assigned one of each pair to intervention or control. In each intervention cluster (average population 7,000); a female facilitator convened nine women's group meetings every month. The facilitator supported groups through an action-learning cycle in which they identified local perinatal problems and formulated strategies to address them. They also monitored birth outcomes in a cohort of 28,931 women, of whom 8% joined the groups. The primary outcome to measure was the NMR. Other outcomes included stillbirths and maternal deaths, uptake of antenatal and delivery services, home care practices, infant morbidity and health-care seeking behaviour.

As per the findings from 2001 to 2003, the NMR was 26.2 per 1,000 (76 deaths per 2,899 live births) in the intervention clusters compared with 36.9 per 1,000 (119 deaths per 3,226 live births) in the control clusters. Stillbirth rates were similar in both groups. The MMR was 69 per 100,000 (two deaths per 2,899 live births) in the intervention clusters compared with 341 per 100,000 (11 deaths per 3,226 live births) in the control clusters. Women in intervention clusters were more likely to have ANC, institutional delivery, TBA and hygienic care than those in the control clusters.

It can be concluded that birth outcomes in a poor rural population improved greatly through a low-cost, potentially sustainable and scalable, participatory intervention with women's groups.

References

Butterfoss, F.D. 2006. 'Process Evaluation for Community Participation'. *Annual Review of Public Health*, 27: 323–40.

Census of India. 2001. Registrar General of India, New Delhi.

Manandhar, D.S., Osrin, D., Shrestha, B.P., Mesko, N., Morrison, J. and Tumbahangphe, K.M. 2004. 'Effect of a Participatory Intervention with Women's Groups on Birth Outcomes in Nepal: Cluster-Randomised Controlled Trial'. *Lancet*, 364: 970–9.

Oakley, A., Strange, V., Bonell, C., Allen, E. and Stephenson, J. and the RIPPLE study team. 2006. 'Process Evaluation in Randomized Controlled Trials of Complex Interventions'. *BMJ*, 332(7538): 413–16.

Rath, S., Nair, N., Tripathy, P.K., Barnett, S., Rath, S., Mahapatra, R., Gope, R., Bajpai, A., Sinha, R., Costello, A., and Prost, A. 2010. 'Explaining the Impact of a Women's Group Led Community Mobilisation Intervention on Maternal and Newborn Health Outcomes: The Ekjut Trial Process Evaluation'. *BMC International Health and Human Rights*, 10:25.

Sample Registration System (SRS). 2009. Registrar General of India, New Delhi.

Tripathy, P., Nair, N., Barnett, S., Mahapatra, R., Borghi, J. and Rath, S. 2010. 'Effect of a Participatory Intervention with Women's Groups on Birth Outcomes and Maternal Depression in Jharkand and Orissa, India: A Cluster Randomized Trial'. *Lancet*, 375: 1182–92.

18

Putting Evidence into Action: Maternal Death Audit/Review

Sutapa B. Neogi and Sourav Neogi

In the past decade increased international attention has been directed to issues regarding maternal and reproductive health. Among the indicators (maternal mortality ratio, maternal mortality rate, the proportion of adult female deaths due to maternal causes and the lifetime risk of maternal death), maternal mortality ratio (MMR) has received the most attention. The safe motherhood initiative launched in 1987 and other initiatives to address the issue have been successful in drawing the attention of policymakers and donor agencies to the tragedy of pregnancy and birth-related deaths and to the 100-fold difference between the best developed country and worst developing country maternal mortality ratios (Hill et al. 1996).

A growing focus on reducing maternal mortality has increased awareness of the need to measure and monitor levels of maternal mortality (Annexure 1). MMR is included among the World Health Organization (WHO)/United Nations Children's Fund (UNICEF) common indicators for monitoring the goals of Health for All and the World Summit of Children. It also figures among the indicators for assessing the Programme of Action of the International Conference on Population and Development (UNFPA 1995). Millennium Development Goal (MDG) 5 relates to maternal mortality and aims to reduce it by 75% between 1990 and 2015.

The medical reasons for maternal deaths are intertwined with social factors such as low status of women, poor understanding by families on when to seek care and inaccessibility of quality health care in rural areas. It is being increasingly realized that these social factors are sometimes more difficult to overcome, but nevertheless must be addressed if India is to achieve MDG 5. India's MMR has declined from an estimated 570 deaths per 100,000 live births in 1990 to 212 (SRS 2011) in 2007–09, which means that the country could come very close to reaching the MDG5 target of 75% decline (from 1990 to 2015). However, a large number of pregnant women or new mothers are still dying every hour from preventable causes.

A key problem in tackling maternal mortality is how to accurately capture data and appropriately monitor it (see Box 18.1). Ascertaining the causes of maternal mortality is difficult even where there is a comprehensive registration of deaths. As most developing countries have weak vital registration and health information systems, they cannot provide an accurate assessment of maternal mortality,

---

Box 18.1: Types of Maternal and Child Death Enquiries

Maternal and child death inquiries have been conducted in many settings. Some examples include: (1) the routine practice of maternal death review by medical practitioners in the United Kingdom for more than 50 years, (2) hospital-based perinatal death reviews encouraged by the American College of Obstetricians and Gynaecologists in the United States, (3) community and hospital inquiry into all maternal deaths required by the Sri Lanka Ministry of Health since 1985, (4) the community verbal autopsy and hospital-based confidential inquiry of maternal deaths encouraged by the Philippines Ministry of Health and (5) maternal death reviews supported by WHO in selected hospitals of Bangladesh, Myanmar and Nepal.

In India, the Tamil Nadu Reproductive and Child Health Programme has reviewed all maternal deaths and a sample of infant deaths since 2003 and the Government of Kerala has reviewed all maternal deaths since 2005 (see Box titled 'An Expert Speaks'). In addition, WHO has supported maternal death reviews at Safdarjung Hospital in Delhi and at Christian Medical College in Vellore.

Source: Pattinson and Hall 2003, Bødker et al. 2009 and Report on Maternal and Perinatal Death Enquiry and Response (MAPEDIR), UNICEF 2008.

---

leave aside its causes. On the other hand, an estimate derived from the more complete vital registration systems such as those in developed countries, suffers from misclassification and under-reporting of maternal deaths.

In this case study, two systems are described for capturing information about maternal deaths and how the information has been used to improve the health system and to empower the community to take appropriate actions:

- Maternal and Perinatal Death Enquiry and Response (MAPEDIR)
- Maternal Death Review (MDR)

An Expert Speaks

'Maternal death in terms of numbers, we don't learn anything. Why the women died at home or on the way to the hospital or in the institution; there are multiple factors for the cause of maternal death; apart from that there are social and economic issues, delay in getting the transport, etc. These three type of delays unless we discuss with the family of the deceased and with the service providers we may not get the whole picture (why women died during the process of labour). To get a whole picture, to identify system deficiencies, social and cultural issues; we need to have a system of reviews involving the various stakeholders.'

Source: Interview with Dr Padmanabhan, NHSRC (PHFI, 2011).

Maternal and Perinatal Death Enquiry and Response

Since 2005, UNICEF has supported the MAPEDIR which is a tool that systematically captures the ground realities of maternal deaths, analyzes the underlying medical, social and systemic factors and finally uses this evidence to generate community and programme action.

Context

MAPEDIR's genesis lies in UNICEF's Maternal Mortality Reduction Advocacy Project, supported by the United Kingdom's Department for International Development (DFID). The MAPEDIR initiative underscores the need for information about the underlying causes of maternal deaths in remote and inaccessible villages (see box titled 'MAPEDIR: Goes beyond Numbers'). It

MAPEDIR: Goes beyond Numbers

'MAPEDIR is much more than only the process of counting maternal deaths, so it starts from counting but goes on from investigating and then sharing it with the community and health systems and taking actions. The process has been simple. The front-line workers and key informants inform about any maternal death in their area; the death gets investigated not only for the medical reasons but also the social circumstances. This information is analyzed and fed back to the communities and to the health systems and subsequently action is taken upon them by the communities or by the system.'

Source: Interview with Dr.Pavitra Mohan, Health Specialist, UNICEF, India (PHFI, 2011).

grew out of UNICEF's decision to support maternal death inquiry as a component of the ongoing second phase of the Reproductive and Child Health Programme (RCH II) and the National Rural Health Mission (NRHM). It emphasizes increasing the demand for quality health care and greater community participation in the planning of public health interventions. Piloted in Purulia, one of the poorest and most backward districts of West Bengal in June 2005, MAPEDIR was implemented in 16 districts in six Indian states with high maternal mortality. These are: West Bengal (Purulia), Rajasthan (Dholpur, Tonk, Udaipur), Jharkhand (Ranchi), Madhya Pradesh (Guna, Shivpuri), Orissa (Nuapada, Koraput, Kalahandi, Bolangir, Sonepur, Malkangiri, Nabarangpur, Rayagada) and Bihar (Vaishali).

The Objectives of MAPEDIR Are Manifold

- Sensitizing communities to maternal and perinatal health issues, including the need for birth preparedness and complication readiness.
- Inquiring into maternal and perinatal deaths by identifying recent maternal deaths and conducting community-based inquiries with close acquaintances of the women so as to find ways by which future deaths might be prevented.
- Sharing the findings of the death inquiries with communities and helping them interpret the data to develop appropriate interventions, as also advocate for improvements in health care to tackle identified problems.
- Using the findings of the inquiries to advocate with policymakers for necessary improvements in health care systems.

The primary scope of MAPEDIR as conceptualized was to examine all maternal and perinatal deaths (i.e., intrauterine deaths from 24 weeks gestation) and each live birth resulting in a neonatal death (up to 28 days of life). In the first stage, only maternal deaths were covered. It was thought that investigation of perinatal deaths might be introduced at a later stage. Secondly, it was originally a scientific investigation tool meant for research. UNICEF adapted it for transforming it also into a tool for action.

What Is MAPEDIR?

MAPEDIR is a tool that systematically investigates maternal deaths. It underscores the logic that it is important to stimulate community participation in probing why women die during pregnancy

Figure 18.1
The MAPEDIR Process

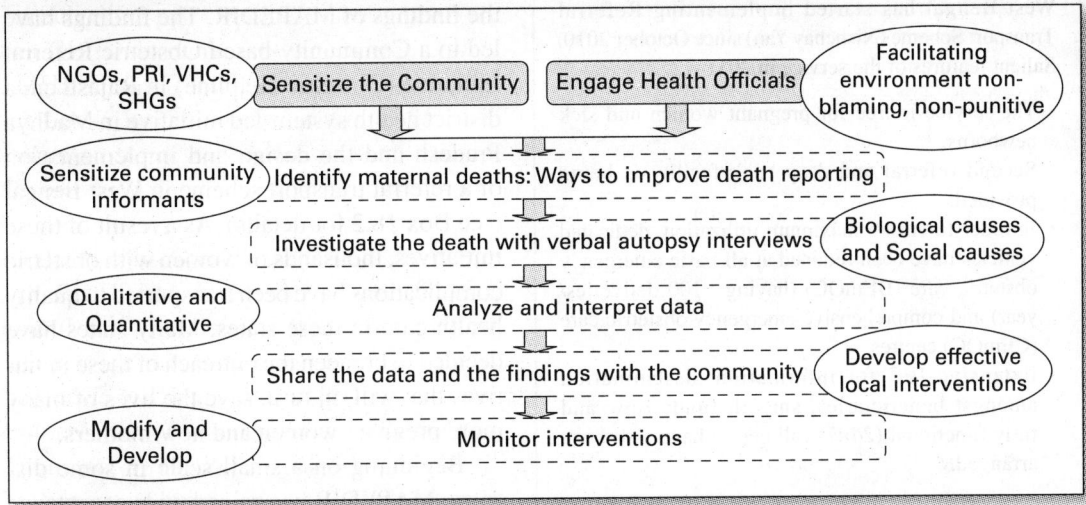

Source: PHFI (conceptual understanding prepared by the authors).

and/or delivery in order to develop feasible solutions. The entire process includes identifying and investigating maternal deaths, sensitizing the community, spurring communities and health systems into action and monitoring and adjusting interventions through continuing inquiries (see Figure 18.1).

The tool is a structured verbal autopsy questionnaire used to interview relatives and/or those who were close to the deceased women. The findings can be aggregated and inferences drawn, corrective action can be taken at the block, district, state and national levels. Such inquiries support evidence-based decision-making.

The inquiry involves ascertaining the personal, familial, social and community factors that led to the mortality without blaming anyone. Interviews at the household level conducted under the MAPEDIR Project in selected districts in India identify the immediate, intermediate and underlying causes of maternal deaths. Typically, medical records capture only the immediate, biological causes of maternal deaths. The personal, familial, socio-cultural, economic and environmental factors contributing to these deaths are left out. MAPEDIR seeks to restore and record these missing links. It provides a confidential, non- threatening environment for the respondent to furnish all the details giving a clearer picture of the sequence of events. The findings of the structured questionnaire (translated into the local language), enquiring minutely into the circumstances of the maternal death, are then widely shared with communities and with local health authorities. The new knowledge stemming from the scrutiny of maternal deaths in rural areas bridges a crucial gap.

Overall Impact of the Model

The report on '*Maternal and Perinatal Death Inquiry and Response—Empowering Communities to Avert Maternal Deaths in India*' published by UNICEF, India 2008, is about the MAPDIER Project

Box 18.2: Overall Impact of the Model

West Bengal has started implementing Referral Transport Scheme (Nishchay Yan) since October 2010. Salient features of the service in 2011–12:

- The service is free for pregnant women and sick newborns.
- Second referral and drop back facility is being provided.
- In order to ensure maximum utilization, dedicated vehicles have been retained at all basic emergency obstetric care (BEmOC) (having >100 deliveries/ year) and comprehensive emergency obstetric care (CEmOC) centres.
- Extensive IEC for information dissemination amongst beneficiaries, smooth funds flow and fully functional (24×7) call centre have also been arranged.

Source: Report on Maternal and Perinatal Death Enquiry and Response (MAPEDIR), UNICEF 2008.

Box 18.3: Actions Following MAPEDIR

In Dholpur, Rajasthan an obstetric helpline implemented in conjunction with a range of interventions to reduce delays in care-seeking is a comprehensive effort at preparing mothers and communities for child birth, enabling transportation, ensuring high-quality facilities and follow-up. The obstetric helpline has been implemented in one block of Dholpur District of Rajasthan and subsequently attempted in the entire district through the government machinery. Key strategies adopted include:

1. Mapping transport facilities.
2. Instituting a toll-free number.
3. Involving an NGO to engage local taxis/transporters and to escort women to the health facility (the community health centre).
4. Negotiate the services and ensure timely payments of financial entitlements.
5. Community mobilization and ownership of government functionaries.

Source: Report on Maternal and Perinatal Death Enquiry and Response (MAPEDIR), UNICEF 2008.

in India. It gives examples of positive changes that took place in the health system because of the findings of MAPEDIR. The findings have led to a Community-based Obstetric Referral Initiative (Obstetric Helpline) in Rajasthan, a district health system-led initiative in Madhya Pradesh and the design and implementation of a referral transport scheme in West Bengal (see Box 18.2 for details). As a result of these initiatives, thousands of women with obstetric complications have been transported to quality health care in these states. Many states have decided to broaden the outreach of these initiatives that will, in turn, save the lives of many more pregnant women and new mothers.

Beginning on a small scale in some districts, MAPEDIR has gained wide acceptance as a viable strategy for preventing maternal deaths by offering much needed data and information. One of the most heartening indicators of its success is community initiated action to ensure safe motherhood. There is greater awareness about the factors leading to maternal deaths as well as the relevance of birth preparedness and complication-readiness. There is also greater willingness to demand service from the health care delivery system. This has been a revolutionary step for rural, remote Indian communities that previously had minimal interface with the health care system. The referral initiative conceived by village leaders in Purulia is one such example. In Dholpur (Rajasthan), village-level transporters (local taxi drivers) have become part of the movement to reduce maternal deaths (see Box 18.3). These are but two examples of the dynamic potential and promise of MAPEDIR. At the institutional level, the MAPEDIR process has spawned new strategic partnerships between government agencies, non-governmental organizations (NGOs), academic institutions and the UN system. A collaborative initiative, it has elicited the involvement of several key institutions and groups including the Government of India, state governments, district administrations, *Panchayati Raj* (village-level) institutions, women's self-help groups (SHGs), local NGOs, medical faculties of Indian universities, the Johns Hopkins Bloomberg School of Public Health (USA), WHO, the United Nations Population Fund (UNFPA) and UNICEF.

Establishment of the above links is generating greater awareness of existing government facilities and schemes for safe motherhood, such as the conditional cash transfer scheme for below poverty line (BPL) women, the Janani Suraksha Yojana (JSY) in rural communities. Even in tribal-dominated districts where community structures may be lacking, MAPEDIR is acting as a catalyst and serving as an alert mechanism. Households deprived of education and other basic amenities are beginning to realize that delays at critical junctures can lead to maternal deaths. In many cases, the arrival of MAPEDIR interviewers in a village has sparked a sense of urgency among local authorities to modernize maternal care facilities by using *Rogi Kalyan Samiti* funds made available by the NRHM. The tool has also underscored the need for better reporting of maternal deaths in states with weak health care systems and infrastructure.

Conclusion

In India, as elsewhere, maternal deaths happen due to a combination of inter-related factors. The initiative helped generate awareness in the community and in turn increased reporting of maternal deaths from the community by grassroots level functionaries. An understanding of the contributing factors has enabled decision-makers and stakeholders to address the obstacles to improving the quality of obstetric care. MAPEDIR also discovers the barriers related to care-seeking for complications that lead to these deaths. It focusses on finding out exactly why mothers die. Despite signs of progress in MAPEDIR pilot districts, hurdles remain. Effective monitoring and supervision are critical tools which must be put in place to ensure the complete success of the initiative. Further, teething problems noticed and which must be addressed, include the reluctance of health workers to report maternal deaths for fear of repercussions, reluctance of families to discuss details of women's care and the varying quality of training and supervision of interviewers.

The innovation can address issues that are high on the policy agenda and also priority for beneficiaries. The project is unique in the sense that it is the first death audit of its kind where community involvement is given due recognition and importance.

Maternal Death Review

Overview

A Maternal Death Review (MDR) provides a rare opportunity for a group of health personnel and community members to learn from a tragic—and often preventable—event. MDRs should be conducted as learning exercises that do not include finger-pointing or punishment. The purpose of an MDR is to improve the quality of safe motherhood programming to prevent future maternal and neonatal morbidity and mortality.

Figure 18.2

Maternal Death Review Process

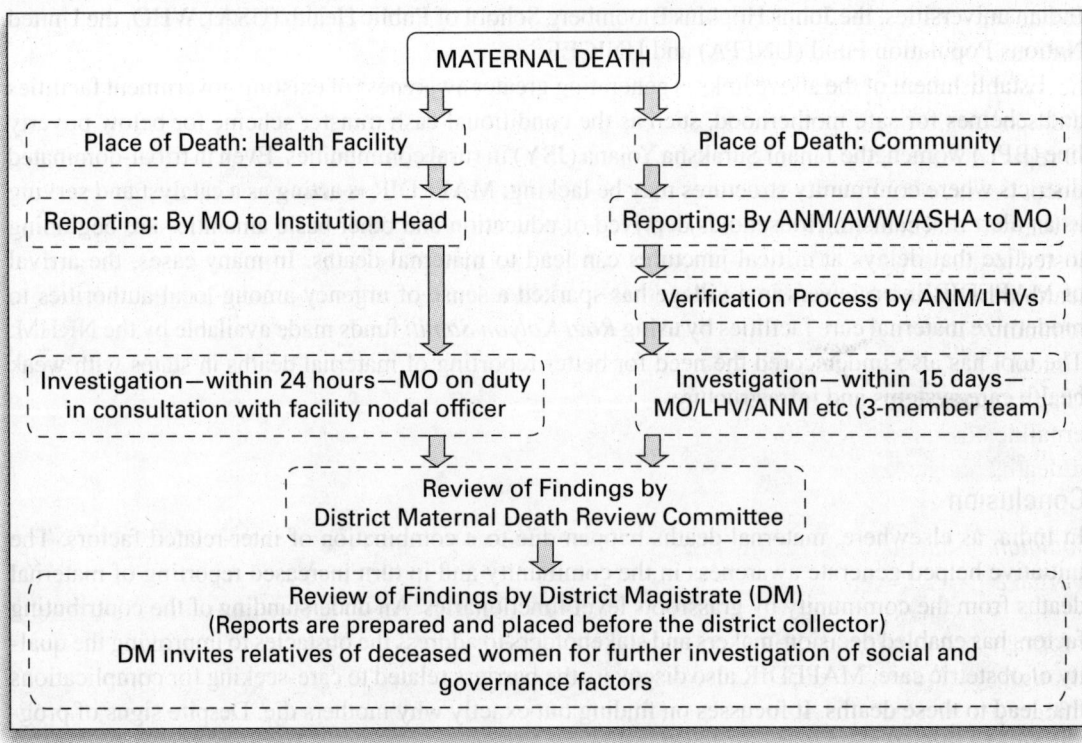

Source: Ministry of Health and Family Welfare, Government of India 2010.

Government is implementing the MDR in two forms—Facility-based Maternal Death Review (FBMDR) and Community-based Maternal Death Review (CBMDR) (see Figure 18.2). FBMDR is a process to investigate and identify causes, mainly clinical and systemic, which lead to maternal deaths in the health facilities and to take appropriate corrective measures to prevent such deaths. CBMDR is a process in which deceased's family members, relatives, neighbours or other informants and care providers are interviewed, by means of a technique called verbal autopsy, to elicit information on various factors—medical, socio-economic or systemic—which lead to maternal deaths, thereby enabling the health system to take the appropriate corrective measures at various levels.

The MDR, a strategy to improve the quality of obstetric care and reduce maternal mortality and morbidity has been spelt out clearly in the RCH II National Programme Implementation Plan document. The importance of MDR lies in the fact that it provides detailed information on various factors at facility, district, community, regional and national levels which need to be addressed in order to improve service and, thereby, reduce maternal deaths. MDR has been conducted as an established intervention for the last few years by some states such as Tamil Nadu, Kerala and West Bengal.

Tamil Nadu Experience and Process

Tamil Nadu is the first state in India which has set-up a system to register all maternal deaths and developed a maternal death audit (Padmanaban et al. 2009 and Malvalankar et al. 2009). The state started compulsory audit of all maternal deaths occurring in the state since 1994 and the system became fully established when the Government of Tamil Nadu issued an order in 2004, stating that all maternal deaths should be audited. It mandates that each maternal death be reported to the Maternal and Child Health (MCH) Commissioner within 24 hours of occurrence, irrespective of place of death—public facility or private nursing home or during the time of transit. Maternal deaths are reported by auxiliary nurse midwives (ANMs), medical officers posted at the periphery, first referral units (FRUs), non-government hospitals, the district public-health nurse and the Deputy Director of Health Services. Investigations are carried out through community-based maternal review (verbal autopsy) and facility-based maternal death review/clinical audit as described in the following paragraphs. The results were encouraging and there was an increase in reporting of maternal deaths from 1994 to 2005. The number of reported maternal deaths increased from 640 in 1995 to 1,600 in 2001, followed by a decline in the number of deaths registered.

Community-based Maternal Reviews (verbal autopsy)

Information on maternal deaths is obtained through telegram/fax/email and medical officers perform the follow-up investigation within 15 days. This investigation tries to document the specific circumstances that led to the maternal death, including the first and the second delay (see Box 18.4 for details) in the community. Members of health staff are reassured that the review of death is not a fault-finding exercise to punish individuals but to improve the system of care.

Facility-based Review of Maternal Deaths

The second part of the review of maternal death is carried out in the facility where the woman was treated and/or died. In the facility-based review, the causes, treatment

---

Box 18.4: Three Delays Model

Phase 1 Delay: Delay in Decision to Seek Care

- Failure to recognize complications.
- Acceptance of maternal death.
- Low status of women.
- Socio-cultural barriers to seeking care: women's mobility, ability to command resources, decision-making abilities, beliefs and practices surrounding childbirth and delivery, nutrition and education.

Phase 2 Delay: Delay in Reaching Care

- Poor roads, mountains, islands, rivers—poor organization.

Phase 3 Delay: Delay in Receiving Care

- Inadequate facilities, supplies, personnel.
- Poor training and demotivation of personnel.
- Lack of finances.

Source: Report on Maternal and Perinatal Death Enquiry and Response (MAPEDIR), UNICEF 2008.

---

given and circumstances of deaths are investigated to see whether these deaths could have been avoided. This addresses the third delay and quality of care in a facility.

The findings of these reviews are placed before the medical death audit committee on a monthly basis. Minutes of the committee meetings are placed before the district reproductive and child health (RCH) committee chaired by the district collector, who also receives relatives of the deceased to give their account of the events. Minutes of the review meetings are sent to the MCH commissioner.

Review of Findings by District Magistrate (DM)

The relatives of the deceased first narrate the events leading to the death of the mother in front of the DM and the service providers who attended the deceased mother. The case histories of each of the selected maternal deaths are heard separately. After the deposition and providing clarifications, the relatives leave. Thereafter the various delays, decision-making at the family level, obtaining transport and institutional delays are discussed in detail. The outcome of the meeting is recorded as minutes and corrective actions are listed with a time line to prevent similar delays in future.

Positive outcomes of the maternal death verbal autopsy system include greater accountability of service providers, advance information to referral centres, better coordination between referring and referral institutions and a very few unrecorded referrals. Reviews of maternal deaths have indicated several problems in the health care delivery system which may lead to maternal mortality. Examples include improper distribution of FRUs in the state, shortage of staff at the FRUs and unnecessary multiple referrals.

Impact on the Health System of Tamil Nadu

Based on the reviews of maternal deaths and other evidence on how to reduce the MMR, the Government of Tamil Nadu has initiated various programmatic improvements as summarized as follows:

1. Enhancement of skilled care providers in rural areas.
2. Attracting doctors and staff nurses to work in rural areas.
3. Increasing availability of specialists at FRUs.
4. Establishment of comprehensive emergency obstetric and newborn care centres with round-the-clock emergency obstetric and newborn services.
5. Special programme for conditional cash transfer to pregnant women.
6. Increasing availability of blood.
7. Birth-companion programme to improve social support during delivery.
8. Maternity picnic.
9. Contracting private anaesthetist, obstetrician and gynaecologist for emergency caesarean section (C-section).
10. Contracting with private partners for ambulances.
11. Certification of CEmOC centres for making the facility accountable for EmOC functions.

MDR has been rolled out across the country. Trainings are being given to the care givers and the teams involved at various levels. A pilot was done in the state of Uttar Pradesh to get some insights into the review process (see Box 18.5 here). MDR has the potential to strengthen the health system but this can only be established once the data starts coming in.

Box 18.5: Community-based Maternal Death Audit (MDA) in a District of Uttar Pradesh

Maternal death audits (MDA), have been shown to contribute to the reduction in maternal deaths, by providing insight into why women die. MDAs have been carried out in the states of Kerala and Tamil Nadu, where they have been identified as an important tool used to achieve one of the lowest MMRs in the country. Keeping in view that UP has one of the highest maternal deaths in the country, the Government of Uttar Pradesh (GoUP) is in the process of initiating MDA in the state, based on the Government of India guidelines, to provide an in-depth understanding of processes and causes leading to maternal deaths, including social-cultural, economic factors and medical causes. The objectives of this study were to identify the operational problems in conducting maternal death audits at community level and their potential solutions, based on government guidelines and to make recommendations to the government on ways to improve maternal health services at the community and or facility level.

The key findings were the following:

1. The major direct causes of the reported deaths were: haemorrhage (38.5%), anaemia (26.3%), sepsis (14%), eclampsia (10.5%) and obstructed labour (7%).
2. Places of maternal death were 16% of the cases in private facilities, 30% in government hospitals, 23% at home and 30% en route to a formal health facility.
3. The mean cost of the transport from home to facility one was ₹254, facility one to facility two was ₹1,042 and facility two to facility three was ₹910.
4. The average cost of the care in facility one was ₹3,044, facility two was ₹10, 319 and facility three was ₹11,900.
5. The mean travel time between facility one, facility two and facility three was two hours

Source: Personal communication with Dr Sunil S. Raj, Additional Professor Indian Institute of Public Health Delhi.

Annexure 1: Evaluating the Delaying Factors Contributing to Maternal Deaths

WHO describes five main approaches to evaluate the delays:

Community-based Maternal Death Reviews

CBMDR are conducted at the community level to ascertain common community factors that may have contributed to the maternal deaths and to act upon the findings.

Definition

A method of finding out the medical causes of death and ascertaining the personal, family or community factors that may have contributed to the death of a woman who died outside of a medical facility.

Requirements

Cooperation from the family of the woman who died. Sensitivity is needed in discussing the circumstances of the death.

Advantages

Provide means to arrive at medical cause of death when a woman dies at home, allows both medical and non-medical factors to be explored and provides the opportunity to include the family's perspective on health services.

Disadvantages

Different assessors may arrive at different causes of death; deaths from indirect causes may be overlooked/underreported.

Facility-based Maternal Death Reviews

FBMDR are conducted at the facilities by the providers as in-depth investigations of the causes of and circumstances surrounding maternal deaths, with the primary objective of improving the quality of care.

Definition

A qualitative, in-depth investigation of the causes of and circumstances surrounding a maternal death at a health facility; the death is initially identified at the facility level but such reviews are also concerned with identifying the combination of factors at the facility and in the community that contributed to the death and which ones were avoidable.

Requirements

Cooperation from those who provided care to the woman who died and their willingness to report accurately on the management of the case.

Advantages

Is a well-understood process in some settings, allows for complete review of medical aspects, provides a learning opportunity for all staff and can stimulate improvements to medical care.

Disadvantages

Requires committed leadership at the facility level, does not provide information about deaths occurring in the community.

Confidential Enquiries[1]

Enquiries that constitute systematic multidisciplinary anonymous investigations of maternal deaths within a region or country. These help to identify the numbers, causes and associated remedial factors (2011).

[1]Mills 2011.

A national or sub-national multidisciplinary committee meets periodically to systematically investigate a representative sample of (or all) maternal deaths to identify the causes and associated factors; the committee then gives written guidelines to health personnel and administrators on how to prevent similar deaths in future. The investigation is carried out in a confidential manner ('No blame, no shame'). It requires a complete and functioning civil registration or health management information system. A sub-national or district-level panel might be more appropriate in countries with high mortality, so that the guidelines issued can be tailored to local situations.

Surveys of Near-misses or Survivors[2]

Surveys of near-misses or survivors of obstetric complications for ensuring improvements in maternal care and programmes with the necessary capacity (UNHCR).

Definition

The identification and assessment of cases in which a pregnant woman survives an obstetric complication; there is no universally acceptable definition for such cases and it is important that the definition used be appropriate to local circumstances to enable local improvements in maternal care.

Requirements

A good-quality medical record system, a management culture where life-threatening events can be discussed freely without fear of blame and a commitment from management and clinical staff to act upon findings.

Advantages

A 'near-miss' may occur more frequently than a maternal death, it is possible to interview the woman herself during the review process and reduce the likelihood of future maternal deaths through quality improvement.

Disadvantages

Requires clear definition of severe maternal morbidity, selection criteria for settings with a high volume of life-threatening events.

Clinical Audit

A quality improvement process that seeks to improve patient care and outcomes through a systematic review of various aspects of the structure, processes and outcomes of care against explicit criteria and ensures the subsequent implementation of change.

[2]Cornier 2010.

The process entails a systematic review or audit of the obstetric care provided to pregnant women against established protocols or criteria, aimed at improving the quality of care. Protocols for the management of obstetric complications will have to be established beforehand in order to ascertain whether cases are being properly managed at health facilities. If properly implemented, it leads to standardized and improved care across health facilities.

Different approaches have been used across the world, including India, to evaluate the delays in both community and facility settings. Experience in the use of these approaches has shown that successful implementation can take place at all levels. A commitment to act upon these findings is a key prerequisite for success.

References

Bødker, B., Hvidman, L., Weber, T., Møller, M., Aarre, A., Nielsen, K.M. and Sørensen, J.L. 2009. 'Maternal Deaths in Denmark 2002–06'. *Acta Obstetricia et Gynecologica Scandinavica*, 88(5): 556–62. DOI: 10.1080/00016340902897992.

Cornier, N. 2010. 'Guideline for Reviewing Maternal Deaths'. Available at http://www.unhcr.org/47f38de12.pdf, accessed on 21 May 2012.

Hill, K., AbouZahr, C. and Wardlaw, T. 1996. 'Strategies for Model-based Estimates of Maternal Mortality Cynthia Stanton'. Prepared for the Seminar on Innovative Approaches to the Assessment of Reproductive Health, organized by the Committee on Reproductive Health of the International Union for the Scientific Study of Population, 24–27 September, Manila, The Philippines.

Mavalankar, D.V., Padmanbhan, P. and Raman, P.S. 2009. 'Maternal Death Audit in Tamil Nadu: Its Impact on Health System'. Available at apha.confex.com/apha/137am/recordingredirect.cgi/id/28053, accessed on 23 June 2012.

Mills, S. 2011. 'Maternal Death Audit as a Tool Reducing Maternal Mortality'. Available at http://siteresources.worldbank.org/INTPRH/Resources/376374-1278599377733/MaternalDeathAuditMarch22011.pdf, accessed on 30 June 2011.

Ministry of Health and Family Welfare, Government of India. 2010. *Maternal Death Review—Guidebook*. Available at http://rrcnes.gov.in/pdf_ppt_zip/mdr_handbook.pdf, accessed on 30 June 2011.

Padmanaban, P., Raman, P. and Mavalankar, D.V. 2009. 'Innovations and Challenges in Reducing Maternal Mortality in Tamil Nadu, India'. *Health Population Nutrition*, 27(2): 202–19; International Centre for Diarrhoeal Disease Research, Bangladesh.

Pattinson R.C. and Hall M. 2003. 'Near Misses: A Useful Adjunct to Maternal Death Enquiries'. *British Medical Bulletin*, 67: 231–43.

Sample Registration System (SRS). 2011. 'Special Bulletin on Maternal Mortality in India 2007–09'. SRS, Office of Registrar General, India. Available at http://www.censusindia.gov.in/vital_statistics/SRS_Bulletins/Final-MMR%20Bulletin-2007-09_070711.pdf, accessed on 21 May 2012.

United Nations Population Fund (UNFPA). 1995. Report of the International Conference on Population and Development, Cairo, 5–13 September. Available at: http://www.refworld.org/docid/4a54bc080.html, accessed on 5 August 2013.

UNICEF. 2008. *Maternal and Perinatal Death Inquiry and Response—Empowering Communities to Avert Maternal Deaths in India*. India: UNICEF.

Social Accountability Initiatives

19

Promoting Social Accountability for Safe Motherhood: White Ribbon Alliance India

Raj Mohan Panda and Sourav Neogi

The White Ribbon Alliance for Safe Motherhood (WRA) is a global movement which builds alliances, strengthens capacity, influences policies, harnesses resources and inspires action to protect the lives of women and newborns around the world. In India, the WRA unites individuals, organizations and communities who are committed to increasing public awareness on how to prevent maternal deaths and promote safe motherhood. The White Ribbon Alliance for Safe Motherhood, India (WRAI) started in 1999 with six organizations and several dedicated individuals who felt a strong commitment to save women's lives. In a span of 12 years, WRAI has grown into a formal and strong national alliance with members across the country, including 152 at national level and over 1,500 organizations at state level (Motihar and Gogoi 2009).

WRAI's approach to improving maternal health is based on utilizing social mobilization strategies to build and strengthen a grassroots movement. Social mobilization activities are undertaken to influence positive behaviour change and create an enabling environment. Purposeful actions must reach, influence and involve all sectors of society from the national to the community level.

Need for Social Accountability Initiatives

Why is there a need for social accountability initiatives in India?

'Social accountability is a very important element when you talk of empowering communities at the grassroots level primarily telling them about their entitlements; you go to any state and look at the policies at the national level; we have wonderful policies on papers, wonderful schemes; but the problem is when we try to roll it out at the grassroots level; the families and communities for whom these schemes and programmes are meant to be; they don't really know about it; they may have 20% information; 50% information and sometime even if they have the information; they do not know what to do with that; don't know what their entitlements are and how they can get their entitlements; that's the reason it is extremely important to work with the communities so that they know what these policies and programmes promise and how they can get those.'

Source: Aparajita Gogoi, Executive Director, CEDPA, India and National Coordinator White Ribbon Alliance, India (WRAI).

The social mobilization approach recognizes that enduring change requires dialogue and partnership among multiple stakeholders (Azad India Foundation 2010) (see box titled 'Need for Social Accountability Initiatives').

This case study documents the various techniques advocated by the WRAI to illustrate the role that the tools of social accountability can play in creating a rights-based mass movement directed towards safe motherhood for all. We conducted several interviews, some in conjunction with research collaborators. Interviewees included government officials involved with health, maternal and child health division heads, beneficiaries, the media, bilateral donors, multilateral agency representatives and academics. Most interviews lasted between one and two hours. Detailed notes were taken during each interview and some were transcribed. Observations at the field sites also helped supplement information. Although some common questions were asked of most interviewees, including their assessment of the political priority for the cause, we did not employ a uniform survey instrument, because each interviewee had unique knowledge about safe motherhood in his/her area. Instead, we asked open-ended questions in an exploratory way to elicit the unique knowledge and experience the diverse constituents had to offer.

Background

In the last decade much has been done to decrease maternal deaths and bring the maternal mortality ratio (MMR) to 212 (SRS 2007–09) per 100,000 live births. Despite this, with a world population share of 17%, India accounts for 19% (WHO, UNICEF, UNFPA and the World Bank 2010) of all maternal deaths worldwide. Experts estimate that 70% of the maternal-related deaths are preventable. Tetanus and anaemia claim a large number of women because mothers get very little or no care in the postnatal period, although anaemia, at least can be managed with appropriate nutrition and supplements (Azad India Foundation 2010). While most maternal deaths are preventable, lack of timely transportation to the nearest hospital, poor health services and scarce resources limit women's access to life-saving, high-quality care. In 2005, India's national flagship health programme, the National Rural Health Mission (NRHM), was launched to provide a strong policy and programme effort to make maternal, newborn and child health and nutrition (MNCHN) related mortality a priority. Recognizing that it is not sufficient to merely strengthen service delivery, community-based monitoring of health services is a key strategy of NRHM to ensure that the services reach those for whom they are meant (see Annexure 1). For this purpose, monitoring and planning committees are set-up at each level. The village-level committee prepares a village report card and facility-level committees prepare facility scorecards. These are aggregated and shared through the village-sharing meetings and through public dialogues at block and district levels. The common review missions of NRHM generally show that community monitoring is weak and many states have not taken up this issue in a structured manner.

Recognizing that progress towards the Millennium Development Goals (MDGs) 4 and 5 requires better coordination and increased global attention, various advocacy efforts have been undertaken to bring together existing maternal health networks and engage new organizations to facilitate global coordination of maternal health programmes. Work in ensuring health provider accountability, however, is missing. Pregnancy and childbirth-related deaths and morbidity still do not occupy priority space in public debate in the country. One reason for this is that there has never been a mass campaign and groundswell to address these issues.

The WRAI's role is to empower communities so that demand side social accountability acts as a monitoring input for better supply of maternal health care. Its campaign for fostering overall social accountability is centered on two important factors—generating greater political will and strengthening social accountability at the grassroots level. These are essential elements which WRAI believes will help fill the existing lacuna at the state, district and block levels. Social accountability consists of actions and mechanisms that citizens, communities, independent media and civil society organizations can use to monitor and hold public officials accountable. It relies on civic engagement where citizens and civil society organizations access information about budgets, expenditures and services and extract accountability. Most social accountability interventions inform citizens of their rights and the performance of services and encourage their participation (Bjorkman and Svensson 2009). Citizens' participation often results in feedback to service providers (the direct channel) or to governments at the higher level (the indirect channel). Therefore, social accountability is often referred to as the demand-side channel for strengthening accountability relationships between communities, local governments, service providers and the state (see Figure 19.1).

Community stakeholders need to understand—and advocate for—their rights to improved maternal and child health services. National and state-level political leaders need to exert greater pressure on their district-level colleagues to make government commitments a reality. Media and other opinion leaders should increase their role as public watchdogs to ensure that funds are being spent on effective interventions that improve maternal and child health. From 2007 onwards, WRAI is making an attempt to create a people-centered accountability initiative at the grassroots level and work with member organizations in building their capacities to demand accountability.

Figure 19.1
A Framework for Accountability Relationships

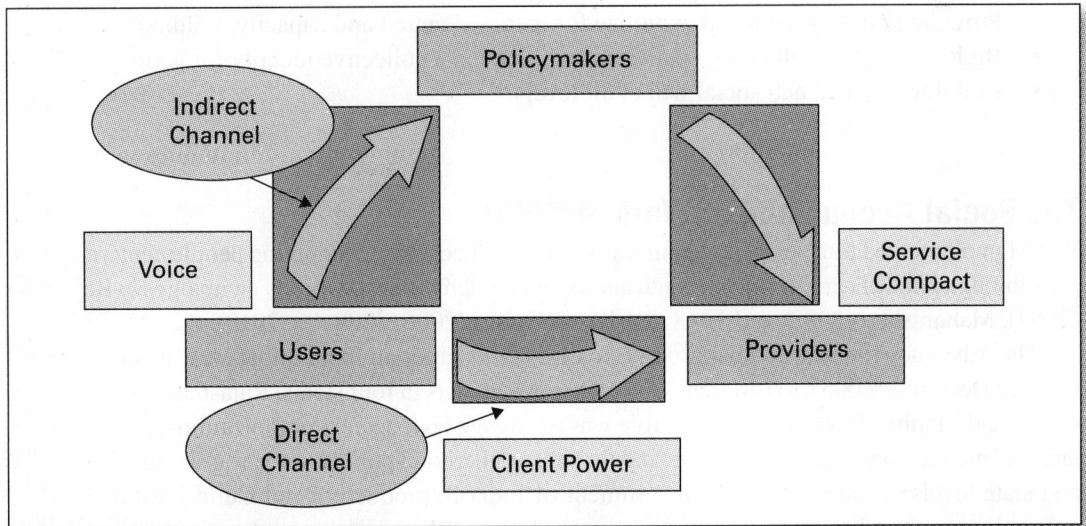

Source: World Bank (2005).

The philosophy behind social accountability centres on the role of empowerment and information in enhancing government commitment and service delivery. Therefore, these initiatives have focussed on three main aspects:

1. Strengthening civic activism to increase demand for maternal health services.
2. Asking for accountability and commitment to deliver maternal health services.
3. Strengthening the capacity of media to address these issues.

Under this initiative, several social watch techniques, i.e., tracking policy implementation, verbal autopsies, national campaigns, public hearings and advocacy through Indian Language Print Media have been used as advocacy tools.

Social Accountability for Safe Motherhood

WRAI believes that joint efforts from organizations/individuals with varied expertise are required to advocate with the government for better performance of the health system. However, collective efforts towards improvement of the system might bring positive results. With this mandate WRAI creates a platform consisting of individuals, organizations and donors to advocate for improvement in the system.

The main strategies used in WRAI campaigns for social accountability are:

* Increasing information equity through sharing of information.
* Promoting evidence-based and promising practices.
* Using events as catalysts for focussed action.
* Involving diverse, multi-sectoral stakeholders.
* Increasing the level of dialogue with multiple stakeholders.
* Providing/pooling technical expertise for focussed action and capacity building.
* Building and strengthening coalitions and creating a collective identity for action.
* Building political and social will at all levels.

The Social Accountability Work of WRAI

WRAI implemented four social watch initiatives using checklists, conducting people centered advocacy through public hearings, verbal death audits and implementing advocacy campaigns in Rajasthan (2007), Maharashtra (2008) and 12+8 districts in Orissa (2006, 2008–09, 2010).

The Advocacy for Safe Motherhood Policy Implementation in India initiative was implemented from 22 December 2005 to 31 March 2007 across 73 districts in four states; Rajasthan, West Bengal, Orissa and Madhya Pradesh. The objective was to engage civil society organizations, parliamentarians and media representatives in advocacy for safe motherhood policies and programmes at national and state levels, as defined in the Government of India Reproductive and Child Health (RCH) 2 policy document and conduct policy advocacy to encourage key decision-makers in state and central governments to improve the status of maternal health services in the country. The partners carried out intensive social mobilization activities across the 73 districts, engaging 437 organizational members. Some 355 media members and 389 elected representatives at all levels (including Members of the Legislative Assemblies and Members of Parliament) who were informed about statistics and issues related to maternal health and received advocacy training. As many as 1,687 advocacy kits were distributed amongst media members, public health officers and elected representatives. At least 53 articles/broadcast spots covered maternal health issues on National Safe Motherhood Day in India. Capacity building of 362 partner members took place and these individuals are continuing the advocacy in their respective areas. The checklist to track policy implementation has proven to be a useful tool and can help the civil movement gather data to back up its demands for better health facilities and policy implementation. During the National Safe Motherhood Day, 2008, there was the launch of 'Deliver Now for Women and Children' in India, with national and state media press conferences to announce the launch.

A national advocacy and consensus development meeting was held on agreement on a common advocacy agenda for maternal, newborn and child health issues.

Social Watch Techniques

Social watch is a tested technique to demand accountability for commitments made. This was adopted by WRAI to create accountability at all levels and to find the gaps requiring further action. Social watch techniques mobilize citizens to demand accountability in the translation of maternal and newborn health commitments and policies into improved access to services (Futures Group 2010).

WRAI conducts orientation sessions and regular capacity building and refreshers trainings for NGOs working in health and other sectors on issues related to women's health, in particular, related to safe motherhood and use of accountability tools for safe motherhood. Similar sessions are also organized for the local media personnel and local elected representatives. Public hearings, national campaigns and engagement of Indian Language Print Media are cornerstones of the advocacy strategy.

Each social watch campaign consists of three steps (see Figure 19.2):

1. **Develop and share tools**: To monitor the maternal health situation and progress on policy implementation. It is also important to build capacities among grassroots level workers and train them to use specific tools for gathering required evidence.
2. **Gather information**: By using tools such as 'tracking policy implementation', conducting 'verbal autopsy' and 'community scorecard'. There is a need to demystify government procedures and actions in order to strengthen citizens' voice and promote social accountability. Information should be relevant, regular and reliable, identify gaps in implementation of the policies and schemes and demand redressal of these gaps.
3. **Spread awareness**: Ensure that civil society has the necessary information about the following:

   - Maternal health situation
   - A women's right to high-quality health care
   - Government policies

Social watch has been successfully implemented by various methods.

Figure 19.2
Social Watch Approach

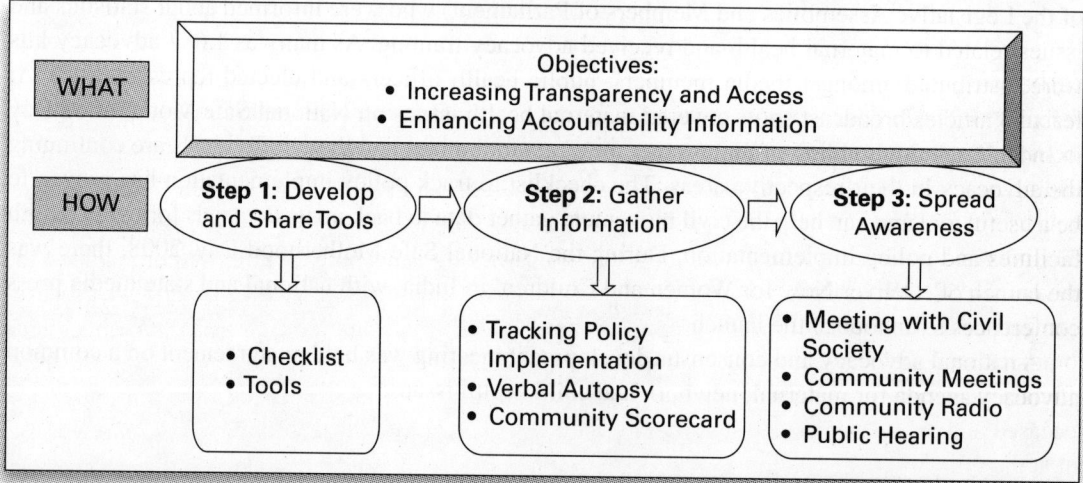

Source: PHFI, 2011.

Community Scorecard

The community scorecard process is a community-based monitoring tool used as an instrument to ensure social and public accountability and responsiveness from service providers. This process can also facilitate the monitoring and performance evaluation of maternal health services, facilities and their service providers. The community scorecard process involves four components: (1) input tracking scorecard, (2) community generated performance scorecard, (3) service providers self-evaluation scorecards and (4) interface meeting between service providers and users to generate a mutually agreed reform agenda.

The community is involved from the very beginning and encouraged to participate in the design of solutions as well as ensure compliance. The strength of the community scorecards in terms of human rights is, therefore, in the area of 'bottom-up participation' (Ackerman 2005). The community is able to discuss its entitlements with regard to maternal health and the reasons for the current situation and examine this in a holistic manner instead of just indulging in a 'blame game', as it is not limited to evaluating the performance of service providers.

Tracking Policy Implementation

An important way to gather information about the health situation and to measure change is to design and implement a mechanism to systematically track policy implementation and maternal newborn and child health (MNCH) budgeting. When members of civil society have access to and are trained in the use of these mechanisms, such as checklists or surveys, the information collected can be used in social watch studies to assess the quality of services provided at various facilities, document progress on the implementation of key policies and provide a picture of the current MNCH situation. Transparency regarding allocations, expenditures and on-ground implementation of policies is analyzed. WRAI then helps share the data gathered during the social watch activities with state governments and health officials at different levels. These reports serve as evidence and provide support for local and national advocacy efforts. Thus participation is not limited to information provision and protest but helps build a movement towards a partnership approach to policy formulation (World Bank 2005).

Verbal Autopsies

Verbal autopsy is a strategy approved by World Health Organization (WHO) to provide information about the causes of maternal death. The verbal autopsy process is a tool to understand the factors leading to maternal deaths and to address household, community and health systems changes that would have prevented such maternal deaths. WRA-Orissa has adopted the verbal autopsy process; the findings have been documented and backed up with evidence and solutions recommended to prevent such deaths in future. An important component of a comprehensive verbal autopsy process is to gather all available information on the maternal death from the relevant health personnel and community members. The team of investigators should include medical personnel, government officials, advocacy groups and members of the media. Team members also visit the family of the deceased and conduct interviews with the family members, particularly with those who were present at the time of death. The team writes a report on the individual maternal death and disseminates it to the community, family members and government officials. Data from the autopsies are then summarized in a report and disseminated widely for sensitization of different stakeholders, including policymakers, to encourage relevant policy changes. Media personnel are engaged in the entire process, whenever possible, to ensure public awareness and encourage public dialogue on the issues identified during the verbal autopsy process. The WRA members facilitate the process and use the evidence to advocate for solutions to address the factors which caused these needless deaths.

Advocacy Campaigns

A key social watch strategy involves sharing information through national campaigns and creating awareness in the community about their maternal health entitlements. After civil society has been engaged in monitoring policy and programme implementation; the broader policy need to be made aware of its findings and issues identified to strengthen accountability. WRAI facilitated national campaigns include actions such as the launch of advocacy campaigns in India, rallies, marches, local events and other activities to attract media attention. In the annual rallies and meetings conducted by WRAI, participants are presented with an advocacy kit or package that outlines key issues the campaign will focus on and what individuals can do to make a difference. Local meetings, workshops and other community-mobilization activities take place throughout the year to spread awareness and build support.

Public Hearings

Public hearings can amplify the voice of women and help in identifying critical implementation gaps. In a public hearing, an ambient environment is created to enable women to raise their voices and invite concerns of the service providers, media and elected representatives.

Public hearings are designed to influence service providers, policymakers, the media, women and their families. The objective of these hearings is that women become aware of their rights, share their stories and demand change from decision-makers (see boxes titled 'A Testimony of an *Anganwadi* Worker' and 'A Women's Testimony during Public Hearing'). During the hearings, community members, elected government officials, media and NGO representatives stand up to call for action to improve women's health. These events often follow a rally in which community members show support for improving MNCH. WRAI-Orissa also supported the media outreach in social mobilization activities and by providing support in generating coverage of the calls for increased implementation of maternal and child health interventions. Generated media coverage was circled back to health decision-makers to make them aware of the spotlight that is shining on implementation of promised maternal and child health interventions. Media representatives were also taken on field trips to interact with health service providers and women directly.

A Testimony of an *Anganwadi* Worker

During an ongoing public hearing during our field trip we found a lady (*Anganwadi* worker) crying and telling a story to the panellist. She said that there was a pregnant lady in her village who was very poor; one day she had severe labour pain; the pregnant lady informed her about the pain; she (*Anganwadi* worker) rushed to the Accredited Social Health Activist (ASHA) of the village; the ASHA took the pregnant lady to the primary health centre (PHC); which is quite far away; the doctor in the PHC without performing any check-up told them that she was 7-months pregnant hence she needs to come later; the pregnant lady came back to her place and delivered a still birth on the next day; she was both physically and mentally affected with the situation and asked her (*Anganwadi* worker) what to do now. Such situations are not acceptable. The doctor should have checked her properly.

Source: PHFI, 2011.

Advocacy through Indian Language Print Media

WRAI, with the objective of involving print media as a channel for advocacy campaigns, trained the local media personnel on maternal and child health issues. The WRA involved the local media officials by inviting them during the social mobilization activities and also supported them to gather information on implementation of maternal and child health interventions in the government facilities. Generated media coverage was circled back to health decision-makers to make them aware of the spotlight on the implementation of promised maternal and child health interventions. Media representatives were also taken on field trips to interact with health service providers and women directly.

A Woman's Testimony During a Public Hearing

'When a maternal death occurs, our family is ruined. You, the collector and the chief district medical officer (CDMO), never feel the sorrow and the pain that our families feel. You are meant to provide us with a quality service but we are not getting it. So whom do we hold accountable for maternal deaths?'

Source: A woman said during a public hearing at Balangir, Odisha (25 June 2008).

Orissa Experience

Although the WRAI implemented the social watch techniques in several states in India, the major success stories have been reported from Orissa. As a part of its Health Policy Initiative, USAID published a report in September 2010 which said that since 2006, 30 public hearings have been organized by WRA-Orissa. With 500–1,300 women taking part in each event, the result was more than 30,000 women participated in these hearings. The platform has been used to inform the participants about their rights and to present their grievances directly to the decision-makers. In these public hearings, elected local government representatives were responsive to community members and answered questions on the concerns raised. Local media covered the hearings, which generated excitement and debate in communities. As a result of successful hearings, media offices in the districts of Orissa had a continuous flow of news on maternal health problems and continued to report on maternal health issues long after the hearings ceased. Citizens of the area become aware of the issues around safe motherhood. The health service delivery system became more responsive and accountable, as demonstrated by the following actions:

- The Government of Orissa has started a new process for the disbursement of payments through cheques, rather than cash, to avoid the misappropriation of funds intended for pregnant women and to better enforce government policies.
- The state health department gave instructions to ensure the presence of auxiliary nurse midwives (ANMs) at all the facilities.
- The chief minister of Orissa declared that women's self-help groups (SHGs) would be involved in the monitoring of maternal health programmes. In some districts, female SHG members were assigned the responsibility of forming a committee to track bribes taken by maternal health care providers.
- In Koraput District authorities pledged to take action against doctors who were found to demand bribes for institutional deliveries. These authorities also committed to ensuring the proper implementation of the Janani Suraksha Yojana Scheme and issued a circular to all service providers calling for health facilities to remain open 24 hours a day.
- Grievance cells have been opened in six district hospitals.

Critical Elements of Success

Discussions with the WRAI officials and representatives of partner organizations highlighted the following elements of success for such a programme.

Large Network of NGOs/Community-based Organizations Empowered

The programme has been implemented in several states in India; however, the intervention has been comparatively more successful in Orissa. In Orissa, WRA membership is spread across the state and covers each district and block. These local WRAs have been quite active in the state. The other states where a similar intervention has been implemented do not have the advantage of a similar member's network.

A large network of WRA members is important for the success of any advocacy campaign. Engagement of these NGOs/WRA members at every stage of the campaign is important to ensure active participation and follow-up with local government authorities on various maternal health issues.

Strong Leadership Skills

During any advocacy campaign the campaigners should have strong leadership skills. Experience shows that advocacy campaigns become difficult at times and continuous persuasion is needed to bring about change. Campaigners who have foresight and strong leadership skills can bring about the desired change.

During discussions with the WRA country officials it was revealed that the intervention in Orissa is successful due to the strong presence of the state WRA team.

Engagement of Media: Long Lasting Impact

In order for each event to have a lasting impact WRA ensures all the major events are covered by the local media officials. This ensures that the discussion lasts beyond the event.

WRAI Experience of Implementing the Social Accountability Approach

WRAI found that

1. The social accountability approaches require a great deal of investment at different levels. Social accountability is more than a process. While methods and tools are important, the institutionalization of social accountability requires a lot of time, money and expertise to implement and be accepted in community. Conflicting interests of different players should be kept in mind while demanding services. Often political differences can cloud genuine issues at hand and it is important to address them from the beginning of the process.
2. Linking supply of and demand for governance. While it is important to build consumer demands for quality of care and entitlements, it is just as important to ensure that the supply side is given equal attention. This includes engagement and advice to governments on creating transparency and accountability. This could cover linking demand-side efforts to public sector reform, anti-corruption and service delivery and promoting participatory policymaking and public information disclosure.
3. Using both sanctions as well as incentives help social accountability in being an effective approach.
4. Skills to implement social accountability interventions are not easily accessible. The skills to implement and carry out such exercises are rigorous and often difficult to build at community level.

Way Forward

Existing evidence on the impact of social accountability approaches is limited. Although there is much anecdotal evidence regarding the success of the approach, impact evaluation and scientific studies on the benefits of social accountability are rare. This is because there have been far too few rigorous impact evaluations. Anecdotal evidence cannot substitute for robust impact evidence and, thus, it is difficult to present social accountability as a tool for advocacy.

Sustainability of Social Accountability Mechanisms

When civil society organizations decide to push for changes they need to be equipped with facts and figures to back their arguments and to have the skills to monitor implementation once policy changes are achieved. However, sustaining the process of mobilization around these issues is another challenge. When designing social accountability, stakeholder analysis can help identify all the relevant players and, thus, identify supporters and build coalitions. Social accountability through community participation is a strategy for strengthening decentralization reforms and adopting rights-based approach to health. To make community participation and accountability work—from both within the system as well as outside—greater resources need to be allocated by the government to build capacities of marginalized groups, NGOs, women's health and human rights groups, elected representatives and providers. Further, a strong tradition of democracy—including electoral democracy, an unbiased judiciary, independent media, space for dissent and strong social movements—is a prerequisite for participation to thrive.

Community participation and accountability strategies cannot be added as simple mechanisms and structures which will work irrespective of context. Thus widening democratic spaces and strengthening a culture of claiming rights seem essential.

Given the power relationships at different levels of the health system, specific interests at local levels may sometimes have greater influence than at the national level. This can lead to conflict in implementation of progressive national policies. Thus evidence-based advocacy at local levels involving political will is essential for achieving outputs. WRAI has made a step in the right direction by empowering member organizations with the skills and techniques for adopting the rights-based approach for demanding the entitlements and benefits that the NRHM principles espouse.

Annexure 1: Community Monitoring Processes under NRHM

Community-based monitoring of health services is a key strategy of the NRHM to ensure that the services reach those for whom they are meant, especially for those residing in rural areas, the poor, women and children. Community monitoring is also seen as an important aspect of promoting community-led action in the field of health.

The provision for monitoring and planning committees has been made at the PHCs, and at block, district and state levels. The adoption of a comprehensive framework for community-based monitoring and planning at various levels under NRHM, places people at the centre of the process of regularly assessing whether the health needs and rights of the community are being fulfilled.

Community monitoring is to review the progress to ensure that the work is moving towards the decided purpose and the purpose has not shifted nor has the work got derailed in any way. Such a review can help to identify obstacles in the work, so that appropriate changes can be made to overcome the obstacles.

Monitoring and Planning Committee

The NRHM proposes a monitoring and planning committee at the village, PHC, block, district and state levels (see Figure 19A.1). The main functions of the committee are:

Figure 19A.1
Flow of Report/Feedback and Necessary Action amongst the Monitoring and Planning Committees

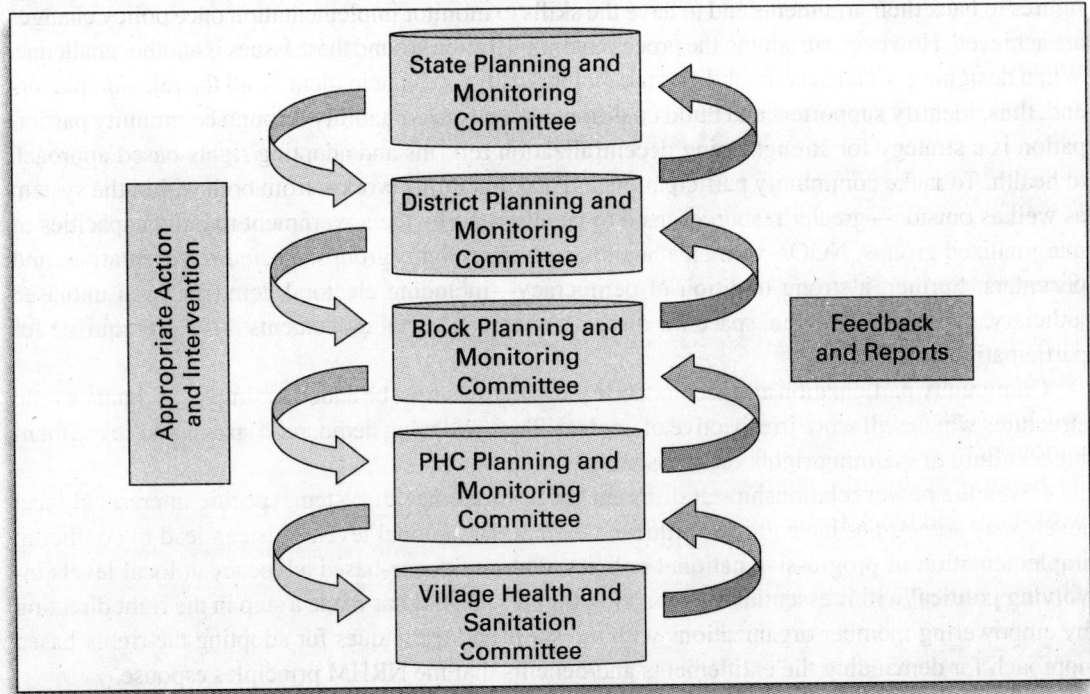

Source: Singh, Das and Sharma 2010.

- To create public awareness about the essentials of health programmes, with focus on people's knowledge of entitlements to enable their involvement in monitoring.
- Conduct participatory rapid assessments to ascertain the major health problems and health related issues.
- Discuss and develop a health plan based on an assessment of the situation and priorities identified by the community.
- Presentation of the progress made at the village level, achievements, actions taken and difficulties faced, followed by discussion on the progress of the achievements of the health facilities.
- Taking cognizance of the reported cases of the denial of health care and ensuring proper redressal.
- Reporting to the monitoring committee at the next level and collating information collected from the lower-level committee.

Processes

The implementation framework includes (see Figure 19A.2):

Orientation of Stakeholders and Strengthening of District/Block NGOs[1]

Orientation of stakeholders is done by means of a state workshop, district workshop, block providers orientation workshop and media orientation workshop, where a shared understanding of the community monitoring process under NRHM is developed and a resolve to work together is taken.

Strengthening of District/Block NGOs

There is capacity building of the district and block NGOs so that they understand the administrative and financial set-up of this programme and the various activities envisaged under it. This capacity building is done by holding state managers' workshops and block facilitator's trainings.

Mobilization of Community

The block facilitator will be familiarized with the village health services. This will aid in compilation

Figure 19A.2
Community Monitoring Processes under NRHM

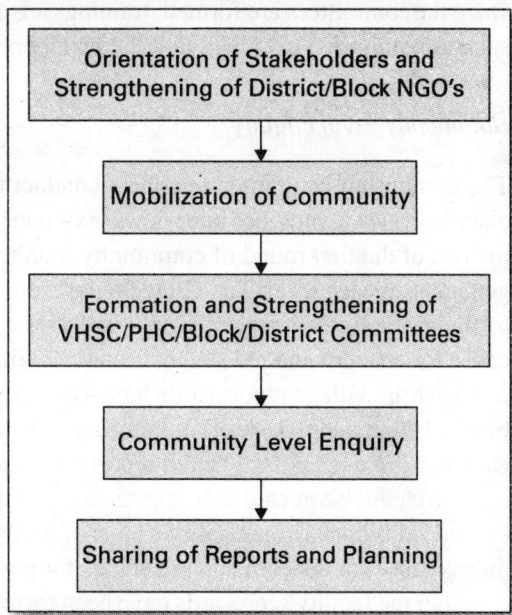

Source: Singh and Morang 2010.

of baseline information to be used for comparison after the community monitoring process is carried out.
Objective of community mobilization:

- To make the communities aware of their health-related entitlements under NRHM.
- To have a shared understanding of the health issues of the community.
- To facilitate the formation or expansion of the village health and sanitation committee (VHSC).
- Building ownership about public health service.
- Developing awareness about determinants of health.

Village Health Services Profile

It is an outcome of the mobilization process. It should be used by the block facilitators and the VHSC members to familiarize themselves before they start with the monitoring process. It will help in comparing the changes that will be brought about after the community monitoring process.

Formation and Strengthening of VHSC/PHC/Block/District Committees

Formation or expansion of committees at village, PHC, block and district levels.

[1] http://www.nrhmcommunityaction.org/, accessed in January 2012.

Strengthening of Committees

Once the committees are formed, trainings are organized for the members at each level on the issues such as monitoring exercises that the members will undertake.

Community-level Enquiry

The monitoring committee members conduct the first round of monitoring by conducting beneficiary interviews, provider interviews, exit interviews, focus group discussions and observations. At the end of the first round of community monitoring, a report card and a cumulative report card are generated at each level. The village report card depicts the status of the issues in question by means of the traffic lights imagery. Green indicates a well-performing village, yellow suggests there is a cause for concern and red suggests that the village is performing badly.

After the village report cards have been created for each village, they are collated by the PHC, block, district and state-level monitoring and planning committees. According to the colour code for each issue in each village health report card, the greens, yellows and reds are added at each level.

The facility scorecard indicates the status of the health facility in the village/block/district. Similar colour codes display the facility's level of performance. Green stands for good performance, yellow means cause for concern and red stands for poor performance.

After the facility scorecards have been formulated for each facility, they are collated by the PHC, block, district and state-level monitoring and planning committees. According to the colour code for each issue in each facility's scorecard, the greens, yellows and reds are added at each level.

Sharing of Reports and Planning

The following items are shared at the village sharing meeting.

- Village scorecard and key findings of the community-monitoring exercise.
- Adverse experiences and adverse outcomes.
- Ways to improve service delivery without finding fault with health care service providers.
- Discussion of key problems and action points suggested.

Jan Samvad (public dialogue)

The following items are dealt with in the *Jan Samvad* which is conducted at the block and PHC levels.

- Presentation of cumulative village report card and facility report card.
- Presentation of denial of care/adverse outcomes.
- Discussion on implementation of outreach services, improving facility-level service utilization and support to denial of care/adverse outcome cases

References

Ackerman, J. 2005. Human Rights and Social Accountability. Social Development Papers—Participation and Civil Engagement No. 86. World Bank. Available at http://www-wds.worldbank.org/servlet/WDSContentServer/WDSP/IB/2005/07/20/000 012009_20050720134205/Rendered/PDF/330110HR0and0SAc0paper0in0SDV0format.pdf, accessed in December 2011.

Azad India Foundation. 2010. Reproductive Health Status of Women in India. Available at http://www.azadindia.org/social-issues/reproductive-health-status-of-women-in-india.html, accessed in 2011.

Bjorkman, M. and Svensson, J. 2009. Scaling up Social Accountability in World Bank Operations. Available at http://siteresources.worldbank.org/EXTSOCIALDEVELOPMENT/Resources/244362-1193949504055/Scalingup.pdf.

Futures Group. 2010. Promoting Accountability for Safe Motherhood, The White Ribbon Alliance's Social Watch Approach, Task Order 1. Futures Group, Health Policy Initiative USA. Available at http://www.whiteribbonalliance.org/Resources/Documents/HPI-WRA-Promoting-Accountability-for-Safe-Motherhood1.pdf, accessed in 2011.

Motihar, R. and Gogoi, A. 2009. 'Catalyzing Collective Action for Saving Women's Lives, The White Ribbon Alliance for Safe Motherhood—India (WRAI) 1999–2009'. Available at http://www.whiteribbonalliance.org/Resources/Documents/09WRA_IndiaRpt5.pdf, accessed in November 2011.

Singh, S., Das, A., and Sharma, S. 2010. Reviving Hopes Realising Rights—A Report on First Phase of Community Monitoring under NRHM. Available at http://internationalbudget.org/wp-content/uploads/Reviving-Hopes.-Realizing-Rights.-A-Report-on-the-First-Phase-of-Community-Monitoring-under-NRHM.pdf, accessed in 2011.

Singh, S. and Morang, D. 2010. National Dissemination Meeting Community Monitoring under – National Rural Health Mission (NRHM). Available at http://www.chsj.org/uploads/1/0/2/1/10215849/cmnationaldisseminationreport.pdf, accessed in October 2013.

WHO, UNICEF, UNFPA and the World Bank Estimates. 2010. 'Trends in Maternal Mortality: 1990–2010'. Available at http://www.unfpa.org/webdav/site/global/shared/documents/publications/2012/Trends_in_maternal_mortality_A4-1.pdf, accessed in September 2011.

World Bank. 2005. 'The Accountability Framework 2005—Making Services Work for Poor People'. World Bank Institute. Available at http://info.worldbank.org/etools/docs/library/230169/Module2Accntblty.pdf, accessed in December 2011.

Section E
Successful Organizations as Innovation Engines

Sub-themes

State Feature
Organization Feature

Section E
Successful Organizations as Innovation Engines

While building the directory of innovations for the purpose of in-depth documentation of innovations in maternal and newborn health, two successful organizations—one government and the other a non-government organization (NGO)—were identified. The State Government selected has generated a large number of innovations and was prominent. The NGO has also been innovating as an innovation engine. Both these different successful innovation engines were addressing multiple areas of maternal and newborn health. What was common between them was a quest to find answers for better health outcomes and a resolution for improved health conditions for mother and child. This section has documented the state-led innovation engine where innovation for maternal child health (MCH) in Tamil Nadu has been documented and the other is the NGO-led innovation platform where Action Research and Training for Health (ARTH) in Udaipur, Rajasthan has been documented.

Action Research and Training for Health (ARTH)—This NGO began its work in Udaipur and is now known for some path-breaking work it has done for MCH in remote parts of Udaipur District. This case study discusses the factors responsible for their interventions being a success. Health delivery, adolescent health and right to reproductive health are some of the interventions discussed.

Tamil Nadu State Health System—In Indian health system, one of the most talked about and better performing states is Tamil Nadu with its inspiring health indicators. The state has achieved such health indicators over the years through a strong public health system. Some of the innovations undertaken by Tamil Nadu are targeted towards improving anaemia, reducing deaths by post-partum haemorrhage and improving the system of drug supply and reporting of maternal deaths.

State Feature

20. Innovative Approaches in Maternal and Newborn Care:
Tamil Nadu Health System

20

Innovative Approaches in Maternal and Newborn Care: Tamil Nadu Health System

Sourav Neogi and Madhavi Misra

It is heartening that the maternal mortality ratio (MMR) of India has declined from 254 in 2004–06 to 212 in 2007–09 (SRS). Still an estimated 56,000 maternal deaths occur each year (WHO 2005). In order to improve the figure, India needs both systemic and innovative health system approaches. Although overall India has made slow progress in reducing maternal mortality, progress in the state of Tamil Nadu has been rapid (Padmanaban et al. 2009).

In terms of basic health indicators (NFHS-3), Tamil Nadu is one of the progressive states in India. Located in the southern part of the country, the state's health system is considered to be the best in the country. Comparison of some major health indicators of Tamil Nadu with all-India figures shows that the state has made impressive progress (see Figure 20.1). Tamil Nadu has shown, over the last two decades, faster reduction in the population growth rate as compared to all other states except Kerala. The annual population growth rate during 1981–91 was 2.14% for all India, while it was 1.43% for Tamil Nadu, second only to Kerala (1.34%) (Human Development Report 2003). As per recently concluded Census 2011 (provisional figures) the decadal growth rate (for 2001–10 period) for India is 17.64%, however, in Tamil Nadu it is 15.60%. The total fertility rate (TFR) for Tamil Nadu showed a sharp decline from 3.9 in 1971 to 2.0 in 1997 (SRS). The most recent National Family Health Survey (NFHS-3) 2005–06 shows a further decline, with Tamil Nadu's TFR to be 1.8, the lowest in the country, surpassing Kerala (1.9) (NFHS-3).

This case study highlights the various innovative initiatives carried out by the state for improving maternal health that resulted in the reduction in the MMR from 380 in 1993 (Sheelarani 2007) to 79 in 2008–09 (State HMIS 2008–09).[1]

It has been a long journey for the state of Tamil Nadu to reach these encouraging figures. During these years the Tamil Nadu health system has innovated in different ways and many of the innovations have later been adopted by the Government of India and other states in the country.

---

[1] Directorate of Health Services, Government of Tamil Nadu, 2011. Available at www.esdproj.org/site/.../MAT-P1_Vaidyanathan_3.7.10.ppt?docID.

Figure 20.1

India and Tamil Nadu Comparison based on NFHS-3 (2005–06) Data

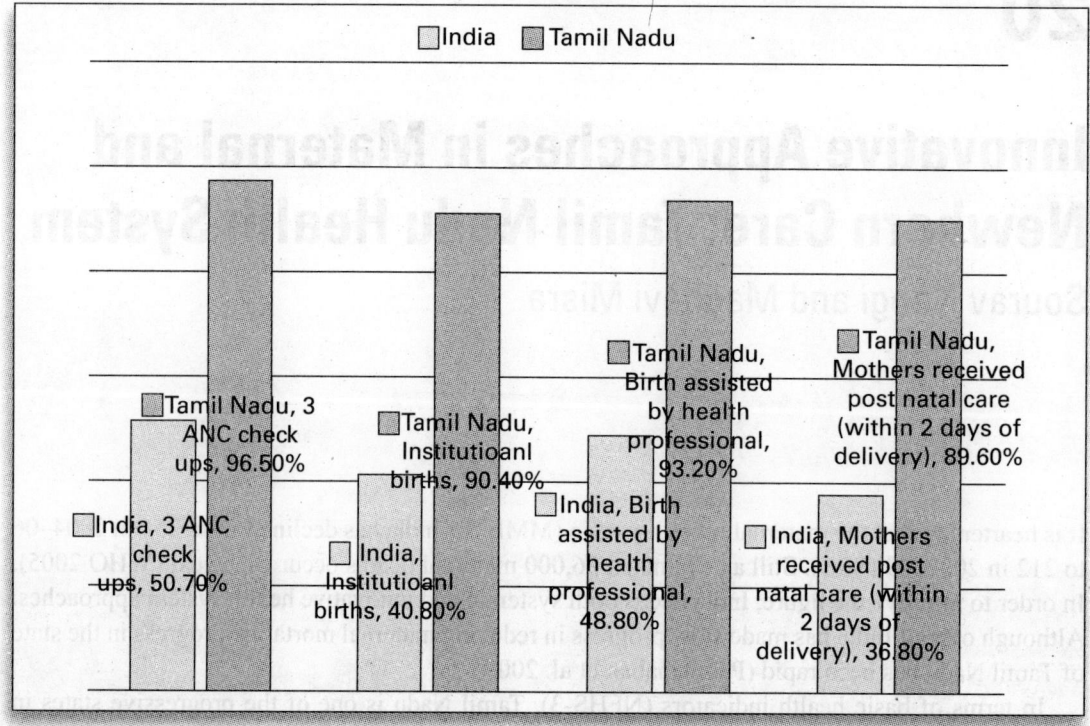

Source: NFHS-3 (2009).

Interview Byte: Girija Vaidyanathan

'Tamil Nadu has always felt that it is very important to focus on health issues and that is one reason why we are doing much better than the rest of the country. The political will to look at health as a priority area has gone back to nearly at least 20 to 30 years and that has reflected in our better indicators and our vital rates have always been better than the country.'

Source: Interview with Girija Vaidyanathan, IAS, Principal Secretary, Department of Health and Family Welfare, Government of Tamil Nadu, Chennai, Tamil Nadu. October 2011.

In this case study we are going to highlight the following aspects of the Tamil Nadu Health System:

1. Systematic changes made by the state of Tamil Nadu to strengthen their health system.
2. State-funded innovations—highlighting some key innovations.
3. What it takes to create a platform for innovative ideas to grow—The Tamil Nadu Experience.

Methodology/Approach

In order to develop this case study, a detailed desk review of relevant literature was conducted. In addition, a visit was made to the state for collecting information on innovations through in-depth

Figure 20.2
A Framework for Health System to Be Innovative

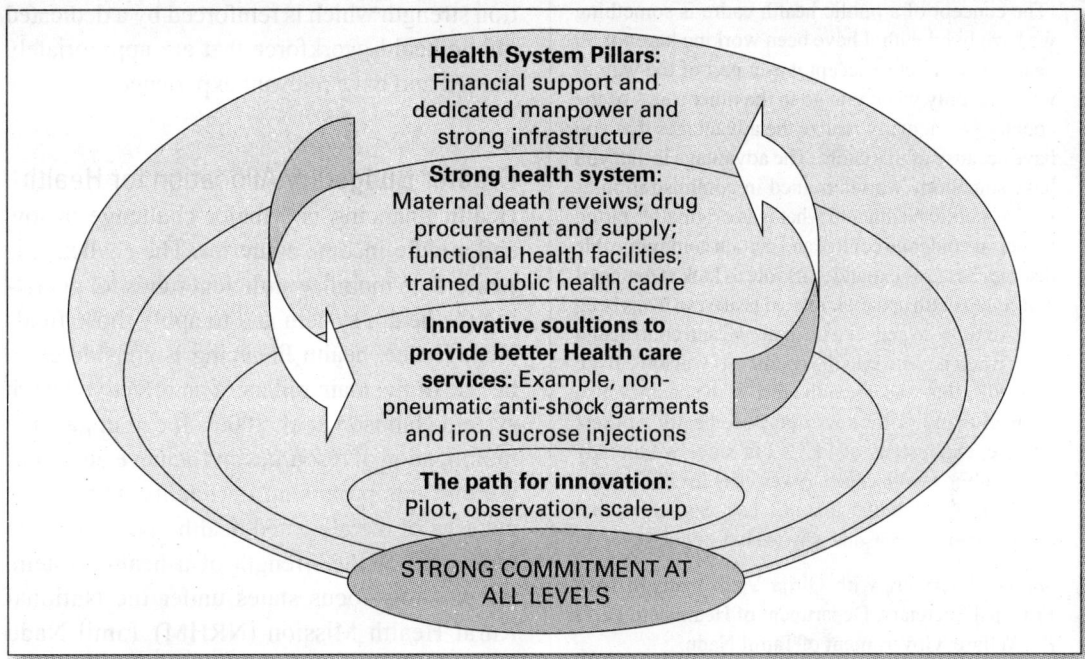

Health System Pillars:
Financial support and
dedicated manpower and
strong infrastructure

Strong health system:
Maternal death reveiws; drug
procurement and supply;
functional health facilities;
trained public health cadre

**Innovative soultions to
provide better Health care
services:** Example, non-
pneumatic anti-shock garments
and iron sucrose injections

The path for innovation:
Pilot, observation, scale-up

STRONG COMMITMENT AT
ALL LEVELS

Source: PHFI, 2011.

interviews with the policymakers, directors and officials at the health department and implementers. Visits were made to some sites and views of the beneficiaries were documented as well.

A conceptual framework for the health system to be more innovative in its approaches is given in Figure 20.2.

Section 1: Pillars/Mechanism of Health System Strengths—Tamil Nadu

How has the state of Tamil Nadu come up with several innovations in the health sector in the last two or three decades? What has led the state to come up with these innovations? In this section, we will try to answer these questions by highlighting some systemic changes that have been the driving force for the state. Without these, innovations could not achieve their desired outcomes. Dedicated Public Health Cadre under the Directorate of Public Health—the health department in Tamil Nadu has three key directorates which are organizationally equal under the health secretary—the Directorates of Public Health, of Medical Services and of Medical Education (Gupta et al. 2010). The Director-ate of Public Health has trained public health managers, who are promoted to the Directorate after years of experience in planning and overseeing public health services in both rural and urban areas. This ensures that the Directorate of Public Health is run by highly experienced staff with a deep understanding of how to run these services (Gupta et al. 2009).

Interview Byte: Girija Vaidyanathan

'The concept of a public health cadre is something we have lived with. I have been working here for 30 years; so you get to accept it as a part of the way of working; only when you go to the other states of the country you actually realize the advantages that you have because of this cadre. The advantage is that you have somebody who is trained in administration as well as public health and what was originally started to look at epidemic control and certain communicable diseases has now expanded its role to look at maternal and child health and their related issues, so it has been easy for us to do and take up maternal and child health work when it came into the country. If you look at the early 80s, this was when the rest of the country also adopted many of the multi-purpose health workers scheme, expansions of PHCs but since we already had a public health cadre, it was easy for us to make this work much better than the rest. So I think that this is one of the reasons why we have done so well.'

Source: Interview with Girija Vaidyanathan, IAS, Principal Secretary, Department of Health and Family Welfare, Government of Tamil Nadu.

One of the reasons why Tamil Nadu is able to achieve good health statistics is its implementation strength which is reinforced by a dedicated public health workforce that are appropriately trained and have relevant experience.

Greater Budgetary Allocation for Health

Health financing is a major challenge in low and middle-income countries. The challenge is twofold: to mobilize sufficient funds for operating the health system and to apply those funds well. Hence, health financing is considered to be one of the main pillars of an effective health system (Jamison et al. 2006). It can impact the mobilization of resources and achieve outcomes without compromising on quality. Utilization patterns of the allocated health budget may be indicative of the strength of a health system. Among low-focus states under the National Rural Health Mission (NRHM) Tamil Nadu is the highest spender (94%) of the allocated NRHM budget.[2]

A strong health system focusses more on primary, preventive and promotive public health care. Along these lines, Tamil Nadu gives focussed attention to the Directorate of Public Health and allocates a dedicated budget to it. The amount allocated to the Directorate of Public Health is large as compared to spending on secondary/tertiary medical care and medical education. The following tables (Tables 20.1 and 20.2) show a comparison of the health allocations among the three Directorates in Tamil Nadu.

Table 20.1

Health Spending (by Directorate), Tamil Nadu Health Department

Directorates	FY 2000–01		FY 2008–09		Compound Annual Growth Rate (Nominal)
	Rs Million	*% Share*	*Rs Million*	*% Share*	*%*
Public Health	4,571	43.4	8,939	38.8	8.7
Medical Services	2,361	22.4	5,303	23.1	10.6
Medical Education	3,595	34.2	8,775	38.1	11.8
Total	1,057	100.0	23,017	100.0	10.3

Source: Gupta et al. (2010).

[2]State Plan Approval and State-wise NRHM Progress—A Snapshot. Figures pertain to financial year 2008–09; also see Kapur and Chowdhury 2011.

Table 20.2
Staff Costs (by Directorate), Tamil Nadu Health Department

	FY 2000–01		FY 2008–09		Compound Annual Growth Rate (Nominal)
Directorates	Rs Million	% Share	Rs Million	% Share	%
Public Health	3,643	46.9	6,497	44.2	7.8
Medical Services	1,718	22.1	2.961	20.2	7.0
Medical Education	2,412	31.0	5,232	35.6	10.2
Total	7,773	100.0	14,690	100.0	8.2

Source: Gupta et al. (2010).

A good example of prioritized budgetary allocation is Muthulakshmi Reddy Maternity Assistance Scheme. In India, most of the states are providing Janani Suraksha Yojana (central-sponsored scheme) money to the mothers who deliver in a health facility. In Tamil Nadu, the state has launched a separate state-funded scheme of conditional cash transfer for institutional delivery, i.e., Muthulakshmi Reddy Maternity Assistance Scheme. This is described in detail in the following paragraphs.

> **Interview Byte: Dr Porkaipandiyan**
>
> 'The budget is very important for any state and the state budget for the health in this year is around 4,761 crores; which is around 841 crores more than the previous year. It is around 20% more than the previous year budget. Since the government allots more funds for the health sector itself, we are able to do more work in the primary health centres (PHCs), even in the hospitals and in the medical college. The budget is definitely more when comparing other states to Tamil Nadu.'
>
> *Source:* Interview with Dr Porkaipandiyan, Director of Public Health, Chennai, Tamil Nadu, October 2011.

Conditional Cash Transfer: Muthulakshmi Reddy Maternity Assistance Scheme

Muthulakshmi Reddy Maternity Benefit Fund Scheme was introduced in 1989. It started by offering a cash incentive ₹500 to pregnant woman. The scheme was initially run by the social welfare department and subsequently handed over to the health department. This particular amount was meant to compensate pregnant woman for wage loss during pregnancy. Subsequently, the amount was increased to ₹2,000 and then ₹6,000. This amount was raised recently to ₹12,000 per pregnancy and is paid by the government for the first two live births. Apart from wage loss compensation, another purpose of giving the money is to provide for additional nutrition to the mother to prevent anaemia and low-birth weight babies. This scheme is only meant for below poverty line (BPL) families (Padmanaban et al. 2009).

This conditional cash transfer scheme to improve institutional delivery was introduced into the health system of Tamil Nadu much before introduction of Janani Suraksha Yojana (JSY) into the health system (introduced in the year October 2007). It is a safe motherhood intervention under the NRHM being implemented with the objective of reducing maternal and neonatal mortality by promoting institutional delivery among the pregnant women. JSY integrates cash assistance with antenatal, intranatal and postnatal care (PNC).

Prioritizing Health: A Political Perspective

Tamil Nadu has a history of social revolution. The insight and commitment of government leaders in Tamil Nadu have made a significant contribution to the health gains in the state. Even though political leaders and parties in power have changed over the years, two aspects of government's approach to strengthening the public health system have remained consistent since the early 1980s. First, health policies and government spending on health have emphasized improving primary care services, especially in rural, poor and disadvantaged communities. Second, political leaders have been committed to implementing innovative interventions, some of which are common across all states and funded by the central government, efficiently and effectively (Balbanova et al. 2011).

Tamil Nadu's neighbour, Kerala, has been long celebrated for its success with health care, education and other social sector programmes. In comparison, Tamil Nadu has received attention only recently in the literature. One reason for this is that the most impressive expansion of public services happened in the state only after the 1970s. There has been some literature since then analyzing the provision of public services. Three prominent explanations of Tamil Nadu's commitment have been: populist leadership, the success of backward caste groups in securing political power and extensive public action at the grassroots for public services. The first two focus on leadership and the third looks at the grassroots action. The extension of public services is seen as the result of the political styles of certain leaders who seek to create mass appeal using an anti-elite rhetoric, thus creating a base of common people as voters in order to secure power. The achievement of power is consolidated by the extension of public services to the non-elite (Srinivasan 2010). This political attention to the health care system over last three decades has helped it to improve and grow.

Public Health Act

Public health service provision in Tamil Nadu is greatly facilitated by the fact that it has a Public Health Act. Such an Act enables proactive measures to avert health threats. A pioneering Act was introduced in 1939, steered by the great scholar and Minister for Health Dr T.S.S. Rajan, which became the first state law for public health enacted in the country. The Tamil Nadu Public Heath Act, 1939, remains as a model till today for the entire country; amendments were made in 1941, 1944 and 1958. The Act was modified in 1970 and it was translated into Tamil in 1986. A few key features of this act are given as follows:

1. Powers of the police officers to arrest offenders.
2. Powers of the executive officers and public health staff to arrest offenders.
3. Act to override other Enactments; 'Public Health Act' is supreme.
4. Power to the government to remove difficulties in implementation of the Act as and when they appear.
5. Powers of the government and of the Director of Public Health and his staff to advise local authorities.

The Act specifies the legal and administrative structures under which a public health system functions, assigns responsibilities and powers to different levels of government and agencies and specifies their source of funding for carrying out these duties. Under the Act, health officers are empowered to detect nuisances/malpractices following a complaint from a citizen or by using their powers for entry and inspection. The Act also provides the legislative basis for all the planning and policy implementation work of the Directorate of Public Health.

The most crucial advantage of the Public Health Act in Tamil Nadu over other available legislation with public health implications is that it includes a very broad definition of a public health 'nuisance'. This includes any situation that poses a credible public health threat, a few examples of which are premises or animals kept in unhealthy conditions, stagnant water or ill-maintained drains, accumulation of refuse and factories that are poorly designed or maintained. This means that the private sector which primarily doesn't work in preventive health also falls under this act.

Strong Infrastructure

A strong PHC infrastructure is also a prerequisite of a strong health system. The central government launched an initiative to expand the number of PHCs and health subcentres (HSCs) in rural areas. Tamil Nadu embraced the concept wholeheartedly and built the facilities much faster than almost all other states. The rate of expansion was remarkable. In the early 1980s there were only about 400 PHCs and 4,000 HSCs across rural areas of the state. By 1990, nearly 1,400 PHCs and about 8,000 HSCs had been opened and Tamil Nadu was very close to achieving the national target of one PHC per 30,000 people and one HSC per 5,000 people. Since then, these achievements have more or less been sustained. In 2005, Tamil Nadu had approximately 1,500 PHCs (one for every 33,000 people) and 8,680 HSCs (each covering a population of 5,100). Very few states have reached this high level of coverage through the primary health care system (Jamison et al. 2006). This strong infrastructure has been used as a platform to promote various preventive health services in rural areas.

The infrastructure described above lays the groundwork for a strong health system, but in order to ensure a strong health system many other structures are also required. A few such innovative structures/frameworks are presented in the next section.

Section 2: Health System Innovations

Tamil Nadu Medical Service Corporation

A major initiative taken by the state government was to set-up a government company in 1995, the Tamil Nadu Medical Service Corporation (TNMSC), with the primary objective of ensuring ready availability of all essential drugs and medicines in all the government health facilities, by adopting a streamlined procedure for their procurement, storage and distribution.

The first step taken by TNMSC was to finalize the list of essential drugs to be procured. Keeping in view the WHO's Model List of essential drugs; the existing list of nearly 900 drugs was reduced to a list of 240 drugs. Now, TNMSC has 271 items of drugs and medicines on its list, accounting for around 90% of the budget outlay for the purpose, leaving other drugs of smaller quantities to be purchased locally by the institutions from out of the remaining 10% of the budget.

Interview Byte: Satyabrata Sahoo

'The basic idea behind creating the TNMSC is to make the drugs, equipment and surgical sutures, all available through a centralized procurement system so that in the entire health system, there is no gap between the availability, maintenance and other related issues. The medical system is so huge, it starts at the public-health level, we reach in each and every village, then there is a secondary medical sector and then the tertiary medical sector; everywhere there is so many requirements of drugs, medicines, sutures, surgical, equipment and maintenance. To provide this through a centralized agency, this was thought of and it started during the year 1994. Through this system, we have been very much able to remove the middleman and delays.'

Source: Interview with Satyabrata Sahoo, Managing Director, TNMSC (PHFI, 2011).

Interview Byte: Dr Padmanabhan (a)

'The accountability of the doctors, nurses, has improved; this is big achievement of the maternal death review. The second important thing is that the findings of the maternal death review give inputs to do advocacy with the political bosses and the bureaucrats. We have evidence in paper to show them. This improved the situation/allocation for health sector; additional nurses, additional specialists, mobilization of the specialists to the primary health centres; all these things happened.'

Source: Interview with Dr Padmanabhan, Advisor, NHSRC (PHFI, 2011).

This innovation of the Government of Tamil Nadu in drug procurement and management has improved availability of drugs in nearly 2,000 government medical institutions throughout the state. The competitive procurement system has resulted in savings in the outlay on drugs to the extent of 36% (Rao et al. 2006) of the allocation. Apart from better budgetary control on drug consumption, medical institutions have become more cost conscious.

Maternal Death Review (MDR)

It is an important strategy to improve the quality of obstetric care and reduce maternal mortality and morbidity. Maternal Death Review[3] (MDR) as a strategy has been spelt out clearly in the RCH II National Programme Implementation Plan document. The importance of MDR lies in the fact that it provides detailed information on various factors at facility, district, community, regional and national levels that are needed to be addressed to reduce maternal deaths. Analysis of these deaths can identify the delays that contribute to maternal deaths at various levels and the information can be used to adopt measures to fill the gaps in service (Government of India 2010).

MDR is contemplated to be implemented in two forms—Facility-based Maternal Death Review and Community-based Maternal Death Review.

To identify the reasons behind maternal deaths, Tamil Nadu started compulsory audit of all maternal deaths occurring in the state since 1994. Sensitization workshops were organized among the health functionaries on the importance of maternal death reporting. The system became fully established when the Government of Tamil Nadu issued an order in 2004, stating that all maternal deaths should be audited.

The reporting itself of the maternal death is the most important step, for as we have seen, many times people do not report maternal death cases. The state mandates that each maternal death be

---

[3]Maternal death is defined as the death of a woman who dies from any cause related to or aggravated by pregnancy or its management (excluding accidental or incidental causes) during pregnancy or childbirth or within 42 days of termination of pregnancy, irrespective of duration and site of the pregnancy.

reported to the Maternal and Child Health Commissioner within 24 hours of occurrence through telegram or fax, irrespective of place of death—public facility or private nursing home or during the time of transit. Multiple sources for reporting are encouraged. Maternal deaths are reported by auxiliary nurse mid-wives (ANMs), the medical officer posted at the periphery, from the first referral unit (FRU) or non-government hospitals, district public-health nurse and Deputy Director of Health Services. Investigations of maternal deaths are carried out through community-based maternal review (verbal autopsy) and facility-based maternal death reviews/clinical audits.

Interview Byte: Dr Padmanabhan (b)

'Almost 30 to 35% of the institutional deliveries are conducted in the PHCs in Tamil Nadu. This has happened due to the provision of services, good infrastructure and the availability of buildings, electricity, toilets and computer stations. This was the first step; followed by (under RCH I Programme), three staff nurses model for the PHCs; a qualified staff nurse has been made available in eight-hour shift. Hence, three nurses are available on a rotational shift which made the PHC to be open for 24 hours. So the 24-hour concept with the three staff nurses' model was really made successful. This helps women as they can walk in any time, during the day or night, to the PHC for services.'

Source: Interview with Dr Padmanabhan, Advisor, NHSRC (PHFI, 2011).

Three Staff Nurse Model: 24×7 Functional PHCs

In the state, 99.8% of all deliveries are conducted in institutions by qualified and trained personnel (Vijay 2011). Tamil Nadu has been able to achieve such encouraging figures due to various policy initiatives which were introduced between 2001–06, one being the 24-hours delivery care service in the PHCs. Tamil Nadu is the first state in the country which introduced the three staff nurse model in the PHCs to make them functional 24×7. This innovation ensures safe delivery services in a PHC to the pregnant women at the onset of labour pains at any point of the day or night.

In the next section of this case study, we will be describing a few innovative technical initiatives undertaken by Tamil Nadu state. It has been recognized that Tamil Nadu has a strong health system which helps it to undertake innovative initiatives. Many models initiated or innovated by Tamil Nadu were later scaled-up across the country. These two innovations are selected based on their potential for scale-up across the country in days to come.

Section 3: Technological Innovations

Iron Sucrose Injections

Anaemia is estimated to affect nearly two-third of pregnant women in developing countries. Iron deficiency anaemia (IDA) is responsible for 95% of anaemia during pregnancy. Over the past years, various oral, intramuscular and intravenous preparations of iron have been used for correction of IDA in the pregnant mothers. However, they are associated with significant side effects and it is not possible to achieve the target rise in haemoglobin (Hb) level in a limited time period when the mother is approaching term.

Interview Byte: Dr Vaidyanathan

'NASG is one part of the full strategy for reduction of post-partum or ante-partum haemorrhage and cannot operate in isolation. In order to manage PPH, the Government of Tamil Nadu initiated training on active management of third stage of labour, followed by availability of safe blood and NASG. The state government realizes that the results of interventions directed towards reduction of PPH can take up to a few years but it is essential to invest in such innovations.'

Source: Interview with Dr Vaidyanathan, Principal Secretary (Health) for Government of Tamil Nadu (PHFI, 2011).

Iron sucrose injection was approved by United States of America Food and Drug Administration (FDA) in November 2000. Iron sucrose is an iron hydroxide sucrose complex in water. It is administered by intravenous (IV) injection or infusion. The recommended schedule is to administer 100 mg intravenously over five minutes, once to thrice weekly until 1,000 mg has been administered. The rate of administration should not exceed 20 mg per minute. A test dose is also not required and is at the physician's discretion (Silverstein and Rodgers 2004).

Iron sucrose complex (ISC) is a relatively new drug; it has been able to raise the Hb to a satisfactory level when used in severely anaemic iron deficient pregnant women. Few state governments in India are conducting initial research on it. The state governments of Bihar, Uttar Pradesh, Karnataka, Tamil Nadu, Maharashtra and Chhattisgarh have allocated resources in their Programme Implementation Plans (PIP) for procurement of iron sucrose for making it available in primary health care settings. The decision to include it has been based on evidence obtained from very small observational studies and on the experience of clinicians who have been using it. Of the above mentioned states Tamil Nadu has implemented the administration of IV iron sucrose in primary health care settings since 2009 (Srinivasan and Ayyanar 2010).

Non-Pneumatic Anti-Shock Garment (NASG)

Worldwide the most common cause of maternal mortality is haemorrhage, but the proportion of deaths due to each different cause varies between regions. MMR in India is estimated at 212 per 100,000 live births (SRS 2009) and post-partum haemorrhage (PPH) accounts for 35 to 56% of these deaths (Kodkany et al. 2004). One of the ways that this can be prevented is by application of non-pneumatic anti-shock garments (NASG) as the immediate first aid treatment for reversing hypovolumic shock in pregnant women suffering from PPH during transportation.

NASG is made of stretchy, lightweight neoprene resembling the bottom half of a wet suit, the garment applies pressure to the lower limbs, pelvis and abdomen via its five velcro closures. The NASG is fairly simple and easy to use by any medical or non-medical person with one-hour training in applying it. Each garment costs only $160 and can be reused up to 50 times. The NASG is safer than traditional anti-shock garments. Because the NASG uses lower pressure, it does not cause compartment syndrome or ischemia.

Pathfinder International initiated the Raksha Project in Bihar, Rajasthan and Tamil Nadu to implement the Continuum of Care philosophy and within that introduced NASG. The way NASG has been scaled-up in Tamil Nadu is different to the way Pathfinder International has scaled it up in Bihar and Rajasthan. Pathfinder International has signed a memorandum of understanding (MoU) with the Government of Tamil Nadu and is committed to providing technical training on the usage of NASG as well as providing a number of garments to the state government.

The Government of Tamil Nadu has incorporated the use of NASG into its protocols for active management of third stage of labour and routinely trains staff at all levels for its use. NASG is now also being kept in all 108 Emergency Management and Research Institute (EMRI) ambulances in Tamil Nadu.

References

Balbanova, D., McKee, M. and Mills A. (eds). 2011. *'Good Health at Low Cost' 25 Years on: What Makes a Good Health System?* London: London School of Hygiene and Tropical Medicine.

Government of India. 2010. Maternal Death Review: Guidebook. Maternal Health Division, Ministry of Health and Family Welfare, Government of India.

Gupta, M., Desikachari, B.R., Shukla, R., Somanathan, T.V., Padmanaban, P. and Datta, K.K. 2010. 'Special Article: How Might India's Public Health Systems Be Strengthened? Lessons from Tamil Nadu'. *Economic & Political Weekly*, xlv(10).

Gupta, M., Desikachari, B.R., Somanathan, T.V. and Padmanaban, P. 2009. 'How to Improve Public Health Systems: Lessons from Tamil Nadu'. Policy Research Working Paper 5073. World Bank Development Research Group, Human Development and Public Services Team.

Jamison, D.T., Breman, J.G., Measham, A.R., et al. 2006. *Priorities in Health*. Washington, DC: World Bank. Available at http://www.ncbi.nlm.nih.gov/books/NBK10265/pdf/ch7.pdf.

Kapur, A. and Chowdhury, A. 2011 'Accountability Initiative – Research and Innovation for Government Accountability'. Budget briefs, NRHM, Government of India, 2011–12. Available at http://www.accountabilityindia.in/sites/default/files/nrhm_goi_2010-11.pdf, accessed on 8 August 2013.

Kodkany, B.S., Derman, R.J., Goudar, S.S., Geller, S.E., Edlavitch, S.A., Naik, V.A., Patel, A., Bellad, M.B. and Patted, S.S. 2004. 'Initiating a Novel Therapy in Preventing Postpartum Hemorrhage in Rural India: A Joint Collaboration between the United States and India'. *International Journal of Fertility and Women's Medicine*, 49(2): 91–6.

National Family Health Survey (NFHS-3) 2005–06. 2007. International Institute for Population Sciences (IIPS) and Macro International. Volume II. Mumbai, India: IIPS.

Padmanaban, P., Raman, P. and Mavalankar, D. 2009. 'Innovations and Challenges in Reducing Maternal Mortality in Tamil Nadu, India'. *Health Population Nutrition*, 27(2): 202–19. International Centre for Diarrhoeal Disease Research, Bangladesh.

Planning Commission. 2003. Human Development Report: Tamil Nadu. Government of India. Available at http://www.planningcommission.nic.in/plans/stateplan/, accessed on 8 August 2013.

Rao, R., Tiwari, Garg and Bansal. 2006. 'Final Report on Impact of TRIPS on Pharmaceutical Prices with Specific Focus on Generics in India'. Project under the work plan of the WHO Biennium 2004–05 and Ministry of Health and Family Welfare, Government of India, p. 73. National Institute of Pharmaceutical Education and Research, Mohali.

Sample Registration System (SRS). 2009. Special Bulletin on Maternal Mortality in India 2004–06; Sample Registration System; Office of Registrar General India. Available at http://www.mp.gov.in/health/MMR-Bulletin-April-2009.pdf, accessed on 8 August 2013.

Sheelarani, C. 2007. 'Splendour in the Grass: Innovation in Administration'. In *Reducing Maternal Mortality and Female Infanticide: Tamil Nadu Experience*. New Delhi: Penguin Books, pp. 91–117.

Silverstein, S.B. and Rodgers, G.M. 2004. 'Parenteral Iron Therapy Options'. Department of Pharmacy Services and Departments of Medicine and Pathology, University of Utah Health Sciences Center, Salt Lake City, Utah.

Srinivasan, A.K. and Ayyanar. 2010. 'Intravenous Iron Sucrose Complex Therapy for Iron Deficiency Anaemia in the Pregnant Women'. Published in Compendium of Scientific Papers presented in TNPHCON 2010 & 2011 and ICONHSS 2010, Department of Public Health and Preventive Medicine, Dharmapuri District.

Srinivasan, V. 2010. 'Understanding Public Services in Tamil Nadu: An Institutional Perspective'. MPhil Dissertation, Maxwell School of Syracuse University, December 2010.

Vijay, V.S. 2011. 'Policy Note on Health and Family Welfare 2011–12'. Health and Family Welfare Department, Government of Tamil Nadu.

World Health Organization (WHO). 2005. 'Improving Maternal, Newborn and Child Health in the South-East Asia Region'. World Health Organization, Regional Office for the South-East Asia. Available at www.searo.who.int/entity/maternal_reproductive_health/documents/SEA-MCH-228/en/index.html, accessed on 8 August 2013.

with the Government of Tamil Nadu and is committed to providing technical training on the usage of RASS as well as providing a number of placements to the state government.

The Government of Tamil Nadu has incorporated the use of RASS into the protocols for active monitoring of third stage of labour and routine intra-partum staff at all levels for its use. RASS is now also being kept in all 106 Emergency Management and Research Institute (EMRI) ambulances in Tamil Nadu.

References

Organization Feature

21. Using Science and Technology for Care: Action Research and Training for Health (ARTH)

21

Using Science and Technology for Care: Action Research and Training for Health (ARTH)

Madhavi Misra

Introduction to the Organization

Action Research and Training for Health (ARTH) is a private, non-profit, research and training organization that was established by a group of professionals in 1997 with the intent to contribute to the improvement of health status among underprivileged communities in India. ARTH focusses on the health needs of marginalized rural and urban slum inhabitants, as well as on those of vulnerable groups such as adolescents, women, migrants and unorganized labour. Its office is located in Udaipur and the field service and surveillance programme operates in two geographic clusters (total population about 60,000) spread over three blocks of southern Rajasthan namely Kumbhalgarh in Rajsamand District and Gogunda and Badgaon in Udaipur District. The southern part of Rajasthan was chosen as the intervention area because this area had the most adverse health indicators in the state.

ARTH focusses its efforts towards the following areas of work.

- Service innovation
- Training
- Research
- Programme support and advocacy

This case study will focus on the service innovation model that ARTH has adopted to carry out its field operations. In its own field area, ARTH has conducted nearly 4,700 deliveries over the past 12 years and also attended to nearly 600 maternal emergencies that came at other times, such as during pregnancy or with post-abortion or post-partum complications.

Motivation/Background to Innovating as an Organization

After its inception, ARTH realized that in order to substantially improve health outcomes of the community of which it was a part, it was essential to begin some form of service delivery and therefore, a service innovation model was adopted by the organization. ARTH then later branched into other areas of research, training and advocacy. It was essential for ARTH to demonstrate that some of its ideas could form the base to generate evidence. ARTH started its work quietly by setting-up a field and health service programme in 10 villages and alongside started an enquiry on how health-seeking behaviour of women in the region, especially for reproductive health issues worked. ARTH started working with a few tribal women in the community who began working as outreach workers. ARTH increased its scope of work from 10 to 18 villages, then reached 49 villages and set-up two health centres.

Dr Sharad Iyengar, the chief executive of ARTH, feels that innovating at the grassroots level forms the very core of ARTH's philosophy. It needs to keep reinventing itself in order to meet the needs of the community. ARTH does not believe in being a large-scale service provider but instead, in demonstrating how innovations can be taken to scale within the government or the private sector. ARTH continuously strives to make services available at a cheaper rate, more conveniently and in a manner that empowers the user. Dr Iyengar believes that there is a role for NGOs to be innovative, to demonstrate, question and criticize. Policymakers should encourage this and learnings from them will then be available to the larger system.

Selected Innovations

Nurse Midwives Run Health Centre

ARTH's first health centre was started in 1997 in one village in the Rajsamand District of southern Rajasthan, with one nurse midwife. At another location closer (25 km) to Udaipur, as part of a drought relief initiative, a second health centre was opened. It was at this point that ARTH realized that if it wished to provide delivery as a care service, it would have to be a 24×7 facility and a 24×7 facility could never rely on the efforts of one professional. Therefore, the number of staff had to be scaled-up and a team set-up. Thus the health centres have two to three nurse midwives at a time, all of whom are trained to provide a 24×7 service.

ARTH now operates three health centres in these villages which cater to a population of about 60,000. The health centres are mainly managed by trained nurse midwives who reside near the health centre premises and are available round-the-clock. They are supported by specialist doctors who come in from Udaipur, once or twice a week to cater to specific problems of women and children. These health centres mainly provide the following services:

- 24×7 delivery services and management/referral for maternal-newborn complications.
- Integrated Management of Neonatal and Childhood Illness (IMNCI) for children and primary health care by nurse midwives.
- Safe abortion services (first trimester).

Figure 21.1
Delivery Conducted by Nurse Midwives at ARTH Health Centres from 2000 to 2011

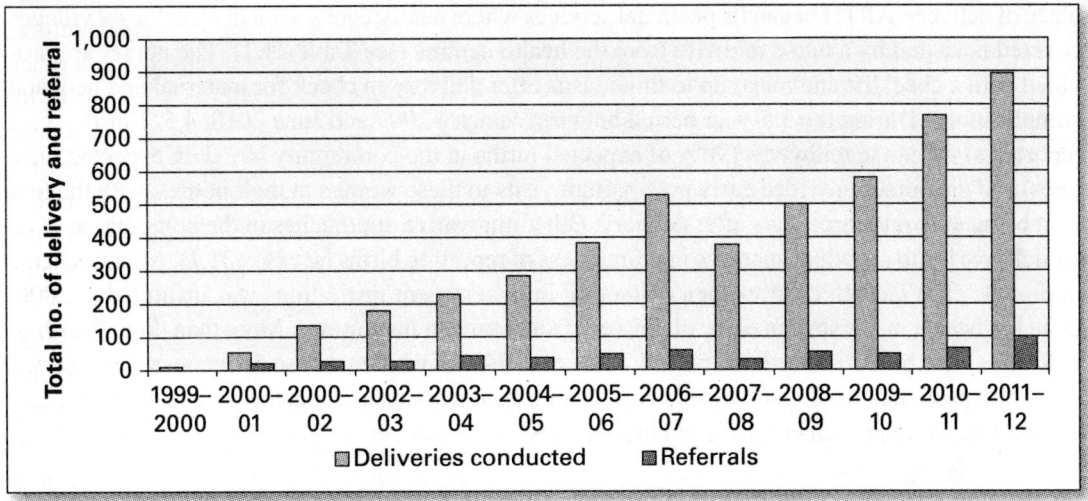

Source: Report provided by ARTH official sources.

- Reversible methods of contraception.
- Gynaecological services, including infertility management.
- Laboratory facilities for basic pathological services.

The nurse midwife-run model is operated with the help of consultant gynaecologists as the nurses consult the doctors on the phone and accordingly take the decision about whether to refer a patient or not. In a study done of the two health centres it was found that from the years 2000 to 2008, 2,771 women in labour and 202 women with maternal emergencies, who were not in labour, were attended by nurse midwives. Of women in labour, 21% had a life-threatening complication or its antecedent condition and 16% were advised referral, of whom two-thirds complied. Compliance with referral was higher for maternal conditions than foetal conditions. Among the 202 women who came with complications antenatal, post-abortion or post-partum, referral was advised for 70%, of whom 72% complied. The referral system included counselling, arranging transport, accompanying women, facilitating admission and supporting inpatient care and led to higher referral compliance rates. According to Figure 21.1, it is evident how the number of women in labour coming to the ARTH health centres increased from 2000 to 2012. ARTH's health centres were accredited under the Janani Suraksha Yojana (JSY) in 2008.

PNC Check-ups at Home

It is usually observed that when a woman has been discharged after delivery of her baby, she is at her most vulnerable. She can suffer disabling consequences and the newborn is at risk of death. ARTH felt that it is imperative to reach women after delivery, i.e., in the postnatal period as most families do not consider this as an important phase for a woman. There are traditional, cultural and even health reasons, why a woman and her newborn are not too mobile at that stage and so ARTH devised the postnatal care (PNC) model where nurse midwives visited every single mother irrespective of her place of delivery. ARTH began its postnatal services where nearly every woman from the 49 villages covered is visited by a nurse midwife from the health centres (see Table 21.1). The nurses are provided with a checklist and make up to three visits after delivery to check for maternal and neonatal complications. During the 3.5-year period between January 2007 and June 2010, 4,521 births were reported to the nurse midwives (90% of expected births in the community based on expected birth rates) and the nurses provided early post-partum visits to these women at their homes, with the first visit being at two to three days after delivery. Other innovative approaches in the home-based PNC model have led to a gradual increase in promptness of reporting births (see Box 21.1). After a scheme to provide cash incentives to women delivering in government institutions was instituted in 2006, there has been a major shift in place of delivery from home to institutions. More than three-fourth of deliveries were by skilled birth attendants. More than 94% of women whose deliveries were reported received a postnatal visit by nurse midwives. Over time it was ensured that the visit occurred as early as possible. An improvement was seen in timeliness of visits over the years.

Access to Reproductive Health at Village Level

Especially in the rural areas, women have little control over their fertility and reproductive health and, besides, are subject to both physical and social mobility constraints. They are unable to travel freely due to lack of low-cost transportation and there are concerns of personal security and social stigma.

The health system's emphasis on female sterilization leaves a high unmet need for reversible contraception among women who wish to delay but not completely prevent the next pregnancy. Women who are adolescents, who have no children, who wish to space their children, who fear the

Table 21.1

Service Package during PNC Period Offered by ARTH

Activities carried out by nurse midwives during post-partum visits	
Mother	*Newborn*
Detailed structured questionnaire, including that for post-partum depression and maternal morbidities.	Enquiry about problems using a structured checklist.
Examination: • General examination including temperature, pulse, blood pressure (BP) and respiratory rate • Haemoglobin test for anaemia • Breast and abdominal examinations • Perineal and pelvic examination if any complaint related to these areas	Examination: • Physical examination including temperature, respiratory rate • Weight • Observation for local infections in eyes, umbilicus • Examination for sepsis
Counselling and information on: • Diet and work • Danger signs and where to go for care • Medications as per the condition • Referral support	Counselling and information of mother on: • Breastfeeding • Bathing, keeping the baby warm • Danger signs • Medications as per the condition • Referral support

Source: Progress Report of ARTH, May 2011.

Box 21.1: Innovations in the Home-based PNC Model

To carry out the home-based PNC visits successfully, there had to be a system of communication whereby ARTH would be informed of deliveries in the area. Thus a system of pregnancy tracking was developed. The system was able to pick up more than 90% of all births in the area. The system using key informants, volunteers and even family members was used whereby, using telephone or other communication means, the nurse midwives were informed of women who had very recently delivered in the area. The challenge is to reach these women within the first couple of days after delivery as there is no point going to a woman's house 10 or 15 days after she has delivered. To overcome this challenge, a small incentive of giving ₹50 for reporting births was used if the birth was reported within 24 hours. A nurse midwife was to visit these women and she would go on a motorcycle and was provided with a chauffeur who would drive her to the locations in order to save time and increase efficiency and productivity. The nurse is provided with a kit with basic diagnostic materials, including some educational material.

Source: Interview transcripts of Dr Sharad Iyengar, August 2011.

---

death of a child or who have unstable marital relationships (and might be concerned that they may eventually have to remarry), may wish to maintain their fertility potential.

While emergency contraception (EC) has become available over-the-counter in cities, women in rural areas yet do not have access to EC. ARTH strongly believed that there is no reason why such a technology should be restricted to the cities and rural women should also have information about and access to EC as a critical step in gaining control of their own fertility.

Again, pregnancy tests have traditionally been available only from specialists or graduate doctors and may cost as much as up to ₹100 in the cities. Due to these conditions, women who are uncertain of their pregnancy status often seek pregnancy tests late and then resort to seeking abortions from untrained providers.

Since June 2007, ARTH has introduced village-level pregnancy advisory services through an initiative called '*gaon pas*' or gpas, whereby village volunteers (accredited social health activists [ASHAs] and village health workers [VHWs]) have been trained to provide awareness of and access to contraceptives, including emergency contraceptives and pregnancy tests (see Box 21.2). This intervention was started almost a year before the Nischay Programme was launched by the National Rural Health Mission (NRHM). In essence, ARTH is utilizing the potential of village volunteers (ASHAs and VHWs) to increase awareness of and access to reproductive health services to enable women to better manage their own fertility.

Uptake of EC was initially slow and increased after about a year and a half. Most EC users were young women with 60% being in the age group of 15 to 24 years. Nearly 17% were unmarried/single. About three-fourth users took EC pills from the health worker in advance, i.e., before unprotected intercourse. Most women took EC either because they forgot to take their contraceptive, had stopped it, used contraceptives irregularly or stayed with the husband only occasionally.

Profile of Pregnancy Test Users

During the three-year intervention period (2007–10) ASHAs and VHWs conducted nearly 3,000 pregnancy tests in the villages and counselled and helped women in seeking services as per their individual needs. The uptake of pregnancy tests was fairly quick. After the first six months, it picked

---

Box 21.2: Emergency Contraception

ARTH introduced the emergency contraceptive pill in 2006 in the community through village volunteers. The product had been around for quite some years before that and is extremely safe. The challenge was on how to promote the use of EC. ARTH, through its surveys and community interactions, understood that there were three scenarios for the use of EC. Firstly, about 40 to 50% of couples in the area are long-distance couples as men have migrated to a city in search of work and the women remain behind in the village. The men make sporadic visits, often sudden, as they do not know when they will get leave from their work. On such occasions the wife is not using any form of contraception and such visits result in unwanted pregnancies. Such unwanted pregnancies are in greater number after festivals or at certain times of the year. ARTH, therefore, positioned EC as something that could be used by a woman if her husband visited her without prior planning. A second scenario is the social custom prevalent in the area where boys and girls are married off young but the girls have not yet started cohabiting with their husbands (which usually occurs after a ceremony of *Gauna*). Before they begin living together there are instances of young, enthusiastic husbands visiting the wife's village and notwithstanding reservations by her parents, they meet the young girl who is the wife when she is out fetching water or firewood, or looking after the cattle and they might have sex and that might result in an unwanted pregnancy. More often the young girl is invited by in-laws' family at the time of any major function in their household and is expected to help in the work for three–four days. This also provides an opportunity for newly married (and yet without the social sanction of *Gauna*) to meet. This pregnancy which has occurred before the official cohabitation phase often creates social embarrassment. ARTH has tried providing access to emergency contraceptive pill either before the cohabitation phase or soon after, in the early months after the marriage. The third scenario is where a woman at any stage faces sexual coercion and would need to use EC. Unfortunately, given the sensitivity of the situation, it has been very difficult to monitor as to whether the pill actually has been used. ARTH's volunteers have provided the emergency pills to several women and adolescents in such situations. However, doubtless, the emergency contraceptive pill has worked as there are anecdotal examples.

Source: Interview transcripts of Dr Sharad Iyengar, August 2011.

---

up to an average level of 50–60 tests per month and then further increased to about 100–120 a month. The intervention was successful in reaching the underprivileged and adolescents. Most women who received pregnancy test services at village level belonged to Scheduled Castes (SCs) or Scheduled Tribes (STs). Nearly 40% were in the 15-to-24-year age group and 70% had either no child or one or two children.

Oral contraceptive pills (OCPs) were the most preferred form of contraception, though we do not know that once initiated, how many of these women continued to use OCPs.

Challenges Faced

When ARTH started its operations from one village; the people were initially sceptical of their work. There was a certain element of suspicion and questioning and it took nearly three to four years before there was a sense of comfort with ARTH. ARTH also faced a challenge while training the village health volunteers as most tribal women were illiterate. Many pictorial aids and hands-on training were used to train village volunteers. During the initial years, it was also difficult to recruit nurse midwives who were willing to stay in the field area to provide 24×7 services.

Managing the 24×7 ARTH health centres was not easy. It is difficult to retain nurse midwives at the health centre for night shifts and especially during the holiday and festival season. The organization

---

Box 21.3: The Introduction and Country-wide Scale-up of Copper-T 380A (The 10-year Copper-T)

The 1991 Census for the area where ARTH started work revealed a female literacy rate among tribals of 0.2%. There has been a big change since then. The ARTH surveys are showing that the fertility rate has come down to 2.4 which is quite remarkable. The fact remains that the ability of women to make their own decisions about when they will have children, when they will get married, about sexual activity and consequences of that sexual activity is still not where it should be in rural Rajasthan. It was observed that family planning was in the form of a directive rather than providing an option and working towards a behaviour change model. In this pursuit, the needs of younger women, adolescents, people who may not have completed a family, couples who may have lost a child or are worried about whether the children will survive, tend to be ignored. Reproductive right is all about enabling people to make decisions and changing decisions. ARTH through its work in health centres started expanding choices in terms of reversible methods of contraception. In 1999, the 10-year Copper T was introduced. This is a Copper T device, which if hygienically provided to the woman, could help her avoid a pregnancy for 10 years. And the logic is that a woman who did not want to have a child for 10 years was unlikely to want one in the 11th or 12th year. Subsequent research showed that this device worked for more than 12 years. It was positioned as an alternative to female sterilization and yet with the advantage of removal, instantly, whenever required by the woman. To ARTH, it appeared like a fixed deposit which had the liquidity of a current account. This method grew in success and we provided it at a nominal rate of ₹50 to 75 per device. Local government officials took note of this achievement as they saw it as something that is affecting the achievement of sterilization numbers. The government (district, state and central) actually helped ARTH to scale-up the Copper T intervention to four blocks of Udaipur District and this was documented. This was noticed by a joint secretary in the Government of India, who on making inquiries, found that the country had the capacity to manufacture this device and in 2004 the whole country switched to the 10-year Copper T. However, while the type of Copper T in the government programme has changed, there has not been adequate attention to providing the reproductive choice to women.

Source: Interview transcripts of Dr Sharad Iyengar, August 2011.

---

has tried to work around this challenge and ensured that the nurses have their residential quarters next to the health centres, so in times of emergency they are available.

It was observed that the community questioned ARTH's operations and were curious about their work. However, the work done by the organization helped ARTH gain the trust of the community. Today, ARTH's reputation in the community allows them to bring in innovative approaches in the provision of health services.

All this ARTH does while staying within the limits of the law.

As Dr Sharad Iyengar puts it, 'We went about our job of providing care'. With this zeal and enthusiasm, ARTH has not just been successfully working in rural communities in Udaipur, but providing innovative ideas for the rest of the developing world to learn. ARTH concedes that innovation is triggered by a sense of restlessness or dissatisfaction with the current state of things. Innovation has resulted from the effort to change and improve the maternal health environment. ARTH has gone through a cycle of testing innovations and successfully scaling them up in their field activities.

Discussion

ARTH has been able to scale-up its activities by influencing policy at the national level (see Box 21.3). For instance, the 10-year intrauterine device (IUD) has been incorporated by the Government of India.

ARTH has also been able to scale-up some of its work by training health workers/officers/medical officers from Rajasthan and across India on various training courses on maternal and child health (MCH).

The dissemination of ARTHs work has been mainly through scientific publications and advocacy at state and national level. ARTH as an organization is seen as an engine which is driving innovations in MCH. There have been a variety of forces affecting the innovative efforts of ARTH as illustrated in Figure 21.2. Funders, beneficiaries, market players, policy environment have all contributed towards ARTH being able to continuously innovate.

Factors such as other competitive players in the market providing similar services (perhaps for a profit), funding opportunities available, policy regulations, technological interventions, clients who visit ARTH's service delivery centre and ARTH's own accountability towards the community it is serving can either help or hinder innovation. In the case of ARTH's innovative engine, these forces have helped ARTH to continue to innovate in the area of MCH and reproductive and child health (RCH).

ARTH has adopted the client-focussed approach where innovations in MCH and RCH have been made more acceptable, of better quality and more affordable. The health-centre model, PNC services and RCH services offered by ARTH have changed the way the clients of these services in

Figure 21.2
Forces Affecting Innovative Efforts of ARTH

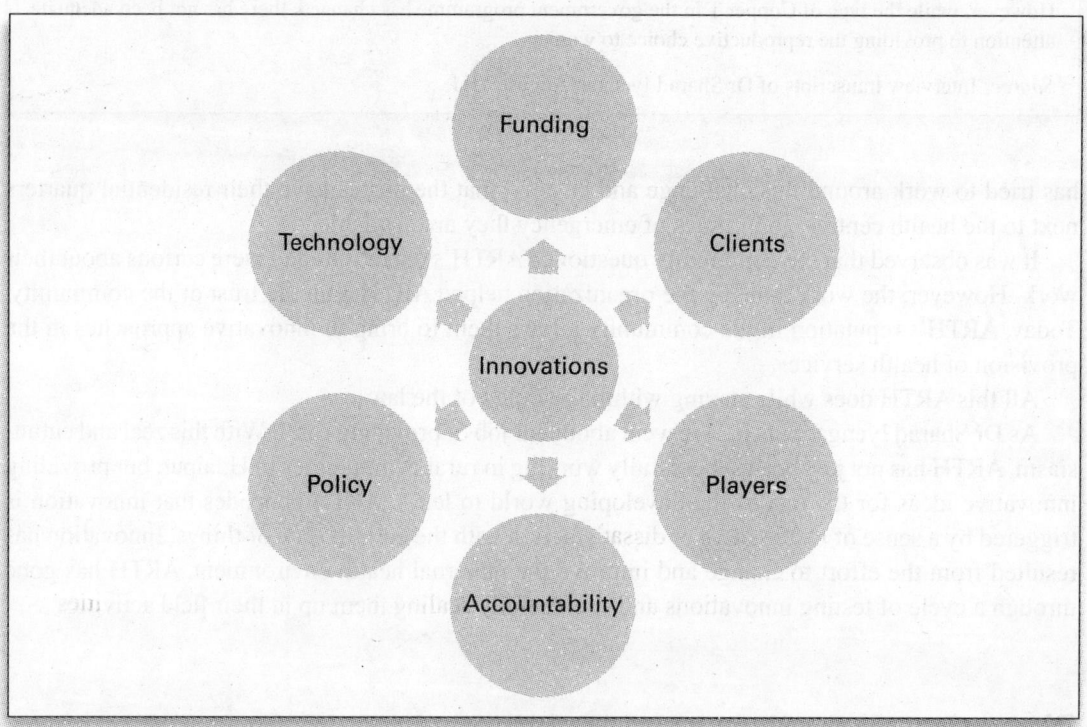

Source: Herzlinger (2006).

Figure 21.3
Attributes of ARTH

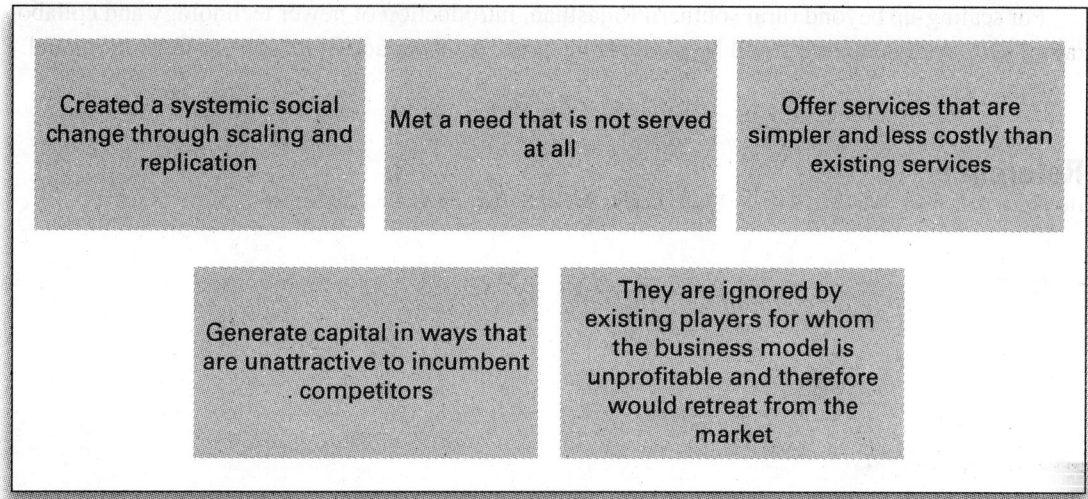

Source: Herzlinger (2006).

the villages of Rajsamand and Udaipur access and use health care. Without these services, the villagers would have to go to quacks or very expensive private providers. Going to the government hospitals was not an option for many. ARTH has provided a more convenient, effective and less expensive treatment option for many. As catalytic innovators, ARTH has been able to meet needs of the communities which are not served at all. ARTH has been able to bring new benefits to most people in the area in which it has been working and has emerged as a strong player from within the established set of players in the area.

As a catalytic player, ARTH has demonstrated the following five qualities as shown in Figure 21.3. ARTH has been able to meet a need of the community which was previously not being addressed; its nurse midwife-led health centre model offering services which were previously not easily accessible to people among other catalytic changes. Many existing players feel that the ARTH model is not profitable and, thus, cease to be competitors to ARTH. The existing competitors rely on the profit model to be able to run their establishment whereas ARTH depends on grants, etc., from donors for services to be given to people. This way to generate capital is unattractive to the incumbent competitors.

Way Ahead

As ARTH has already demonstrated its successes and disseminated its findings in a scientific way. Going forward, technological innovations seem to be a route for ARTH to adopt. Using technology-based health solutions in the field for improving health coverage and health outcomes might prove beneficial for ARTHs growth and impact. Piloting and testing some field-based health technologies with the community and scaling them up will provide robust evidence for the use of phone and information technology-based interventions.

For scaling-up beyond rural southern Rajasthan, introduction of newer technology and collaborating with external partners will help ARTH in spreading the reach of its service-delivery model.

Reference

Herzlinger, R.E. 2006. 'Why Innovation in Health Care Is So Hard?' *Harvard Business Review*, 84 (5, May): 58–66.

About the Editors and Contributors

Editors

Jay K. Satia is Senior Vice President of the Public Health Foundation of India (PHFI), New Delhi. He holds a PhD in Industrial Engineering from Stanford University, USA. He was professor at the Indian Institute of Management, Ahmedabad (IIM-A) for more than 20 years and served as its dean during 1987–89. At IIM-A, he worked on operations management as well as on management of health, population and nutrition programmes.

During the period 1993–2008, Professor Satia was the executive director of the International Council on Management of Population Programmes (ICOMP), a Malaysia-based international NGO dedicated to seeking excellence in management of population programmes.

He has several publications to his credit. He has also received research grants from numerous organizations and has been a consultant to many governments and international agencies including the World Bank and the United Nations Population Fund (UNFPA). He has served as a member on the board of several organizations.

Madhavi Misra is currently Research Scientist and Adjunct Assistant Professor at PHFI. She is a trained social worker and completed her Masters in Social Work from Tata Institute of Social Sciences in Mumbai. She has also completed her Masters of Public Health from University of Warwick in the UK. Additionally, Misra has completed a certificate course in Tobacco Control from Johns Hopkins Bloomberg School of Public Health and a certificate course in Global Health Diplomacy from Graduate Institute of International and Development Studies, Geneva.

She is a public health professional with work experience of more than seven years in the field of maternal and child health. She has had experience of working with the marginalized population of Maharashtra, Andhra Pradesh and Orissa and has conducted large baseline study on maternal and child health, nutrition, communicable diseases and health systems.

Radhika Arora is presently enrolled in the Master of Public Health Programme at the Institute of Tropical Medicine, Antwerp. She is an alumnus of the Indian Institute of Public Health, Delhi, where she earned a Postgraduate Diploma in Health Economics, Financing and Policy. She has previously worked at the Public Health Foundation of India (PHFI) towards developing audio-visual case studies on innovative programmes in the area of maternal and child health being implemented in India. Before joining PHFI, Arora worked as a features writer with Outlook Traveller and Time Out, Delhi. She has a Masters in Broadcast Journalism and almost six years of experience in both print and broadcast journalism, as well as development communications. She has worked with NDTV and CARE India. Her interest in public health, developed after she worked, briefly at Delhi-based public relations firm, Imprimis PR, which specialized in health communications. Her present work assignment at PHFI allows her to apply her past work experience in broadcast journalism to health.

Sourav Neogi is working with Ernst & Young in the Development Advisory Services. He is a postgraduate in Health and Hospital Management from Indian Institute of Health Management and Research, Jaipur. He is currently working with Ernst & Young Pvt. Ltd as a consultant in the Development Advisory Group.

His prior work experience includes project on 'Developing Case Studies of Innovations in Public Health for Competency Strengthening and Advocacy' at Public Health Foundation of India (PHFI) as a research associate for 2.5 years. Neogi also worked with Action Research and Training for Health (ARTH), Udaipur as programme manager and the public health team in Medica Synergie Pvt. Ltd. He worked as an independent consultant to support State Health Society, Bihar for Preparation of State Programme Implementation Plan (PIP) under National Rural Health Mission (NRHM) for the year 2008–09.

He has seven years of experience in the health sector and his understanding of the development sector has enabled him to gain experience in areas such as health system strengthening, documenting innovative initiatives, microfinance, reproductive child health, preparation of health action plans, biomedical waste management and hospital acquired infection. Neogi worked with the grassroots level NGOs, for-profit organizations, government and international donor agencies.

Contributors

Sanghita Bhattacharya has an MPhil and PhD in Population Studies from Jawaharlal Nehru University, India. She has a decade of experience in working on issues such as maternal and child health, gender-based violence, etc. Her expertise includes conducting operation and evaluation research. At present, she is engaged in a number of research projects in maternal and child health in different states of India and serves as a senior public health specialist at Public Health Foundation of India (PHFI).

Sutapa B. Neogi has an MBBS from Nil Ratan Sircar Medical College, Calcutta and MD from Postgraduate Institute of Medical Education and Research (PGIMER), Chandigarh and Diplomate of National Board (DNB) in Maternal and Child Health. She received the 'Kataria Memorial Gold Medal' for being the best outgoing student of PGIMER, Chandigarh.

Neogi is a public health specialist actively engaged in research and teaching at the Indian Institute of Public Health, Delhi, as associate professor. She has rich experience in public health, starting a career as a resident followed by consultancy for United Nations Children's Fund (UNICEF) and IC Health.

Raj Mohan Panda is a preventive medicine specialist who has trained in public health at Emory University in the USA. He has previously worked as a primary health care doctor in the Orissa State Health Department. His various other stints have been at CARE India, the American Cancer Society and Tobacco Technical Assistance Consortium at Emory in Atlanta.

Dr Panda currently leads many research projects at Public Health Foundation of India (PHFI) and serves as a senior public health specialist.

Index